SMALL ANIMAL SURGICAL NURSING

Skills and Concepts

SMALL ANIMAL SURGICAL NURSING

Skills and Concepts

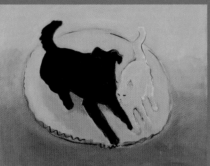

Sara J. Busch, DVM

Professor
Manor College
Program of Veterinary Technology
Jenkintown, Pennsylvania

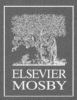

ELSEVIER
MOSBY

ELSEVIER
MOSBY

11830 Westline Industrial Drive
St. Louis, Missouri 63146

SMALL ANIMAL SURGICAL NURSING: SKILLS AND CONCEPTS
Copyright © 2006 by Mosby, Inc.

NOTICE

Knowledge and best practice in this field are constantly changing. As new research and experience broaden our knowledge, changes in practice, treatment and drug therapy may become necessary or appropriate. Readers are advised to check the most current information provided (i) on procedures featured or (ii) by the manufacturer of each product to be administered, to verify the recommended dose or formula, the method and duration of administration, and contraindications. It is the responsibility of the practitioner, relying on their own experience and knowledge of the patient, to make diagnoses, to determine dosages and the best treatment for each individual patient, and to take all appropriate safety precautions. To the fullest extent of the law, neither the publisher nor the author assumes any liability for any injury and/or damage to persons or property arising out or related to any use of the material contained in this book.

ISBN-13: 978-0-323-03063-2
ISBN-10: 0-323-03063-7

Publishing Director: Linda L. Duncan
Managing Editor: Teri Merchant
Publishing Services Manager: Patricia Tannian
Senior Project Manager: Anne Altepeter
Designer: Julia Dummitt

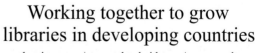

Working together to grow
libraries in developing countries

www.elsevier.com | www.bookaid.org | www.sabre.org

ELSEVIER | BOOK AID International | Sabre Foundation

Printed in China

Last digit is the print number: 9 8 7 6 5 4 3 2

CONTRIBUTORS

Marta Bates, CVT
Orthopedic Nurse, Surgery
Matthew J. Ryan Veterinary Hospital
University of Pennsylvania
Philadelphia, Pennsylvania

Sara Busch, DVM
Professor
Manor College
Program of Veterinary Technology
Jenkintown, Pennsylvania

Mel Chambliss, DVM
Alfred State College
Alfred, New York

Paula Emma, BA, CVT
Endoscopy Nurse
Matthew J. Ryan Veterinary Hospital
University of Pennsylvania
Philadelphia, Pennsylvania

Gail Hartman, DVM
Manager of Veterinary Services
Becker College
Leicester, Massachusetts

Paige A. Jones, BS, RVT
Instructional Technologist
College of Veterinary Medicine
Purdue University
West Lafayette, Indiana

James Q. Knight, DVM
Director of Animal Sciences
Becker College
Worcester, Massachusetts

Michael McCallum
Operating Room Veterinary Nurse
Matthew J. Ryan Veterinary Hospital
University of Pennsylvania
Philadelphia, Pennsylvania

Teri Raffel, CVT
Instructional Assistant
Madison Area Technical College
Veterinary Technician Program
Madison, Wisconsin

Zoe Ramagnano, BS
Operating Room Tech/Pending VMD (2005)
Matthew J. Ryan Veterinary Hospital
University of Pennsylvania
Philadelphia, Pennsylvania

Marissa Richio, CVT
Ophthalmology Nurse
Matthew J. Ryan Veterinary Hospital
University of Pennsylvania
Philadelphia, Pennsylvania

Mary Scherer, LVT
Veterinary Teaching Hospital
Michigan State University
East Lansing, Michigan

Nancy Shaffran, CVT, VTS (ECC)
Pfizer Animal Health
New York, New York

Pat Weinmann
Director of Central Supply
Veterinary Teaching Hospital
College of Veterinary Medicine
Purdue University
West Lafayette, Indiana

This book is dedicated in loving memory to Elizabeth Rockershousen.

PREFACE

Simply put, the role of the veterinary surgical nurse is to assist the veterinary surgeon in the performance of surgical procedures. However, to be a valued and appreciated surgical nurse, one must rise above the minimal requirements and become a staunch advocate for the patient. Assuming the responsibility of being the patient's advocate gives veterinary technicians the confidence to speak up when they might not otherwise. Veterinary technicians, whether because they are new graduates with little experience, or have years of experience but are starting a new job working with a surgeon who may be intimidating, are often reluctant to speak up for themselves. However, when their attitude is one of looking out for the patient's best interest, technicians often find the necessary resolve to demand the best health care for their patients. This, in turn, makes them an effective surgical nurse and an indispensable member of the surgical team. Once a technician has become an appreciated and valued member of the surgical team, the technician has more reason to expect and more leverage to request commensurate compensation. This is the classic case of where attitude is everything.

Once the veterinary surgical technician adopts an attitude of being the patient's advocate, the technician frequently experiences increased job satisfaction and a desire to continue life-long learning. With medical technology growing as rapidly as it is, it is important for veterinary technicians to continue to develop their skill sets to stay current with the ever-changing and expanding field of veterinary medicine. With an increased skill set, veterinary technicians assume more responsibility in surgical cases. Generally, the veterinary surgeon is responsible for diagnosing the surgical problem and for knowing what surgical procedure is indicated for the specific problem and how to perform the surgery. The veterinary surgical nurse, on the other hand, must be able to perform all of the perioperative responsibilities associated with each surgery. These responsibilities include the following:

- Taking a history
- Performing a thorough physical examination
- Explaining to an owner/guardian the details of the procedure and collecting a signed consent form
- Collecting and analyzing (as opposed to interpreting) preanesthetic diagnostics
- Working with the veterinarian to select the best premedications for the specific case
- Cleaning and setting up the surgical area
- Implementing pain management protocols to reduce the surgical patient's pain
- Placing intravenous catheters
- Intubating the patient with an endotracheal tube
- Inducing, maintaining, and monitoring anesthesia
- Preparing the surgical site for surgery
- Scrubbing-in and assisting in surgery
- Circulating in and out of the operating room as a circulating nurse
- Recovering the patient from anesthesia
- Writing a surgical report
- Providing postoperative nursing care and at-home care instructions once the patient is ready to leave the hospital

Phew!

So much to do and so little time! And that is where there is a need for a textbook that explains in a logical progression the details involved with performing all of the job responsibilities the small-animal surgical technician is expected to know. *Small Animal Surgical Nursing: Skills and Concepts* covers all of those responsibilities and identifies the patient's needs at every step along the way.

The contributors who wrote this book are dedicated veterinary technician educators and talented practicing veterinarians and veterinary surgical nurses. Every effort was made to make the book clear and detailed so that it can be used as a teaching aid and as a reference for the practicing veterinary surgical nurse. With all of that said, the goal of this book is to help the veterinary surgical nurse (student and practicing nurse, alike) become the patient's strongest advocate, earn a respectable salary, and enjoy the profession.

Sara J. Busch

ACKNOWLEDGMENTS

I thank Dr. Joanna Bassert at Manor College for giving me the opportunity to write this book, and Teri Merchant at Elsevier for not letting me pass up the opportunity. Sincere thanks to Mike McCallum at the University of Pennsylvania, whose help was indispensable in pulling this work together. And many thanks to Paul van Rijn at Manor College, for his computer expertise.

CONTENTS

PART III

POSTOPERATIVE CONSIDERATIONS

**Chapter 8 The Postoperative
          Patient, 287**

PART I

Preoperative Considerations

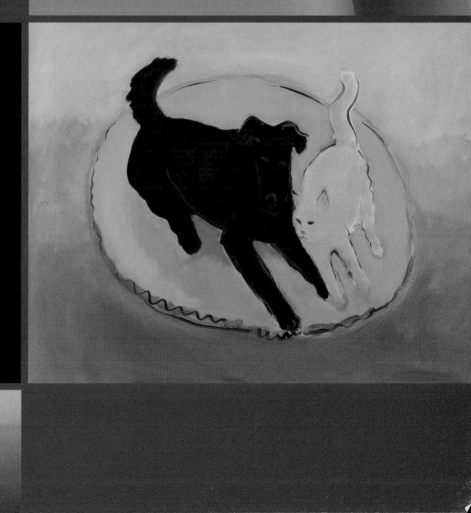

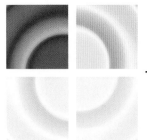

CHAPTER 1

The Preoperative Patient

Sara Busch, Mel Chambliss, Teri Raffel,
Nancy Shaffran

LEARNING OBJECTIVES

After studying this chapter, the reader should be able to do the following:

- Collect and record a patient's history in the medical record.
- Understand the importance of and be able to perform a complete physical examination on the day of a scheduled surgery.
- Know the legal significance of a signed surgical consent form.
  - Explain to clients the details in a surgical consent form.
- Collect and analyze preanesthetic diagnostic tests.
  - Describe what is considered a minimum database for particular patients.
  - Bring the veterinarian's attention to any abnormal or invalid results.
- Understand the reasons for premedicating surgical patients.
- Explain the importance of preemptive analgesia.
- Describe the drug options available for preemptive analgesia.
- Explain the mechanisms of action of the different types of analgesics.
- Discuss the indications for placement of an intravenous (IV) catheter.
- Identify appropriate sites for placement of IV catheters.

- List the supplies required for IV catheter placement.
- Discuss the technique for IV catheterization of peripheral vessels.
- Identify the components of an endotracheal (ET) tube.
- Discuss factors considered for determining ET tube size.
- List supplies required for endotracheal intubation.
- Identify the anatomic structures of the larynx.
- Discuss the differences between the one-person technique and the two-person technique of performing endotracheal intubation.
- Discuss methods of assessing proper ET tube placement.
- Describe hair removal protocols for a variety of soft tissue, orthopedic, neurologic, and miscellaneous surgical cases.
- List antiseptic products available for use when preparing patients for surgery.
- Discuss different patterns used in applying materials for the surgical preparation.
- Discuss potential patient reactions from clipper or chemical irritation.

3

HISTORY TAKING

The ability to collect a history that is both concise and chronologically accurate is a skill that takes practice. After the client (owner, guardian) and patient (animal) have been brought into the examination room and introductions have been made, a good starting point for collecting the history is to confirm the patient's *signalment.* Confirming the patient's age, gender, and breed with the owner, then comparing this information with the patient's medical record, will ensure the record's accuracy and clarify any confusion should a discrepancy be found.

Once the patient's signalment has been established and verified, ask the client about the chief complaint (or reason for the visit). This is usually a brief but complete description of the current problem; for example, "HBC [hit by car] 2 days ago and fractured right femur." Once the chief complaint has been established or confirmed, ask the client to explain the sequence of events, starting from the beginning of the particular problem.

While collecting a history, it is important to avoid asking leading questions. Leading questions make the client feel compelled to answer a certain way; for example, "You don't feed your dog anything other than dog food, do you?" The owner feels compelled to answer in the negative because the question is leading toward or encouraging a specific answer. Formatting the question in a different way encourages the owner to answer the question truthfully, without prejudice. "What do you feed your dog?" is a nonleading, nonthreatening question and usually yields more useful information than the first example. Follow-up questions should be asked when appropriate. If there is a concern regarding the dog's nutritional status or body condition, it would be appropriate to ask *how much* and *how often* the dog is fed, in addition to *what* the dog is fed. A concluding question for the specific topic is often revealing as well. A final question about the dog's diet could be asked as follows: "Is there anything else your dog eats?" Again, this is a nonleading question and allows the owner to share information that may be helpful or even significant.

During the history it is important to review what other treatments have been tried to address the current problem, including any attempts by the owner to treat the problem at home. In addition, it is important to establish the nature of the treatment and the patient's response to each treatment. A review of the current medications and supplements that the animal may be given, including both "over the counter" (OTC) and prescription medications, is an important part of the history. Certain medications and supplements may interact with diagnostic tests or premedications and anesthetic drugs.

Once the history of the current problem has been thoroughly investigated, a general question about any previous medical problems is appropriate. If a patient has had surgery or medical treatment in the past, additional follow-up questions may be in order. A good way to conclude the history-taking session is to ask the owner if there is anything else that would be helpful to know but that was not addressed. Occasionally, this general question will remind clients about something else that is relevant to the situation or that they wanted to ask.

Allowing the animal to explore the examination room at will (e.g., letting the cat out of the carrier) during the history taking helps to determine the patient's general attitude and condition, without even touching it. In addition, most animals will take this opportunity to familiarize themselves with the scents and sounds of the hospital, and they may even relax if given a chance to explore the exam room on their own terms. An observant technician can establish a first impression of the patient's personality and degree of anxiety during the history.

After the history has been collected, the details need to be recorded in chronologic order in the medical record.

PHYSICAL EXAMINATION

The veterinary technician should be adept in the performance of the physical examination (PE), even though veterinarians may elect to perform the PE themselves. The veterinary medical team will consult the PE findings when determining the appropriate anesthetic and surgical protocols for the patient. The owner's presence during the PE allows for ongoing communication between the technician or veterinarian and the owner in regard to the findings and provides a historical perspective to unusual findings. This is especially true for any physical findings that might impact the surgical procedure or anesthetic protocols (e.g., retained testicles, pregnancy).

The complete PE should become a *routine* for the veterinary technician. This routine should be carried out in the same manner every time the PE is performed (e.g., head to tail or by body systems). This minimizes the possibility of forgetting to check a vital system and helps to ensure patient safety. Being able to perform a complete PE is the first step in being the patient's advocate. The PE reveals the needs of the patient more than any other diagnostic procedure, and knowing their needs is the only way to advocate for patients.

General Body Condition and Mentation

The patient's general body condition (e.g., "strong and healthy" or "weak and emaciated") and mentation (e.g., "bright, alert and responsive" [BAR] or "dull and depressed") should be observed and noted during the history taking. The patient's ability to see and hear is assessed during the history taking as well. If the patient is clearly distressed or aggressive, it is appropriate to request an assistant and use a restraint device (e.g., muzzle) before the "hands-on" portion of the PE. If the patient is scared and timid, a slow, calm, and soft-spoken approach may sufficiently relax and calm the patient to allow for a thorough PE. Any gait abnormalities (lameness, ataxia), muscle atrophy, or asymmetry should be noted while observing the animal during the history taking and should be examined more closely during the hands-on examination.

Head and Neck

Gently restrain the patient's head to examine the eyes, nose, ears, and throat. The eyes should be bright and shiny. The pupils should be equal in size, and both pupils should constrict when light is shined into one eye (pupillary light reflex, PLR). The sclera of the eyes should be white, and the conjunctiva of each eye should be pink. There should be no ocular discharge. The nose should be moist and pliable, with no nasal discharge. The ears can be quickly examined by gently lifting the pinna up and away from the base of the ear. The ear canals should be clean and dry.

If the patient is willing, gently work the lips and cheeks apart to view the premolars and molars on one side of the mouth. Observe the moisture and color of the gums (gingivae), and check the capillary refill time (CRT). Normally the gums are moist and pink. If the gums are sticky or tacky, the patient may be dehydrated. CRT can be assessed by gently pressing on the pink gingiva to blanch it, then counting how many seconds it takes for the color to return. CRT should be less than 2 seconds. A prolonged CRT suggests problems with the cardiovascular system. Quickly scan the teeth and gingiva for any chipped, fractured, or missing teeth. Note any dental tartar that tends to accumulate on the buccal surfaces of the cheek teeth. Inspect the gingiva for any increased redness and inflammation.

Perform the same inspection on the other side of the mouth, and finish by opening the mouth wide to examine the entire length of the tongue and both the hard and the soft palates. Opening a dog's or a cat's mouth often causes it to pull the tongue farther back into the mouth, making it difficult to examine its entire length. The tongue can be extended farther out of the mouth by placing a thumb under the mandible and gently pushing up just caudal to the mandibular symphysis. This procedure is useful to check the base of a cat's tongue for any possible linear foreign body (e.g., string) that may be wrapped around the base of the tongue.

Examination of the neck includes feeling for submandibular lymph nodes in dogs and cats and palpating the thyroid gland in cats (Figure 1-1). To palpate the submandibular lymph nodes, milk the skin ventral to the ramus of the mandible while feeling for any tissue to "blip" between the folds of skin being massaged. Healthy, normal, palpable lymph nodes are generally not tender and are usually small, soft to firm swellings between the skin folds under the mandible. To palpate the thyroid gland, gently extend the cat's head toward the ceiling and run an index finger and thumb down either side of the extended trachea, feeling for any protrusions. An enlarged thyroid gland may indicate hyperthyroidism, and the cat should have a blood test to check its thyroid levels.

Tenting the skin on the dorsal surface of the neck is a quick way to assess the patient's hydration status. A well-hydrated patient's skin should quickly return to its normal shape and position after it has been tented. A dehydrated patient's skin will have a delay and will remain tented before returning to its natural position.

Finish examining the neck by gently taking the neck through a complete range of motion (ROM) exercise. Gently assist the neck into ventroflexion by pointing the nose toward the floor. Then assist the neck into dorsiflexion by pointing the nose toward the ceiling. With the head and neck back in neutral alignment, gently flex the neck to the left and then to the right. Any resistance to these assisted maneuvers by the animal may indicate pain in the cervical vertebrae or neck region.

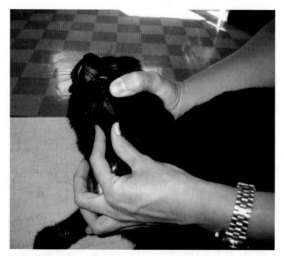

Figure 1-1   To check for an enlarged thyroid gland on a cat, one hand gently grasps the head and extends the neck while the thumb and index finger of the other hand palpates along either side of the extended trachea. An enlarged thyroid gland will bulge or protrude from the trachea.

Chest and Front Legs

With one hand on either side of the patient's neck, gently slide the flat surfaces of the fingers down the neck to the cranial edge of the scapula. Gently work the flat surfaces of the fingers (not the fingertips) into the prescapular muscles to palpate for the prescapular lymph nodes. Then, place one hand on either side of the thorax and gently squeeze and release the ribs toward each other to check chest compliance. There should be some "give" in the ribs of an animal with healthy lungs and ribs, and this procedure should not elicit a cough or any discomfort.

This point in the PE is a good time to auscultate the thorax with a stethoscope (Figure 1-2). Place the stethoscope into the ears with the ear pieces forward into the auditory canals, not toward the back of the head. Next, check which part of the chest piece of the stethoscope is "active." With the ear pieces placed correctly in the ears, gently tap on the diaphragm of the chest piece. If the diaphragm is the active side, a clear tap will be heard as the diaphragm is tapped. If the bell piece is the active side, a muffled tap will be heard as the diaphragm is tapped. Swiveling the chest piece will switch which side is the active, listening side. Generally, the diaphragm is used to auscultate the chest of most dogs and cats.

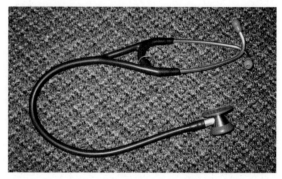

Figure 1-2   Typical stethoscope, with both diaphragm and bell in chest piece. Swiveling the chest piece determines whether the diaphragm or bell is used for auscultation. Note the curvature in the stems of the ear pieces. The stems should be placed in the ear canals pointing toward the nose.

However, some technicians and clinicians may prefer to use the bell piece to auscultate chests.

Thoracic Auscultation

Thoracic auscultation requires using a stethoscope to listen to the chest for both heart and lung sounds. The heart and lungs are heard best with the animal standing still on all four legs. A talented veterinary technician will quickly learn how to keep a cooperative animal standing quietly while auscultating the thorax without an assistant (Figure 1-3). Occasionally it is necessary to prevent a dog from panting or a cat from purring. To stop a dog from panting, use the hand with the wristwatch to extend the neck by gently lifting up on the dog's mandible using the top surface of the hand, while the other hand holds the stethoscope to the patient's chest. Clamping the mouth shut to try to prevent a dog from panting (Figure 1-4) frequently results in excessive movement as the dog tries to wriggle out of the technician's grip. Most dogs will tolerate a gentle lift of the mandible with the top of the hand better and will stand quietly long enough to count a heart rate. To stop a cat from purring, it may be necessary to restrain the cat firmly near a sink and turn on the water to a slow stream.

The heart is located on the left, cranioventral thorax. Begin auscultating the heart by placing the diaphragm of the stethoscope's chest piece just caudal to the point where the dog's left elbow meets the chest. For cats a more ventral placement of the chest piece may be necessary to hear the heart best. One heartbeat normally has two sounds; that is, the "lub-dub" is two sounds but one heartbeat. Once the distinctive lub-dub heart sounds have been identified, time 15 seconds on a watch and count the number of heart sounds heard. To determine the heart *rate,* multiply the number of beats heard in 15 seconds by 4; this number is the heart rate in beats per minute. Systolic murmurs are usually heard as a swishing sound between the lub-dub ("lub-shh-dub"). Moving the stethoscope one rib space cranially or caudally may amplify the sound of the murmur. The rib space where the murmur is heard the loudest is the *point of maximum intensity* (PMI). The rib space can be identified by counting backward from the last (13th) rib. Keep in mind that some murmurs are heard loudest on the right side of the chest. The presence of a murmur and the PMI of the murmur should be noted in the medical record.

The lungs should fill up the pleural space when fully expanded during maximum inhalation. Normal lung sounds should be distinct but soft and free of any wheezing, crackling, or

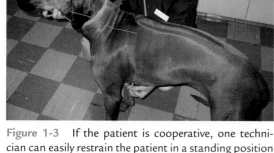

Figure 1-3   If the patient is cooperative, one technician can easily restrain the patient in a standing position while auscultating the thorax.

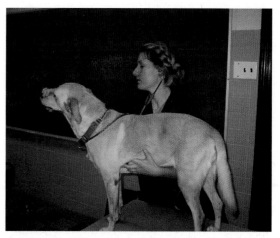

Figure 1-4   Preventing a dog from panting by gently closing the mouth while auscultating the thorax helps the examiner hear heart sounds over breath sounds.

popping sounds. Normal lung sounds should be heard equally well on both the left and the right side of the thorax. Be sure to listen to both sides (cranial and caudal, dorsal and ventral) for lung sounds. One breath is a two-part movement: inhalation and exhalation. To determine the respiratory *rate* (number of breaths per minute), count the number of breaths in 15 seconds and multiply that number by 4. Any increased effort by the animal to breathe (dyspnea) and any increased or absent lung sounds need to be noted in the medical record and addressed. Usually, addressing respiratory abnormalities includes giving the patient supplemental oxygen.

Range of Motion Evaluation of Front Legs

While supporting the standing patient to help it balance on three legs, gently flex all the joints of one front leg, taking care to keep the limb in an anatomically neutral alignment to avoid "torquing" or twisting the joints out of alignment. While supporting the elbow and carpus, gently extend all the joints of the front leg cranially and then caudally. Note any crepitus (popping or crunching felt or heard in joints or around tendons and ligaments), muscle atrophy, resistance, flinching, or inability to flex or extend the leg fully. Check both front legs. Note the animal's ability or reluctance to balance on three legs during the ROM exercises. Weak or ataxic patients may need to be in lateral recumbency for this procedure. A good time to inspect the toe pads and toenails is while the leg is flexed.

Abdomen and Haunches

Abdominal Palpation

Abdominal palpation can be performed with the animal standing or in lateral recumbency. In either case, it is important that the fingernails of the person palpating the abdomen be shorter than the tips of the fingers, and that the flat surfaces of the fingers, not the fingertips, be used to palpate the abdomen. Some healthy cats will resist any attempts at abdominal palpation. If a dog resists abdominal palpation, however, this may indicate pain or discomfort in the dog's abdomen.

Place one hand on either side of the chest, then slide the hands caudally off the last rib and gently work the fingers cranially under the last ribs to find the liver and begin the abdominal palpation. A systematic palpation of the abdomen usually involves working from the cranial to the caudal abdomen and from the dorsal to the ventral abdomen. In general, the flats of the fingers should almost be able to "feel" each other through the mid-abdomen of most animals in good body condition. The bladder with urine should be soft and feel like a water balloon in the caudoventral abdomen. Loops of intestines with gas may crinkle like bubble wrap on palpation. Fecal balls may be palpable in the descending colon of dogs and cats.

To palpate the kidneys in the cat, a dorsal approach to the abdomen is taken. Walking the fingers off the dorsal surface of the last ribs, work the flats of the fingers underneath the last ribs and gently squeeze the fingers toward each other. This will readily identify the left kidney in most cats. The left kidney tends to be a little farther caudal and not as tightly associated with the abdominal wall as the right kidney. Finally, palpate along the patient's navel to check for an umbilical hernia and palpate along the groin to check for any enlarged inguinal lymph nodes or inguinal hernias.

If the patient is a male dog, the prepuce should be inspected at this time. Note any abnormalities. Any tensing of the abdominal muscles or flinching during any part of the abdominal palpation may indicate pain or discomfort. A more gentle approach should be taken, and the tensing should be noted in the medical record.

Range of Motion Evaluation of Hind Legs

Support the patient in a standing position and gently flex all the joints of one rear leg, noting the degree of flexion the patient tolerates. Support the stifle with one hand and the metatarsals with the other, and gently extend all the joints of the rear leg into full cranial extension and then full caudal extension. Note any crepitus in the joints or luxation of the patella ("kneecap") out of its femoral groove. Repeat the flexion and extension ROM exercises with one hand over the coxofemoral (hip) joint. Note any crepitus or resistance in the hip. Repeat the flexion and extension ROM exercises on the other rear leg. Note the animal's ability or reluctance to balance on three legs while performing the ROM exercises. Inspect the toe pads and toenails of the rear legs as well.

Taking the Temperature

A well-lubricated thermometer is used to take the patient's temperature. Some patients strongly resist this part of the PE, and therefore taking the temperature should be saved for the end of the examination so that the patient may be more cooperative for most of the PE. Some states no longer allow the sale or purchase of mercury thermometers, but it is still important that every veterinary technician can read a mercury thermometer (Figure 1-5). Place the mercury thermometer on a flat surface with the name facing down; inspect the thermometer by locating where the silver column of mercury ends on the numbered scale. Careful rotation of the thermometer may be necessary to see the silver column of mercury. Before placing the thermometer in the anus, be sure all the mercury is below the lowest reading on the thermometer by carefully shaking the thermometer with a snap of the wrist. Most mercury thermometers require 90 to 120 seconds to record the patient's temperature (check the manufacturer's recommendation). Most digital thermometers emit a series of audible beeps within 60 seconds to

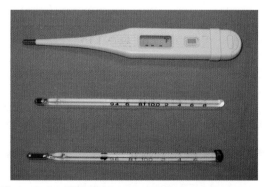

Figure 1-5 Digital thermometer *(top)* and two mercury thermometers. Note the differing ranges between the lower and upper limits of the two mercury thermometers (94°-108° and 96°-106° F).

indicate the final temperature has been recorded (see Figure 1-5).

While the thermometer is incubating, inspect the hair and skin near the base of the tail for the presence of any fleas or flea dirt. This is also a good time to palpate gently the medial thighs and perineal area. Intact male dogs and cats should have both testicles descended in the scrotum, and both testicles should be about the same size and freely movable in the scrotum. The vulva of female dogs should be examined at this time. In addition, the perineum can be inspected for any hernias, masses, or enlarged anal glands. The popliteal lymph nodes can be found in the caudal aspect of the rear legs, directly behind the patella, and should be palpated at this time.

Integument

One final full-body palpation can be performed by gently caressing the hands all along the animal's body from head to tail. Check for any lumps, bumps, or skin lesions.

Any abnormalities or noteworthy findings found during the PE need to be recorded in the medical record and brought to the attention of the attending veterinarian. Even if the animal was seen recently, it is imperative that a thorough PE is performed **the day of the surgery, ideally with the owner present.**

CONSENT FORM

A consent form is a piece of paper that identifies the patient (name, signalment, and descriptors such as hair coat color and body weight), the specific procedure(s) to be performed along with the potential risks to the patient, the physician(s) who will perform the procedures, and the signature of the owner consenting to the procedure(s). Frequently, the receptionist merely hands the consent form to the owner to sign when the animal is brought to the hospital on the day of the scheduled surgery. Because the consent form contains such important information, however, the veterinary technician familiar with the surgical procedure should review the form in detail with the owner at completion of the PE. This gives the owner the opportunity to ask any last-minute questions about the procedure before the animal is admitted to the hospital. Open and clear communication is essential to avoid any confusion and to prevent miscommunication that could lead to legal complaints later. Many legal complaints originate with poor or rushed attempts at client communication.

The procedures should be written out and should be all inclusive; that is, *everything* that will be done to the animal needs to be listed. This form also should document whether or not the patient was fasted appropriately, should include a notation that the owner received an estimate for the procedure(s) to be performed, and should provide a way of contacting the owner during the time the procedure(s) will be performed. It is extremely important that the owner can be contacted during the procedure, should the need arise.

PREANESTHETIC DIAGNOSTIC TESTS

With the ever-increasing standards of care in veterinary medicine and the owner's expectations for the surgical patient's optimum health care, the minimum preanesthetic diagnostic database, or *minimum database* (MDB), is continually increasing in scope. Information collected in the history and PE will help determine which diagnostic tests should be performed before anesthetizing the patient. What is considered the MDB for an elective surgical procedure on a young, healthy animal will be different than the MDB for a surgery on a geriatric patient with preexisting health problems. The MDB results may suggest additional diagnostics may be indicated, or that the original anesthetic protocol may need to be amended.

Minimum Database

The four parameters that constitute the minimum preanesthetic diagnostic testing to evaluate a young and healthy surgical patient are the packed cell volume, total solids, blood glucose, and blood urea nitrogen. These four tests should be considered a starting point, and other diagnostic tests should be performed if any of these four basic parameters cause any concern. These tests are generally easy to run, can usually be performed as "point of care" or "in-house" tests, and require only a small amount of blood. With minimal time and effort, much useful information can be gained from these four tests.

Packed Cell Volume (Hematocrit)

The *packed cell volume* (PCV), or hematocrit (Hct), is the percentage of whole blood that is made up of red blood cells (RBCs). Low PCVs are found in cases of decreased RBC production (as in chronic renal failure), decreased RBC life span (as with some autoimmune diseases and parasite infections), and blood loss (secondary to trauma, blood-clotting disorders, or gastric ulcers). Increased PCV may indicate dehydration (common) or absolute polycythemia (rare). Any values outside the normal range need to be brought to the attending clinician's attention.

Checking a PCV requires microhematocrit tubes, a tube sealant (e.g., Critoseal), a centrifuge, and a hematocrit card reader (Figure 1-6). If whole blood is collected in a syringe without an anticoagulant, heparinized microhematocrit tubes should be used for this test. If blood is collected into a heparinized syringe or placed in a Vacutainer tube with anticoagulant (EDTA) in it, a plain microhematocrit tube should be used. Glass microhematocrit tubes are generally easier to work with than the plastic variety.

After spinning the microhematocrit tube for the appropriate time in the centrifuge (Figure 1-7), the tube is placed on the card reader. Line up the top of the clay with the "0%" line on the card reader. Roll the tube across the card until the top of the plasma lines up with the 100% line on the card. Read the percent line that crosses the point where the packed RBCs are separated from the plasma, at the "buffy coat," and this percent is the PCV (Figure 1-8). The buffy coat usually appears as a small column of white between the packed RBCs below it and the clear plasma above it. The buffy coat contains white blood cells (WBCs) and platelets.

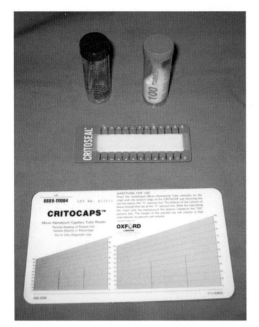

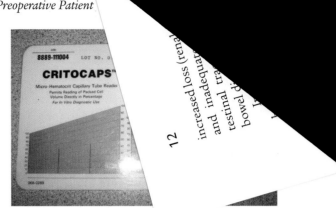

increased loss (renal...
and inadequa...
testinal tra...
bowel d...

Figure 1-8   To read packed ... volume (PCV) on a card, line top of the clay plug on 0% line, and line top of the plasma on 100% line. PCV is read on the line where plasma and packed red blood cells meet. On this sample, PCV is approximately 40%.

Figure 1-6   Heparinized *(red)* and plain *(blue)* microhematocrit tubes, packed cell volume (PCV) card reader, and clay to seal blood in microhematocrit tube.

Plasma is the liquid (noncellular) component of blood and separates out from the packed RBCs after whole blood is placed in a microhematocrit tube, sealed with the clay, and spun in a centrifuge. Normally, plasma is clear and colorless. If the plasma has any color, the color should be noted next to where the PCV percent is recorded in the medical record and brought to the attention of the veterinarian.

Total Solids or Proteins

Total solids (TS) or total proteins (TP) provide information on the animal's plasma protein levels. There are three major plasma proteins: albumin, globulin, and fibrinogen. These levels have a direct effect on serum oncotic pressure. The lower the TP, the lower is the serum oncotic pressure. Changes in serum oncotic pressure directly affect changes in the patient's fluid shifts between the interstitium and the vasculature. With a low serum oncotic pressure, fluid tends to accumulate in the interstitium, resulting in edema. On the other hand, with a high serum oncotic pressure, fluid shifts out of the interstitium and back into the vasculature (blood vessels).

Elevated plasma proteins are associated with dehydration, malignancies (e.g., lymphosarcoma), and infections. Decreased plasma proteins are associated with inadequate production (albumin is made in the liver), inadequate intake (starvation),

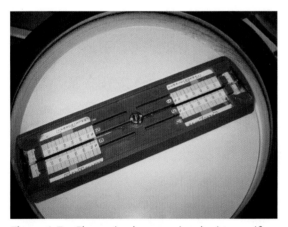

Figure 1-7   Place microhematocrit tube in centrifuge with clay plug toward the outside.

The area just above the buffy coat can be examined under a microscope to do a heartworm screening for live microfilaria.

Normal Range of Packed Cell Volume (PCV)
- Canine: 37% to 54%
- Feline: 27% to 48%

disease, blood loss, parasites), absorption from the gastrointestinal tract (pancreatic disease, inflammatory bowel disease).

In addition, plasma protein levels are important because some anesthetics (some barbiturates) are highly bound to proteins. If a patient is hypoproteinemic, more free drug (not bound to plasma proteins) will be available to function as an anesthetic, effectively increasing the dose. Therefore the animal's protein levels should be noted when deciding which anesthetics to use, or the anesthetic dose may need to be adjusted accordingly.

Supplies needed to check plasma proteins include a refractometer (Figure 1-9) and microhematocrit tubes. After the PCV level is checked, the glass microhematocrit tube can be snapped in the area of the plasma column. Take care not to touch or scratch the glass platform of the refractometer with the sharp edges of the microhematocrit tube. The plasma is allowed to drip onto the refractometer out of the microhematocrit tube. The TS level is read on the scale seen in the refractometer.

Normal Range of Total Solids (TS)
- Canine: 5.5 to 7.5 g/dl
- Feline: 6.5 to 8.2 g/dl

Blood Glucose
Blood glucose (BG) levels indicate carbohydrate metabolism and measure the endocrine function of the pancreas. Eating raises BG levels, and fasting decreases BG levels. Stress will elevate BG levels in cats. Juvenile patients and diabetic patients may need to have their BG values checked intraoperatively and postoperatively if the procedure is especially long.

Glucometers are available at most pharmacies and are easy to use (Figure 1-10). Usually, only a drop of fresh whole blood is required. Some glucometers (e.g., Roche's Accu-Chek Advantage) can determine BG levels using blood collected in ethylenediaminetetraacetic acid (EDTA) or heparin, two types of anticoagulants, but they will not accurately measure BG in serum. It is important to use blood recently collected because glucose values will be affected the longer the blood sits before it is analyzed. Likewise, it is important to follow the manufacturer's guidelines and directions. Any invalid results should be addressed (e.g., repeat with another sample) and any abnormal results should be brought to the attending veterinarian's attention and addressed.

Normal Range of Blood Glucose (BG)
- Canine: 80 to 130 mg/dl
- Feline: 70 to 180 mg/dl
- Both canine and feline: less than 40 mg/dl indicates hypoglycemia.

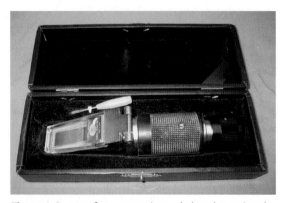

Figure 1-9   A refractometer is needed to determine the total solids in plasma.

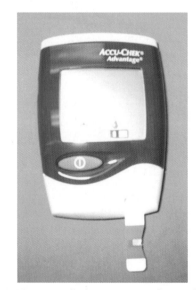

Figure 1-10   A small glucometer can be purchased at most pharmacies.

Blood Urea Nitrogen

Urea is a nitrogenous compound that is a product of amino acid breakdown in the liver. Blood urea nitrogen (BUN) levels are used to evaluate the kidney's ability to remove nitrogenous wastes (urea) from the blood. If the kidneys are not working properly, sufficient urea will not be removed from the plasma and will result in increased BUN levels.

An estimate of the patient's BUN value can be assessed quickly using a reagent strip (e.g., Bayer's Azostix; Figure 1-11). Blood mixed with the anticoagulants EDTA or heparin (as long as it does not contain an ammonium salt) will not affect the estimated BUN of an Azostix; however, neither serum nor plasma should be used for this test. Supplies needed to check BUN on a reagent strip include the reagent strip, fresh blood sample, watch with second hand, and a strong stream of water to rinse the strip. The color change on the reagent strip is compared with the color scale on the bottle for the strips. The corresponding color match between the reagent strip and the bottle indicates the estimated BUN (Figure 1-12).

Some anesthetics are primarily metabolized by the kidneys, and if there is any question of the patient's renal function, choosing a drug that is not primarily metabolized by the kidneys ought to be considered. Further diagnostic tests assessing kidney function (e.g., urinalysis) should be considered as well.

Normal Range of Blood (BUN)

- Canine: 5 to 35 mg/dl
- Feline: 5 to 35 mg/dl

Additional Tests

Other diagnostic tests specifi_____ patient's history and PE findings should be performed before any surgery. Generally, preanesthetic diagnostics are noninvasive and may eliminate ("rule out") the need for more invasive procedures. However, these diagnostic tests may support the need for additional, more invasive diagnostics or procedures. For example, the logical progression of diagnostic testing for a puppy with vomiting and diarrhea would start with an intestinal parasite test ("fecal") and a "parvo" test, followed by abdominal radiographs, then an abdominal ultrasound, and finally an abdominal exploratory procedure. In addition, the puppy with vomiting and diarrhea should have a complete blood count (CBC) and serum chemistry panel and electrolyte panel submitted to aid in determining what type of intravenous fluids or additional support (e.g., antibiotics, parenteral nutrition, plasma transfusion) is indicated.

It is important to note that preanesthetic diagnostic tests will not be the same for every patient and that not all preanesthetic diagnostics are limited to blood tests (e.g., CBC; serum chemistry, electrolyte, thyroid, and clotting panels; heartworm and feline leukemia virus tests; blood

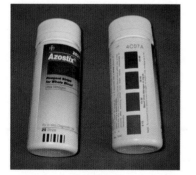

Figure 1-11   Bottle of reagent strips (Azostix) used to estimate blood urea nitrogen (BUN); color scale is used to estimate BUN value.

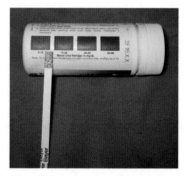

Figure 1-12   Comparing sample reagent strip with color scale on bottle provides estimated BUN level.

). For example, intestinal parasite tests, graphs, diagnostic ultrasounds, urinalyses, d electrocardiograms may need to be performed before surgery on certain patients, depending on the history and PE findings.

Once all the preanesthetic diagnostic tests have been performed and analyzed, if the results still indicate surgery is necessary and is the appropriate next step, the patient is premedicated for anesthesia.

PREOPERATIVE MEDICATIONS (PREMEDICATIONS)

Surgical patients are routinely premedicated with a combination of agents, including analgesics, sedatives, and at times anticholinergics. The purpose of administering these agents before induction is threefold. First, the patient is more relaxed, allowing a less stressful transition to anesthesia. Second, pain management is provided at the optimum time, before surgical tissue trauma occurs. Third, appropriate premedications ("premeds") ease the transition out of anesthesia, facilitating a smooth recovery. Anticholinergics may be added to prevent some of the undesired effects of the analgesia and sedation, mainly bradycardia.

Principles of Pain Management

The basic principles of current pain management involve (1) preemptive (preventive) analgesia, (2) multimodal analgesia (using different classes of drugs simultaneously to interrupt the pain pathway at various points), and (3) appropriate follow-up analgesia (postoperative and at home; see Chapter 8). Using this strategy, veterinarians design an analgesic plan for each patient that maximizes pain control, maintains patients on an analgesic plane, and reduces unwanted side effects.

These simple principles have evolved from our current understanding of the pain pathway, or *nociception.* Pain signaling occurs in a distinct pathway that begins at the onset of a noxious stimulus. The stimulus may be tissue trauma, surgical incision, or even heat. When tissue is traumatized, the first phase of the nociceptive pathway is triggered, and the event is converted

to a signal that can be sent to the central nervous system (CNS) for processing. This phase is called *transduction.* The second phase, *transmission,* is the propagation of the impulses up toward the spinal cord. Once in the spinal cord, pain signals may undergo a number of different effects. Some signals are handled locally by the release of endogenous opioids, whereas others are sent to the brain for further processing. This sorting process is called *modulation,* the third phase; pain signals are said to be "modulated" in the spinal cord. The fourth and final phase of nociception, *perception,* occurs only in the conscious patient. Perception is "knowing" that pain is present and usually results in such reactions as withdrawal, vocalization, and in some cases aggression. Anesthesia interrupts the perception phase *only.* It is important to remember that interfering with perception alone does not address transduction, transmission, or modulation. Patients who undergo surgery only with anesthesia have essentially no pain management; the spinal cord is continually bombarded by pain signals, which will become evident as soon as the animal wakes.

The four distinct phases of the pain pathway allow pain to be interrupted at more than one juncture. Pain management specialists believe that interrupting nociception or pain perception can be achieved most effectively by targeting multiple points along the pathway. The analgesic drugs currently available target one or more of the nocicepetive phases, although each class of agents exerts a major effect on one of the four phases (Figure 1-13). This is the rationale for combining different analgesics as premedications for surgery, a process called *multimodal analgesia.*

Analgesics

Optimum premedication for surgery is likely to include several agents, as just discussed. Four classes of drugs can be effectively used to deliver preemptive analgesia: opioids (e.g., butorphanol, buprenorphine, morphine, fentanyl), nonsteroidal anti-inflammatory drugs (e.g., carprofen, meloxicam, deracoxib), local anesthetic agents (e.g., bupivacaine, lidocaine), and alpha$_2$-adrenergic agonists (e.g., medetomidine, xylazine). (Appendix A

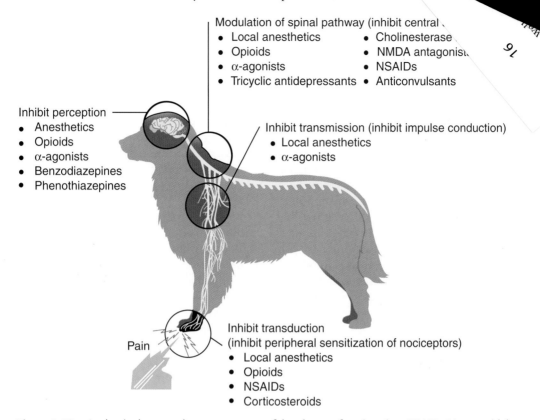

Modulation of spinal pathway (inhibit central ...
- Local anesthetics
- Opioids
- α-agonists
- Tricyclic antidepressants
- Cholinesterase
- NMDA antagonist.
- NSAIDs
- Anticonvulsants

Inhibit perception
- Anesthetics
- Opioids
- α-agonists
- Benzodiazepines
- Phenothiazepines

Inhibit transmission (inhibit impulse conduction)
- Local anesthetics
- α-agonists

Pain

Inhibit transduction
(inhibit peripheral sensitization of nociceptors)
- Local anesthetics
- Opioids
- NSAIDs
- Corticosteroids

Figure 1-13   Analgesic drugs work at one or more of the phases of nociception. *NSAIDs,* Nonsteroidal anti-inflammatory drugs; *NMDA, N*-methyl-D-aspartate.(From Tranquilli WJ, Grimm KA, Lamont LA: *Pain management for the small animal practitioner,* Jackson, Wyo, 2000, Teton New Media.)

provides complete dosage information.) The most effective time to administer analgesia is before tissue trauma or damage occurs. *Preemptive analgesia,* the anticipation of pain and treating in advance, is a critical pain management strategy. Most patients require less anesthesia and actually experience less pain on recovery with smaller doses of analgesics when effective preemptive analgesia is administered.

Opioids

Opioids, the mainstay of acute pain management, provide analgesia by binding to specific opioid receptors in both the CNS and the peripheral nervous system (PNS). Opioids work at several locations along the pain pathway, affecting nociceptive signal transduction, modulating signals at the spinal level, and inhibiting perception of pain. In addition to providing analgesia, opioids help reduce anxiety and nonpainful distress.

Almost every patient expected to experience pain is a candidate for opioid analgesia. As a class, opioids produce minimal side effects in animals. The only cases in which opioids may be contraindicated are patients with head trauma, because even mild respiratory depression associated with opioids may worsen potential intracranial pressure. Opioids are most effective when administered before the onset of pain. Opioids can be administered through the conventional intravenous (IV), intramuscular (IM), and oral (PO) routes. Other, less common but effective routes of administration include transdermal (e.g., fentanyl), epidural, and intra-articular, as

...ell as by constant-rate infusion. Buccal administration has become a popular route for buprenorphine in the cat, whose unique oral pH allows for excellent absorption by this route. (See Appendix A for an in-depth description of these techniques).

How Opioids Work

Opioids bind to opioid receptors in the spinal cord. The mu (μ) and kappa (κ) opioid receptors are primarily responsible for producing analgesia, with the μ receptor producing the most profound analgesia. The κ receptors produce much milder analgesia. Both receptor types are also responsible for producing respiratory depression, euphoria, sedation, and miosis. An opioid can interact with one or more types of opioid receptor. Drugs that bind to a receptor and cause expression of activity are called *agonists*. Drugs that bind to receptors and block their action are called *antagonists*. There are further subclassifications into full (pure) agonists, partial agonists, and mixed agonist-antagonists. The opioid drugs are classified by these subdivisions, which describe their potential action and duration.

Pure agonists (e.g., morphine, hydromorphone) bind and stimulate all types of opioid receptors, causing maximum analgesia. They are extremely effective but of only moderate duration, typically about 4 hours. Full agonists are also the most likely to cause side effects.

Partial agonists function much the same as full agonists, but the interaction occurs with less-than-full activity at the receptors. Buprenorphine is a μ partial agonist. Although buprenorphine only partially binds to the μ receptor, it does so with great affinity. Therefore, although it provides analgesia of less intensity than morphine, buprenorphine has a much longer duration of action, up to 8 to 12 hours.

Agonist-antagonist opioids (e.g., butorphanol) bind to more than one type of opioid receptor, causing an effect at one type but blocking effects at another receptor. Butorphanol binds and activates κ receptors to produce analgesia and sedation; it also binds with μ opioid receptors, blocking (antagonizing) the receptors. For this reason, butorphanol is considered a mild analgesic with extremely short duration, less than

1 hour in most cases. Butorphanol does produce profound sedation for up to 2 hours, outlasting the analgesia provided. Co-administration with butorphanol may result in reversal of the μ effects of full opioid agonists.

Antagonist opioids fully or partially reverse the effects of opioid agonists. Naloxone is a pure opioid antagonist that completely reverses the effects of all opioid agonists at all receptor sites. Butorphanol can be used as a partial reversing agent, reversing μ activity but not κ effects.

Side Effects

Opioids produce few clinically significant cardiovascular effects, other than bradycardia, in dogs and cats when administered at recommended doses. However, opioid-induced bradycardia is responsive to anticholinergics and can be reduced if a patient is pretreated with an anticholinergic. Respiratory depression is a common side effect with opioids in humans but rarely is clinically significant in veterinary patients. Emesis (vomiting) is a common side effect of some opioids, particularly morphine and hydromorphone. Vomiting typically occurs once when opioids are used as a premedication rather than when administered to an animal already in pain. Panting is a fairly common side effect of many opioids, especially at higher doses. This potential side effect may not be clinically important, but it can make patient monitoring difficult postoperatively because it is difficult to differentiate between panting as a sign of pain or as a reaction to an opioid (see Chapter 8).

Nonsteroidal Anti-Inflammatory Drugs

Nonsteroidal anti-inflammatory drugs (NSAIDs) have been used in human and veterinary medicine for many decades to treat fever, inflammation, and pain. More recently, NSAIDs have been shown to be quite efficacious for treating inflammation and pain associated with surgery, and several NSAIDs have been approved for preoperative use in dogs. NSAIDs can be incorporated into premedication protocols to control mild to moderate pain associated with surgery. For maximum effect, NSAIDs should be administered preoperatively, up to 1 to 2 hours before tissue trauma. When used in this way, controlling inflammation before it begins, dramatic results can be observed in the postoperative period. Patients who receive preemptive NSAIDs tend to recover with significantly less pain and often require less postoperative analgesia than those who do not. This class of drugs can be safely combined with opioids to provide excellent multimodal analgesia. NSAIDs are available in several formulations, including oral tablets, chewable forms, liquids, and injectable solutions.

How NSAIDs Work

When cells are damaged as a result of trauma, surgery, or disease, fatty acids such as arachidonic acid (AA) are released from cell membranes. The release of AA triggers a cascade of biochemical activities that ultimately produce prostaglandins, which serve many functions in the body; some prostaglandins are essential for normal homeostasis, and some result in inflammation and pain. The enzyme cyclooxygenase (COX) metabolizes AA to prostaglandin and is the target of NSAIDs. To date, two forms of COX enzymes have been identified. These enzymes are closely related and are now known as COX-1 and COX-2. Each converts AA to prostaglandins, although the prostaglandins produced by each COX enzyme appear to serve very different functions. COX-1 is continuously present in most cells, and it is important for normal body functions. In the stomach, COX-1 plays a key role in maintaining integrity of gastric mucosa. In platelets, COX-1 is essential for thromboxane A_2 production. In contrast, COX-2 is not readily present in the cells, but it is rapidly synthesized in response to various inflammatory stimuli. Once induced by tissue injury, COX-2 converts AA into prostaglandins that create inflammation and pain. Both COX-1 and COX-2 play a vital role in the kidney as important mediators of salt and water balance, rennin (chymosin) release, and vascular tone. NSAIDs exert their antiinflammatory effects by inhibiting activity of COX-1, COX-2, or both. This inhibitory activity varies between NSAID compounds and between animal species.

Side Effects

As a class, NSAIDs are associated with specific types of potential side effects. Some of these are species specific and drug specific, as in the case of acetaminophen metabolism in cats. Possible side effects associated with NSAIDs include gastrointestinal tract damage, hepatopathy, renal toxicity, impaired platelet function, and cartilage destruction. Administration of NSAIDs should be restricted to the well-hydrated, normotensive animals with normal hepatic and renal function, no hemostatic abnormalities, and no evidence of gastric ulceration.

Alpha$_2$-Adrenergic Agonists

Alpha$_2$-adrenergic agonists (α_2-agonists) are short-duration sedative/analgesic/muscle relaxants that can be rapidly reversed with α_2-antagonists. This characteristic makes these drugs suitable for procedures requiring short-term restraint and analgesia as well as premedication for longer surgical procedures. Use of α_2-antagonists as premedications may result in substantial reduction in both induction and inhalant anesthesia dosages. Alpha$_2$-agonists are non-narcotic and nonscheduled agents. Medetomidine and xylazine are the two α_2-agonists currently approved for use in dogs in the United States. Medetomidine is a dose-dependent sedative-analgesic often used as a preanesthetic agent in healthy animals. Onset of effect is 5 to 15 minutes depending on route of administration (IV or IM), and sedation can last up to 90 minutes. Alpha$_2$-agonists are administered intravenously (IV) or intramuscularly (IM).

How α_2-Agonists Work

Alpha$_2$-agonists inhibit release of the excitatory neurotransmitter norepinephrine to produce analgesia and sedation. Alpha$_2$-agonists interrupt the pain pathway by inhibiting nerve impulse transmission, modulating nociceptive signals in the spinal cord, and inhibiting perception within the brain. Because α_2-adrenoceptors are found in various sites throughout the body, α_2-agonists normally induce a number of physiologic changes in addition to sedation, analgesia, and muscle relaxation. Administration results in physiologically normal peripheral vasoconstriction, which creates a transient increase in blood pressure. Because the normal cardiovascular response to these events is a reflexive decrease in heart rate, patients are expected to become bradycardic. All cardiovascular parameters smoothly return to presedation levels on reversal with atipamezole.

Side Effects

Alpha$_2$-agonists can have profound effects on the CNS and cardiovascular system, but using low dosages can minimize these adverse events. Bradycardia and vomiting are the most common side effects with α_2-agonists. All α_2-agonists are associated with potential side effects, including hypertension, bradycardia and heart block, respiratory depression, excessive CNS depression, vomiting, increased urine production, and peripheral vasoconstriction.

Candidates for α_2-agonist administration should be healthy, have sound cardiovascular systems, and be exercise tolerant. Do not administer an α_2-agonist to an animal with a compromised cardiovascular or respiratory system.

Local Anesthetics

Local anesthetics are inexpensive to use and quite effective in blocking the transmission of nociceptive signals at the source. Use of local anesthetics offers three major benefits. First, local anesthetics produce *true* analgesia, that is, a complete absence of pain. Second, they are nonscheduled agents, requiring no cumbersome paperwork. Third, the techniques used to administer local anesthetics are relatively easy to perform. Most blocking techniques are well within the skill level of licensed veterinary technicians. Local anesthetics can and should be used in any surgical patient with an identifiable site for nerve blockade. For example, local anesthetics can be used effectively in patients undergoing thoracotomy, elbow surgery, maxillomandibular procedures, local excisions, feline declawing, and knee or cruciate repair. Anesthetic agents can be administered in the following ways to create local and regional anesthesia and analgesia:

- *Field block,* such as an incisional line block, produces regional anesthesia.
- *Infraorbital nerve block* provides anesthesia and analgesia to the upper lip and nose, the dorsal aspect of the nasal cavity, and the skin ventral to the infraorbital foramen.

- *Mandibular nerve block* provides anesthesia of the teeth, skin and mucosa of the lower lip, and chin.
- *Intercostal block* provides analgesia after thoracotomy and for desensitizing the area around broken ribs.
- *Intra-articular administration* of a local anesthetic provides analgesia to a joint before and after a surgical procedure.
- *Circumferential ring block* provides anesthesia and analgesia around a given area, such as a foot or claw.

In addition, local anesthetics are most often the drugs of choice for epidural anesthesia and analgesia. This technique is a good alternative to general anesthesia or as an adjunct to inhalant anesthesia, especially for patients at high risk during general anesthesia and those undergoing painful orthopedic surgeries of the hind limb. Finally, an IV constant-rate infusion of a local anesthetic can provide sustained pain control in a variety of patients undergoing extensive nerve trauma, such as limb amputation. (See Appendix A for dosing information.)

Lidocaine and bupivacaine are the agents most often used for dogs and cats. Lidocaine is characterized by rapid onset (5-10 minutes) but short duration (45-90 minutes). In contrast, bupivacaine has a longer onset (15-20 minutes) but provides up to 6 hours of analgesia.

How Local Anesthetics Work

Local anesthetics act by inhibiting transduction and transmission of nerve impulses and by modifying the signals at the spinal cord. Local anesthetics inhibit generation and transmission of nerve impulses by blocking sodium channels in the neuron's cell membrane. This slows the rate of depolarization of the neuron cell membrane and prevents the threshold potential from being reached.

Side Effects

When administered at an appropriate dose, local anesthetics have relatively few, if any, adverse side effects. The potential systemic side effects of local anesthetics involve the CNS and cardiovascular system. Other potential side effects include development of methemoglobinemia, nerve and skeletal muscle toxicities, and allergic reactions, including hypersensitivity or anaphylaxis.

Table 1-1 summarizes the side effects of analgesics. Note that not all the agents described in Table 1-1 and earlier are approved for use in veterinary patients. Some are approved for use in dogs but not cats, and some are approved for use as single agents rather than in combination with other drugs. However, although the U.S. Food and Drug Administration (FDA) has not approved all the previously cited analgesics for use in veterinary medicine, the Animal Medical Drug Use Clarification Act of 1994 (AMDUCA) permits veterinarians to use them on an "extralabel" basis.

Sedation and Tranquilization

Sedatives alone do not possess any analgesic properties but are an important adjunct to premedication protocols. Sedation should be incorporated into preoperative regimens to reduce stress, fear, and anxiety, all of which exacerbate pain, and vice versa. However, sedatives alone (with the exception of α_2-agonists) should never be administered to an animal without analgesia when pain is anticipated. Sedation alone may decrease the animal's ability to express pain and give the false impression that the animal is pain free. The most frequently used sedatives for premedication include the tranquilizing agents phenothiazines (acepromazine) and benzodiazepines (diazepam, midazolam).

Anticholinergics

Anticholinergic drugs such as atropine and glycopyrrolate are sometimes added to premedication protocols that are expected to produce profound, sustained bradycardia. For example, anticholinergics are frequently given to patients who receive opioids and are expected to have a long gas anesthesia time. Anticholinergics are given to reduce bradycardia and to dry oral secretions. Atropine sulfate has a quick onset of action and rapid elimination and can be given subcutaneously (SQ), IM, or IV at a dose of 0.04 mg/kg to prevent or to treat bradycardia and to dry oral secretions. Glycopyrrolate can be given SQ, IV, or IM at a dose of 0.011 mg/kg, although onset of action is substantially increased when given IV. Glycopyrrolate is typically used to prevent rather than treat bradycardia once it has occurred. The effects of glycopyrrolate are much longer lasting than with atropine.

Anticholinergics can increase the incidence of cardiac arrhythmias and sinus tachycardia. Increasing heart rate is not always beneficial to the patient because higher heart rates do not necessarily translate into better perfusion. Whether or not an anticholinergic should be routinely

TABLE 1-1	Side Effects of Analgesics	
AGENT	ADVERSE EFFECTS	MONITORING
Opioids	Sedation, low blood pressure, respiratory depression	Mentation, blood pressure, respiratory rate and quality
Local anesthetics	None unless given by CRI With CRI: nausea, vomiting, neurologic signs, seizures	Observe regularly for muscle tremors and GI upset.
NSAIDs	GI disturbances, GI bleeding, renal disturbances	General observation, hydration status, stool quality, urine production
Alpha$_2$-agonists	Bradycardia, cardiac arrhythmias, hypertension, peripheral vasoconstriction	Palpate femoral pulse rate and quality; auscultate heart; monitor blood pressure.

CRI, Constant-rate infusion; *GI,* gastrointestinal; *NSAIDs,* nonsteroidal anti-inflammatory drugs.

administered in conjunction with drugs that lower heart rate (e.g., α_2-agonists) has been the subject of considerable scientific debate. Initially, treatment of α_2-agonist–induced bradycardia was thought to be beneficial. Currently, however, anticholinergic drugs are *not* generally recommended to prevent periods of expected transient bradycardia. Bradycardia that is considered life threatening because it is associated with poor perfusion can be rapidly corrected with atropine. The most practical approach may be to avoid "routine" use of anticholinergics, administering them on a case-by-case basis only to patients in need.

INTRAVENOUS CATHETERS

After the patient has received the appropriate premedication, an IV catheter is usually placed. In addition to the analgesic benefits provided by premedicating the surgical patient, premedication also makes for a more sedate and cooperative patient when the catheter is placed.

The placement of an IV catheter offers many benefits to the surgical patient. Once an IV catheter has been placed, it is easier for the veterinary technician to administer, as well as less stressful for the patient to receive, multiple IV medications. Puncturing through the skin and vein (venipuncture) for every injection is unnecessary when an IV catheter is in place. Also, with an IV catheter the patient is not poked with a needle every time an IV medication is administered. Likewise, the veterinary technician does not need to find a "good" vein for every drug administered intravenously. Many drugs needed by a surgical patient are intended to be, and some can only be, administered intravenously, and the IV catheter allows for easier administration of these drugs. For example, induction agents for general anesthesia, analgesics, antibiotics, fluids, and emergency drugs may need to be given to the surgical patient at some point during its hospital stay. Having established access to the vascular system through an IV catheter aids in the efficiency of administering these medications.

The type and placement site of the catheter greatly influence its capabilities. Peripheral catheters

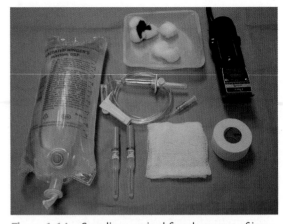

Figure 1-14 Supplies required for placement of intravenous (IV) catheter and administration of IV fluids. *From left,* IV fluid bag (1-L bag of lactated Ringer's solution shown), cotton balls and scrub product, IV fluid administration set, IV catheters, gauze squares, tape, and clippers.

are completely adequate for short-term use (1-3 days), anesthetic induction, and medication administration. However, for long-term use (>3 days), extended fluid therapy, or systemic monitoring, a central line should be placed.

Peripheral catheters are most often placed in the following sites:

> *Canine:* cephalic and lateral saphenous veins
> *Feline:* cephalic, medial saphenous, and femoral veins

Almost any palpable vessel can be used when placing a catheter. Regardless of the site, the basic supplies needed to place the catheter remain the same (Figure 1-14).

Supplies

Catheter
Many styles of catheters are available for use. The three most common styles are the over-the-needle catheter, the through-the-needle catheter, and the butterfly catheter (Figure 1-15). The choice of catheter style is primarily determined by the site of placement and the intended use. The over-the-needle type is typically used for short-term

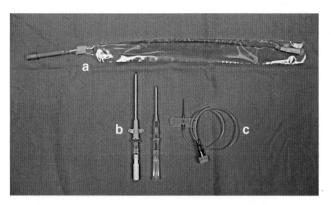

Figure 1-15   Examples of IV catheters: *a*, through-the-needle catheter; *b*, over-the-needle catheters; *c*, butterfly catheter.

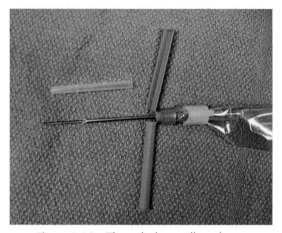

Figure 1-16   Through-the-needle catheter.

and surgical catheters and is usually placed in a peripheral vein (e.g., cephalic vein). The butterfly catheter is useful when vascular access is required for medications that need to be administered once (as in outpatient treatments) and slowly (i.e., over 1-3 minutes). Butterfly catheters are sharp and rigid and are not intended to remain in a patient that is not being directly monitored (i.e., with hands-on monitoring). Through-the-needle catheters are often placed in the jugular veins of animals that will need intensive nursing care postoperatively (Figure 1-16).

The choice of catheter size is primarily influenced by five factors: (1) site of placement, (2) length of time the catheter will be needed, (3) reason for placement, (4) diameter of the vessel, and (5) length of the vessel working area.

Catheter diameter *(gauge)* should be chosen after evaluating the vessel's size and the reason for placement. The length of the catheter needs to be considered after the vessel has been chosen so that the length of the working area is known. For example, a 2-inch catheter placed in the cephalic vein of a dachshund is inappropriate because once completely seated, the catheter would be proximal to the patient's elbow and would be more likely to kink every time the leg was bent. Table 1-2 provides guidance in making appropriate catheter selections based on the factors listed.

Injection Caps, T-Ports, and Fluid Administration Sets

Injection caps may be placed on the catheter if occasional injections or blood sample collections are anticipated (Figure 1-17). Injection caps allow for repeated punctures through the cap without resulting in damage to or leaking from the cap. Needle-less styles of injection caps are available and are a good option because they reduce accidental needle punctures of workers.

T-ports (or T-sets) serve the same purpose as an injection cap and also allow easier access to the catheter (see Figure 1-17). The short tubing incorporated into the design of the device allows sample collection or medication administration to be done more easily. A fluid administration set of the appropriate size should be used if continuous infusion of fluids or IV medications is anticipated, and the set can be connected to the T-port.

Usually an administration set of 15 or 20 drops per milliliter is used for patients weighing greater

TABLE 1-2   Intravenous Catheter Selection Guidelines

PATIENT SIZE (POUNDS)	VEIN	TYPE OF CATHETER	CATHETER DIAMETER (GAUGE)	CATHETER LENGTH (INCHES)
Canine				
0-5	Saphenous/cephalic	Over the needle	24	3/4
5-25	Saphenous/cephalic	Over the needle	22	1-1 1/4
25-80	Saphenous/cephalic	Over the needle	20	1-2
80 and up	Saphenous/cephalic	Over the needle	18	1-2
0-5	Jugular	Through the needle	21	11 1/2
5-25	Jugular	Through the needle	18	11 1/2
25-80	Jugular	Through the needle	16-18	11 1/2
80 and up	Jugular	Through the needle	16	11 1/2
0-5	Saphenous/cephalic	Butterfly	24-23	3/4-1
5-25	Saphenous/cephalic	Butterfly	22	3/4-1
25-80	Saphenous/cephalic	Butterfly	20	3/4-1
80 and up	Saphenous/cephalic	Butterfly	18	3/4-1
Feline				
0-4	Femoral/cephalic	Over the needle	24	3/4
4 and up	Femoral/cephalic	Over the needle	22	1
0-4	Jugular	Through the needle	21	11 1/2
4 and up	Jugular	Through the needle	18	11 1/2
0-4	Cephalic	Butterfly	24	3/4
4 and up	Cephalic	Butterfly	22	3/4

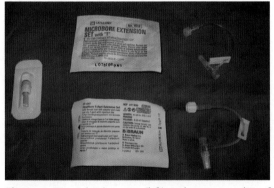

Figure 1-17   Injection cap *(left)* and two examples of T-ports or T-sets.

than 7 kg. Sets with 60 drops/ml are used for patients weighing less than 7 kg for more accurate fluid administration. For extremely small patients, a Buretrol administration set can be employed for the most accurate measurement of fluids administered, and it is especially useful if

an electric fluid infusion pump is not available (Figure 1-18).

Extension Sets
An extension set may be used in conjunction with an administration set to allow for better animal mobility in the cage postoperatively. The administration sets are often not long enough to be practical, so extension sets may be used.

Tape
One-inch white tape is needed to secure the catheter to the patient. A 1-inch-wide piece of tape long enough to encircle the patient's limb or neck, depending on where the catheter is placed, will be needed. Two additional pieces of 1/2-inch-wide tape, the same length as the 1-inch-wide piece, will be needed to secure the catheter further in place.

Catheter "Prep" Materials
Clippers with a number 40 (No. 40) blade or a No. 50 blade are required for hair removal from the

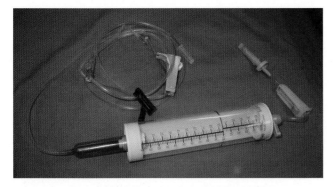

Figure 1-18   Buretrol administration set can be attached to bag of IV fluid and the chamber filled with amount of fluid to be administered. These sets are generally used on small (e.g., pediatric) patients when an electric infusion pump is not available.

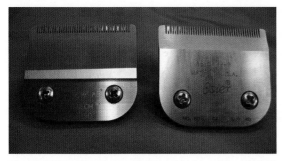

Figure 1-19   Two types of clipper blades, a No. 50 *(left)* and a No. 40 *(right)*, that can be used to clip hair in preparation for surgery or when placing an IV catheter.

catheter site (Figure 1-19). The amount of hair to remove depends on the catheter site and the patient's size. In general, for peripheral veins a margin of 1½ to 2 inches on all sides of the proposed puncture site is appropriate (clipping an area of this size often requires clipping the entire circumference of the limb). Catheters placed in the jugular vein should have a larger area clipped.

"Prepping" materials include cotton balls saturated with either dilute (50:50) povidone-iodine scrub or chlorhexidine scrub for the cleansing step and cotton balls saturated with 70% isopropyl alcohol for the rinsing step. Jugular catheter sites may be prepared with saturated gauze sponges instead of cotton balls.

Fluids or Heparinized Saline

Either continuous infusion of IV fluids or regular flushing of the catheter with heparinized saline is necessary to maintain patency of the catheter once it is placed. If fluids are used, 0.9% sodium chloride (NaCl) or lactated Ringer's solution (LRS) is most often used.

Heparinized saline ("hep saline") can be made by adding 5 units of heparin per milliliter of saline in the bag (or bottle) of sterile saline. For example, a 250-ml bottle of sterile saline should have 1250 units of heparin (1.25 ml of 1000-unit/ml concentration of heparin) added to it. The bottle should be labeled and dated as such. Shelf life of the hep saline is 72 hours at room temperature. If using 0.9% saline that contains a bacteriostatic agent, however, the expiration date on the bottle is the shelf life.

Bandage Materials

Bandage materials are needed if the catheter is to remain in place after the surgical procedure is completed. Antibiotic ointment, elastic gauze, and elastic tape (or Vetrap) are the materials of choice. Usually, 1-inch widths of all materials work best, given the area that will be bandaged on most dogs and cats, but personal preference eventually becomes the determining factor. Tegaderm is a sterile, transparent, breathable adherent dressing used to cover the insertion site of the catheter. This dressing is impervious to liquids and bacteria and therefore is effective in maintaining a catheter. Other sterile wound dressings may be used depending on the indication for and placement site of the catheter.

Even with aseptic placement and appropriate bandaging, peripheral catheters should only remain in place for 3 days. Daily evaluation of the catheter and insertion site helps to prevent phlebitis and to detect any problems early.

Placement Technique

Box 1-1 details the placement of IV catheters in a peripheral vein.

Jugular Catheters

Some surgical patients require intense postoperative critical care. If part of this care requires central venous pressure (CVP) measurements or long-term fluid therapy, a jugular catheter (central line) should be placed.

Supplies

The supplies required for placement of a jugular catheter are similar to those used for a peripheral vein catheter. Jugular catheters are longer, usually

---

BOX 1-1   Technique for Placement of a Peripheral Intravenous Catheter

1. It is difficult to define a set area of the patient's limb that needs to be clipped for placement of the catheter because of the many variables involved (e.g., size of animal, vessel being used, type of catheter being placed). Expect to clip an ample amount from the area where the catheter is to be placed. Bear in mind that no component of the catheter and no accessories (e.g., injection cap, end of fluid line) should be resting in hair once the catheter has been placed. When in doubt, shave more than would seem necessary. To avoid surprises when the owners see the animal, be sure to inform them that the hair will be removed for placement of the catheter.
2. After clipping, remove all loose hair from the tabletops and dispose of it in the waste can. The clipped area should be cleansed using a surgical scrub product and rinsing agent combination, either povidone-iodine/70% isopropyl alcohol or chlorhexidine/70% isopropyl alcohol (Figure 1-20). Cotton balls are best used to help prevent depositing excessive amounts of fluid on the area. The target pattern should be used when preparing the area. Begin at the proposed puncture site and move in a circle progressively toward the hair margins. Cotton balls that have left the center of the area must never return to the center. A rinsing agent should be used in the same manner to remove the scrub from the skin. A minimum of three "cycles" of scrub/rinse should be performed. If, however, after the third rinse the skin is still dirty, continue cleansing until the skin is clean. No final prep solution is necessary unless the catheter will be left in place after the surgery is completed. In this case, apply the solution using the target pattern as previously described.
3. Before beginning the placement of the catheter, be sure all supplies are available and readily accessible. To begin, the restrainer should occlude the vessel to be catheterized (Figure 1-21). Proper restraint must be used to prevent contamination of the prepped catheter site.

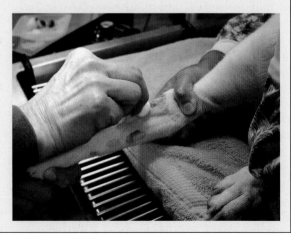

Figure 1-20 Scrubbing clipped area before catheter placement.

BOX 1-1 Technique for Placement of a Peripheral Intravenous Catheter—cont'd

4. Open the catheter using aseptic technique. Remove both the injection plug at the end of the catheter and the cover on the catheter. Break the seal on the stylet and catheter by quickly sliding them apart and then returning them to the original position. Take care to avoid touching the exposed catheter.

5. Place the thumb of the nondominant hand parallel to, but not touching, the prepped vessel. The hand should be holding the leg in extension as well.

6. Hold the catheter at the junction of the catheter and stylet with the thumb and index finger of the dominant hand (Figure 1-22).

7. Ensure that the bevel of the stylet is facing up.

8. Using a 10- to 20-degree angle, quickly penetrate the skin with the catheter and then insert it into the vessel.

9. Check the stylet for blood flow (Figure 1-23). If present, advance both the catheter and the stylet 1 to 2 mm. Check the stylet again. If blood flow is still present, grasp the stylet with the hand that is holding the leg. Using the other hand, advance only the catheter into the vessel (Figure 1-24). Be sure to advance the catheter all the way to the hub. If blood flow is not present, redirect the catheter until blood flow is established.

10. With the hand holding the stylet, grasp the hub of the catheter.

11. Using the other hand, quickly remove the stylet and connect either an injection cap, a T-port, or a fluid administration set to the catheter hub (Figures 1-25 and 1-26).

12. If using a fluid administration set, be sure to turn on the fluids to maintain a patent line. If using an injection cap or a T-port, flush the catheter with 2 ml of heparinized saline.

13. Use a dry gauze sponge to remove any blood on the clipped area or hair near the catheter.

14. Begin securing the catheter by using a ½-inch-wide piece of tape long enough to encircle the limb at least once. Place the tape, sticky side up (Figure 1-27), under the hub of the catheter all the way up to the puncture site. Bring the long side of the tape over the hub (Figure 1-28) and tape all the way around the leg, leaving a tab of tape folded over (Figure 1-29) to aid in removal of the tape when the catheter is removed later. This piece should be snug, but not occlusive, because it is the "anchor" for keeping the catheter in place.

15. Take a 1-inch-wide piece of tape and place it, sticky side down, under the catheter all the way up to the first piece of tape (Figure 1-30). Bring the long side of the tape over the catheter hub and around

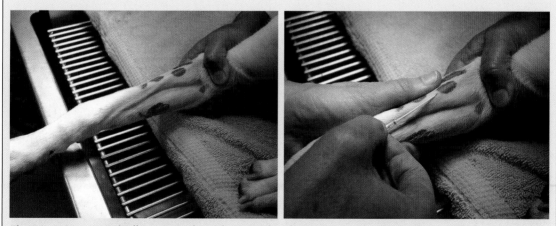

Figure 1-21 Aseptically prepped and properly restrained catheter site.

Figure 1-22 Properly holding catheter and appropriate approach to vessel.

Continued

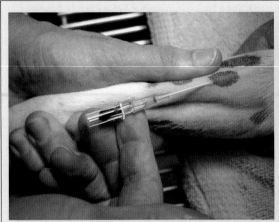

Figure 1-23   "Flash" of blood in stylet of catheter ensures proper placement in vessel.

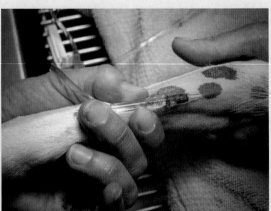

Figure 1-26   Attached fluid line.

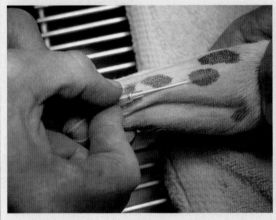

Figure 1-24   Advancing catheter into vessel.

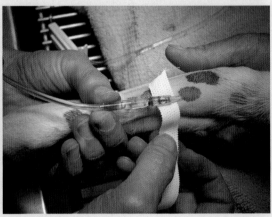

Figure 1-27   Place ½-inch piece of tape, sticky side up, under hub of catheter.

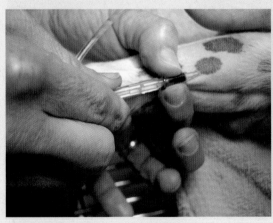

Figure 1-25   Attachment of injection port, T-port, or fluid administration set to catheter hub. Note hand placement to stabilize hub.

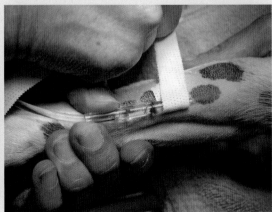

Figure 1-28   Bring long piece of tape over hub and around leg.

BOX 1-1   Technique for Placement of a Peripheral Intravenous Catheter—cont'd

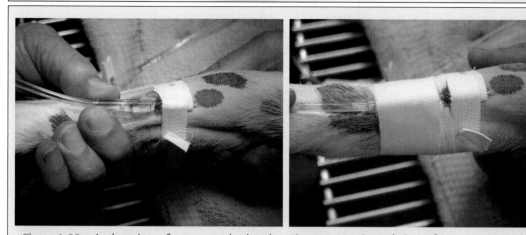

Figure 1-29   Anchor piece of tape properly placed.

Figure 1-31   Second piece of tape securing catheter.

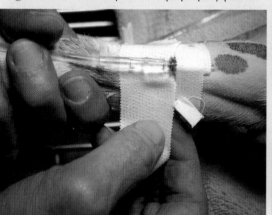

Figure 1-30   Place 1-inch piece of tape, sticky side down, under catheter.

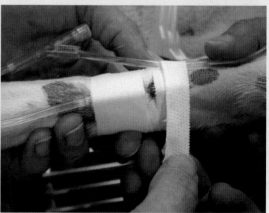

Figure 1-32   A stress loop is made by carefully folding a length of the IV fluid line and taping it securely to patient's leg. Stress loop relieves direct pressure at the connection between catheter (or T-port) and fluid administration set should patient exert tension on administration set. Stress loop makes it less likely that patient will pull its catheter out while shifting positions and moving about the cage.

the leg, securing the hub of the catheter. Be sure the connection of the fluid line and the catheter is not covered (Figure 1-31).

16. The final step in securing the catheter is to use a second piece of ½-inch-wide tape to secure the fluid line with a stress loop (Figure 1-32). When making the stress loop, be sure not to kink the line to impair or obstruct the flow of fluid. Tape the loop to one of the other pieces of tape to ensure that it is secure.

17. Ensure the catheter is still patent by checking the limb for any swelling or "blebs." Generally the fluids will not run if the catheter is not in the vessel. The drip chamber of the fluid administration set can also be observed to see that the fluid is flowing. Another trick to check catheter placement is to lower the bag of fluid lower than the patient's heart and see if blood flows back into the catheter.

8 to 12 inches, and can be single lumen or double lumen. The extra length is needed to ensure placement of the catheter close to the right atrium of the heart, which is required to measure CVP. Because they are long-term catheters, jugular catheters should always be secured with a sterile bandage in addition to the tape. Antimicrobial ointment, elastic gauze, and elastic tape can be used for the bandage.

Placement

With the animal in lateral recumbency, a large area is clipped over the ventrolateral neck to reveal the jugular vein. The site is aseptically prepared as done for a peripheral catheter. Because these catheters are generally left in place for a longer time, a final paint is applied after the last rinse. The person placing the catheter should wear sterile gloves, and a sterile drape should cover the prepared area. Different catheters will need to be inserted with different techniques, so it is best to consult and follow the manufacturer's recommendation for placement.

After the catheter has been placed and is secured, it is essential to maintain the patency of the line. The administration of fluids will aid in ensuring line patency. If fluids are not being administered, hep saline should be used to flush the line at regular intervals (e.g., every 6 hours).

Sample Collection

Sample collection from the catheter is easily accomplished and much less stressful on the patient than performing a venipuncture each time a sample is needed. Initially, 4 to 6 ml of blood should be aspirated through the catheter. This sample should be discarded rather than being used to run the test because it is diluted by the fluids being administered through the line. Next, a sample for the test can be aspirated into a new syringe. After the sample has been collected, the catheter must be flushed with hep saline before the fluids are reattached to maintain patency.

Central Venous Pressure

CVP monitoring is done to assess how well blood is returning to the heart as well as how effectively blood is pumped from the heart. This procedure is helpful in monitoring a patient with right-sided heart failure because blood backs up into the vena cava in these patients. CVP monitoring also helps to assess overhydration with fluids because as blood volume increases, CVP increases as well. A water manometer is connected to the catheter to determine the measurement. A normal reading for cats and dogs is less than 8 cm H_2O.

ENDOTRACHEAL INTUBATION

Endotracheal (ET) tubes are an important piece of anesthetic equipment. ET tubes are used for two main reasons: administration of oxygen and inhalation anesthetics and assistance with resuscitative needs.

Components of Tube

All ET tubes have several components (Figure 1-33). It is important to know each of these components

Figure 1-33   Endotracheal tube: *a,* hose connector; *b,* body; *c,* cuff indicator; *d,* cuff; *e,* Murphy eye.

in order to use the tubes properly and evaluate the integrity of each tube before use.

1. The *hose connector* is found at one end of the ET tube. It connects the tube to the Y-piece, non-rebreathing system, or Ambu bag.
2. The *body* is the major portion of the ET tube. Several numbers may be found on the tube body. The length measurements are in 2-mm increments and identify the length of the tube. The manufacturer's name may also be seen on the body. The large bold number is the size of the internal diameter in millimeters. The most common tubes are available in sizes ranging from 3.0 to 12.0 mm in 0.5-mm increments.
3. The *cuff indicator* is used to determine the pressure of the cuff on the trachea once air has been infused into the cuff.
4. The *cuff* is present to permit the creation of a leakproof system. Air is infused into the cuff, via the cuff indicator, to ensure a seal between the ET tube and the lumen of the trachea. The cuff prevents the patient from inhaling room air, which would dilute the gas delivered to the patient during anesthesia. The cuff also prevents the patient from exhaling anesthetic gas into the operating room and from aspirating any vomitus while intubated.
5. The *Murphy eye* is found at the tip of the ET tube. It allows airflow in the event the end of the tube should become occluded with respiratory secretions (mucous plugs).

Box 1-2 explains how to check an ET tube for leaks before using it in a patient.

Selection of Proper Tube Size

When intubating a patient, the largest size of ET tube possible, without being traumatic, should be used. Generally, tube size is based on a patient's weight, although palpation of the trachea and experience will aid in this decision. Table 1-3 is provided as a reference. Because of the variability in patient size, multiple tubes should be set aside for possible use and checked for leaks with every patient. An acceptable practice is to choose the size thought to be needed, in addition to a tube 0.5 mm smaller and a tube 0.5 mm larger.

Supplies

Using the proper supplies in the proper manner will significantly increase the success rate of intubation (Figure 1-34).

BOX 1-2   How to "Leak Check" an Endotracheal Tube

The endotracheal (ET) tube must be checked for leaks each time it is used.

1. Completely submerse the tube in a pan of clean water.
2. Attach a syringe to the cuff indicator.
3. Fully inflate the cuff and observe for any bubbles. Bubbles in the water, seen coming from any spot on the tube, indicate a leak in the tube.

The ET tube may be thrown away, or it may be kept and identified as a leaky tube if that type of equipment would be needed (e.g., tracheostomy tube).

TABLE 1-3   Approximate Sizes for Endotracheal Tubes Based on Body Weight

BODY WEIGHT (kg)	INTERNAL DIAMETER (mm)
Canine	
2	3-4
5	5-6
10-12	7-8
14-16	8-9
18-20	9-10
>20	11 and up
Feline	
2	3.0-3.5
4-5	3.5-4.0
>5	4.0-4.5

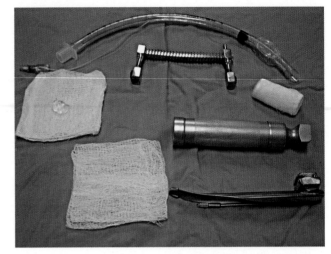

Figure 1-34   Supplies needed for endotracheal intubation.

Endotracheal Tube

Both clear and colored ET tubes are available. Although both types work equally well, the clear tubes have two distinct advantages. First, any type of occlusion in the tube (e.g., blood, mucus) is more easily identified in a clear tube than in a colored or nonclear tube. Second, clear tubes allow visualization of the fog that moves along the lumen of the ET tube as the patient breathes. This is another useful means of quickly confirming that the patient is breathing.

Rolled Gauze

Rolled gauze is used to secure the ET tube to the patient once proper placement has been established. Any width can be used, although 2-inch gauze is most often used. The gauze is placed on the tube to indicate the depth of placement of the ET tube in the patient. Proper depth of insertion is determined by measuring the tube before placement. Box 1-3 describes the procedure for measuring the tube for proper placement in the patient.

Sterile Lubricant

Sterile lubricant is needed to lubricate the tip and cuff of the ET tube to permit easier passage of the tube through the larynx. The lube should be placed on a clean gauze sponge or clean paper towel and then applied to the tube.

BOX 1-3   Measuring an Endotracheal Tube for Proper Placement in Patient

1. Position the patient in sternal recumbency if possible.
2. Identify the thoracic inlet and the larynx. The ramus of the mandible may be used as a landmark for the larynx.
3. Without touching the tube to the patient's hair coat, place the tip of the endotracheal (ET) tube halfway between the larynx and the thoracic inlet.
4. Identify where the tube is just caudal to the canine tooth.
5. Place the gauze tie on the tube at the point where the tube is just caudal to the canine tooth.
6. Ideally the connector end of the tube should be at the incisors. If too much tube extends beyond the incisors, the ET tube may need to be cut to decrease the "dead space."

Cuff Syringe

The cuff syringe is needed to inflate the cuff of the ET tube. Generally, a 6- or 12-ml syringe is used. It should be readily available throughout the procedure, but the syringe should not be placed in a pocket, out of sight. Taping a syringe

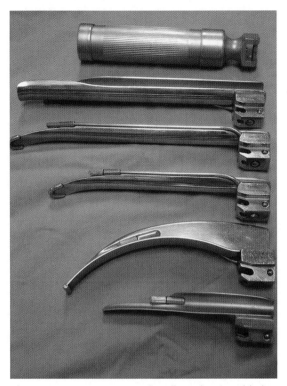

Figure 1-35   Laryngoscope handle and various blades.

case to an accessible area of the anesthesia machine provides reliable storage for constant availability.

Laryngoscope or Light Source

The use of some type of light source significantly enhances the process of intubation. Easy visualization of the larynx permits greater success at first attempts to intubate. Laryngoscopes are composed of two major parts: the blade and the handle (Figure 1-35). The *blade* houses the light bulb and can be curved or straight. Curved blades are commonly identified as Miller blades, and straight blades are often called Wisconsin blades. The numbers included in the identification process refer to the length of the blade. The higher the number, the longer is the blade. Often, "0" blades work well with cats, No. 1 blades for small dogs, No. 2 for medium-sized dogs, and No. 3 blades for large breed dogs. The *handle* houses the batteries that power the laryngoscope. Alternative light sources include floor lamps and overhead lights.

Mouth Speculum

The use of a mouth speculum is not necessary, but its use has definite advantages. First, the mouth can be opened wider to allow better visualization, therefore increasing success rates for endotracheal intubation. Second, the speculum prevents the patient from biting the ET tube should the patient transition into a lighter stage of anesthesia. Third, the speculum helps the restrainer to keep the mouth open. Also, in an emergency, the speculum allows for single-person intubation.

Tube Placement

Patient Anatomy

Proper knowledge of the anatomy of the throat is critical when placing the ET tube. Proper recognition of structures assists in the detection of abnormalities and helps to ensure proper placement of the tube. Figure 1-36 displays the anatomy of the throat. When viewing the throat, the following structures can be seen: vocal folds, epiglottis, and glottis. The *vocal folds* are the most lateral structures, located on the lateral edges of the glottis. The *epiglottis* is a triangular flap of tissue that covers (or protects) the glottis when in the "up" or most dorsal position. The epiglottis must be lying down for intubation to be accomplished. The vocal folds are located on the lateral edges of the glottis. The *glottis* is the most ventral opening in the throat. The esophagus runs along the dorsal surface of the trachea, just left of center.

One-Person Technique

Box 1-4 describes the technique for performing single-person endotracheal intubation.

Two-Person Technique

Box 1-5 describes the technique for performing two-person endotracheal intubation.

Laryngospasms

Certain species, most often cats and rabbits, experience the phenomenon of laryngospasm during endotracheal intubation. If excessively stimulated, the muscles of the larynx will spasm, and the vocal folds will clamp shut. Application of

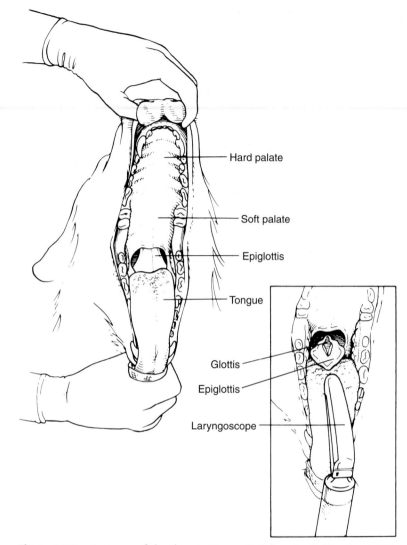

Figure 1-36   Anatomy of the throat. (From McKelvey D, Hollingshead KW: *Veterinary anesthesia and analgesia,* ed 3, St Louis, 2003, Mosby.)

0.05 ml of 2% lidocaine to each vocal fold (drip the lidocaine out of a tuberculin syringe onto the vocal folds with the needle removed) just before attempting intubation will significantly decrease the occurrence of laryngospasm. Another tactic to avoid laryngospasm is good technique. Repeated stimulation of the area may cause the muscles to spasm, so avoiding unnecessary touching of the area until actually passing the tube will be beneficial.

Confirmation of Proper Tube Placement
The following methods are used to confirm proper placement of the ET tube:

1. *Cough.* Many animals will cough as the tube is passed into the trachea. Although fairly accurate, this method can be deceiving because as the animal coughs, the ET tube may move off the glottis and into the esophagus as it is advanced.

BOX 1-4   Single-Person Endotracheal Intubation

1. Place the animal in sternal recumbency.
2. Place the mouth speculum in the mouth.
3. Position floor lamp or overhead light if being used.
4. Holding the mandible with the nondominant hand, fully extend the tongue and hold it in place with the thumb. The thumb should be caudal to the canine tooth, and the rest of the hand should be on the ventral surface of the mandible.
5. Visualize the glottis. If the epiglottis is lying dorsally, it will need to be pulled down with the endotracheal tube to ensure visualization of the glottis.
6. Pass the lubricated tube through the glottis to the predetermined length, as indicated by the gauze tie placed on the tube.
7. Secure the tube to the patient.
   a. For dogs, tie the gauze tie in a bow on the muzzle, just caudal to the canine teeth.
   b. For cats, tie the gauze in a bow behind the ears at the base of the skull.
8. Leave mouth speculum in place until the patient has reached a surgical plane of anesthesia, to avoid accidental biting of the tube.

BOX 1-5   Two-Person Endotracheal Intubation

1. The restrainer holds the patient in sternal recumbency.
2. Place the mouth speculum, if being used. If no speculum is used, the restrainer opens the mouth by holding the maxilla in one hand and the mandible in the other hand.
   a. Dogs should have the maxilla held caudal to the canine teeth.
   b. Cats should have the maxilla held just caudal to the ear pinna so that the skull is in the palm of the hand.
3. The hand holding the mandible grasps the tongue and fully extends it over the mandibular incisors (Figure 1-37).
4. The restrainer lifts the head and extends the neck to aid the intubator's visualization.
5. Using the laryngoscope, illuminate the larynx for proper visualization (Figure 1-38).

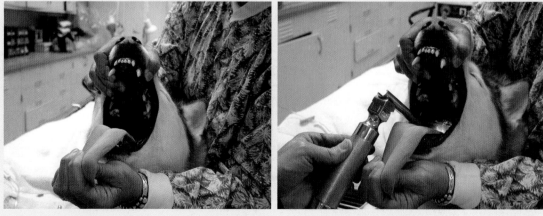

Figure 1-37 Proper positioning for endotracheal intubation.

Figure 1-38 Placement of laryngoscope.

Continued

BOX 1-5   Two-Person Endotracheal Intubation—cont'd

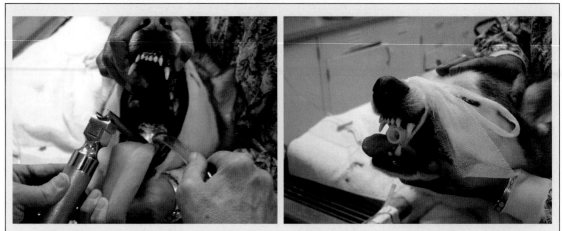

Figure 1-39   Passing endotracheal tube.

Figure 1-40   Endotracheal tube tied in place.

6. Visualize the glottis, and pass the tube between the vocal folds into the glottis (Figure 1-39).
7. Advance the tube to the predetermined depth, as indicated by the preplaced gauze tie.
8. Secure the tube to the patient.
   a. For dogs, tie the gauze in a bow on the muzzle (Figure 1-40). The gauze should be snug but should not constrict circulation.
   b. For cats, tie the gauze in a bow caudal to the ears at the base of the skull.
9. The speculum should be left in place, although the tension may be reduced, until the patient reaches a surgical plane of anesthesia, to avoid accidental biting of the tube.

2. *Fogging in the tube.* When an ET tube has been properly placed in the trachea, there should be fogging of the lumen of the tube with each expiration. This method can be employed only if using a clear tube.
3. *Blowing of gauze or hair.* A few strands of gauze or hair placed at the connector end of the ET tube will blow away with each expiration if the tube is correctly placed. A disadvantage is that the hair may move from the tube because of excessive movement of room air rather than expiration.
4. *Air movement.* If the ET tube is in the trachea, forced air should be felt at the connector end of the tube with each expiration. Bilateral chest compressions can be used with this method to ensure placement. Care must be taken to avoid compressing the abdomen, because an incorrectly placed tube may provide a false-positive assessment.
5. *Palpation.* Palpation of the ventral neck should result in the identification of one "tube."

If the ET tube is in the trachea, only one firm, tubelike structure should be felt. If the ET tube is in the esophagus, however, two firm, tubelike structures will be palpated.

Whatever method is used to ascertain correct tube placement, it should be done before connecting the patient to the anesthesia machine. Once the patient is connected to the machine, a double check of placement can be done. Movement of the flutter valves and the rebreathing bag with each inspiration and expiration will confirm proper placement.

Once the patient is successfully intubated, the intended surgical site can be prepared.

PATIENT PREPARATION

Proper preparation ("prepping") of the surgical patient is a critical part of the surgical process. The veterinary technician should be the primary staff member responsible for this task, either as the performer or the supervisor.

Before the actual prepping of the surgical site, the following preoperative considerations are addressed:

- The technician needs to verify that food and water have been withheld from the patient. Solid food should be withheld for at least 6 hours before surgery.
- If possible, the animal should be walked outside before the surgery. Exercising the animal will encourage bowel and bladder evacuation, thereby decreasing the potential for this type of contamination in the operating room (OR).
- Extremely dirty patients may require a bath before surgery. The bath will decrease overall body soil and will aid in reducing the risk of postoperative complications from iatrogenic contamination. However, the patient's hair coat must be completely dry before inducing general anesthesia. Wet animals are at an increased risk of developing hypothermia while under anesthesia.
- A double check (with the neck ID band, cage card, and medical record) and triple check (with the surgeon) of the patient's correct identity and exact surgery are confirmed. Cross-check that the consent form has been signed by the client for the correct procedures. If the surgery is an amputation, double-check (with the record and consent form) and triple-check (with the surgeon) that the correct limb is being prepared. Any radiographs taken before anesthesia should be in the OR and hung on the view boxes.

Hair Removal

Once the patient has been stabilized under anesthesia, the process of clipping may begin. It is ideal to have the patient positioned for the preparation in the same way as for the procedure (Figure 1-41). Although this may be easily accomplished (for an exploratory laparotomy) or may be more of a challenge (perineal surgery), it is an important step to ensure an appropriate "prep" of

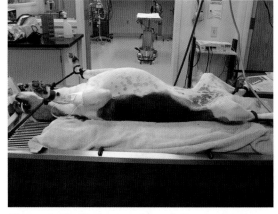

Figure 1-41 Patient positioned for ovariohysterectomy (OHE, "spay").

the surgical area can be accomplished. Except in an emergency, it is recommended that the anesthetist be comfortable with the patient's level of anesthesia before any manipulation begins. Emergency cases are more critical and time is of the essence; therefore the anesthetist may not have the patient at the ideal anesthetic depth before the prep begins. While waiting for the nonemergency patient to stabilize at the appropriate anesthetic level, the surgery technician (frequently the circulating nurse) can complete some of the prep tasks, such as securing the leg ties to the patient and manually expressing the bladder.

The hair clipped needs to be neat, tidy, and symmetric (Figure 1-42). The client's impression of the clip's appearance may influence the client's impression of the entire clinic and staff. Clipping should only be done with a surgical clipper blade. This design of clipper blade has close-set teeth to achieve the closest possible shave. When clipping, the person performing the clip needs to hold the clippers in a pencil grip (Figure 1-43). This grip will permit the greatest amount of control and maneuverability. Other grips will prove to be cumbersome and may strain the wrist and arm. The clipper should be held flat against the skin for the closest shave. The hand not holding the clipper can tense the skin to encourage as easy a movement as possible for the clipper (Figure 1-44). Hair should be removed by clipping *against* the grain of the hair. Clipping with the grain will

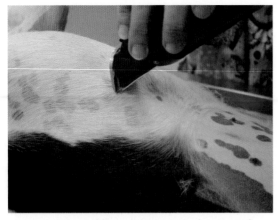

Figure 1-42   Holding clipper at 90-degree angle to skin creates an even, neat margin for clipped area.

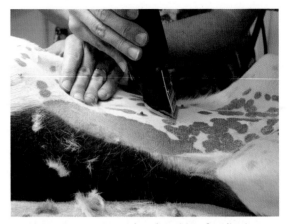

Figure 1-44   Proper hand position for clipping.

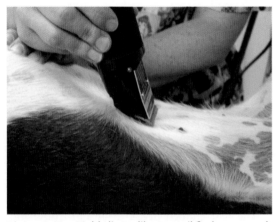

Figure 1-43   Hold clipper like a pencil for best control.

remove the hair but will leave long enough stubble to cause a problem. At this point, shaving back against the grain of the hair will not provide a close enough shave, and hair stubble may be deposited into the wound when the incision is made.

The use of alternative hair removal products is not routinely done in veterinary surgery. Depilatories generally are not effective given the length of the hair. Using a razor after the initial clipping may provide a close shave, but there is a high risk of causing skin trauma.

The amount of hair to be removed depends entirely on the surgery being performed. For general soft tissue surgery, a good rule of thumb is to clip two (2) clipper blade widths in every direction

from the proposed incision site. However, depending on the size of the animal, its length of hair, and the procedure being done, the clip may be altered. For example, a gastrotomy will require a very different clip than a prostatic biopsy. The technician should be sure to check with the surgeon for any special circumstances or anticipated additional procedures. Preoperative clipping and prepping need to include preparations for any ancillary procedures that may be done (e.g., chest tube placement, drain placement, feeding tube placement). Table 1-4 provides clipping guidelines for specific procedures.

Orthopedic preps use the rule of thumb of clipping the limb from the joint distal to and the joint proximal to the surgical incision. The limb needs to be clipped circumferentially to allow complete limb draping and manipulation. As with soft tissue cases, the rule for clipping may need to be adjusted based on the patient's size, the surgeon's preference, and additional procedures to be performed (e.g., bone graft harvest, drain placement). Tables 1-5 (forelimb) and 1-6 (hindlimb) provide clipping guidelines for most orthopedic procedures.

Neurologic surgical patients are usually quite easy to clip, especially when the surgical site is a caudal thoracic or lumbar vertebral space. Clipping two vertebral spaces cranial and two vertebral spaces caudal to the affected site is usually adequate. As with other surgical cases, communication with the surgeon is critical to ensure

TABLE 1-4   Clipping Guidelines for Selected Soft Tissue Surgical Cases

SOFT TISSUE PROCEDURE/AREA	GUIDELINES
Exploratory laparotomy	Mid-sternum to pubis; laterally to edge of ribs
Gastric, liver, splenic	Mid-sternum to pubis; laterally to edge of ribs
Urinary bladder	Umbilicus to caudal pelvis; laterally to edge of ribs
Kidney	Mid-sternum to pubis; laterally to edge of ribs
Prostate	Umbilicus to caudal pelvis, including prepuce; laterally to edge of ribs
Uterine, ovarian	Xiphoid to pubis; laterally to edge of ribs
Ventral neck	Cranially to mid-mandible; caudally to thoracic inlet; laterally to commissure of lips

TABLE 1-5   Clipping Guidelines for Selected Forelimb Orthopedic Cases

FORELIMB AREA	GUIDELINES
Digit	Nails to mid-humerus; use towel clamp through nail to suspend limb
Metacarpal	Nails to mid-humerus; use towel clamp through nail to suspend limb
Carpus	Second metacarpal to mid-humerus.
Radius, ulna	Mid-metacarpals to shoulder; ventrally to midline; cranially to thoracic inlet; caudally to seventh rib
Elbow	Carpus to dorsal midline; ventrally to ventral midline; cranially to thoracic inlet; caudally to seventh rib
Humerus	Carpus to dorsal midline; ventrally to ventral midline; cranially to base of neck; caudally to seventh rib
Scapula	Mid-radius to 2 clipper-widths past dorsal midline; cranially to base of neck; caudally to tenth rib

TABLE 1-6   Clipping Guidelines for Selected Hindlimb Orthopedic Cases

HINDLIMB AREA	GUIDELINES
Digit	Nails to mid-femur; use towel clamp through nail to suspend limb
Metatarsal	Nails to mid-femur; use towel clamp through nail to suspend limb
Tarsus	Second metatarsus to mid-femur
Tibia, fibula	Mid-metatarsals to hip; ventrally to midline; cranially to last rib
Stifle	Tarsus to hip; cranially to last rib; caudally to tuber ischii
Femur	Tarsus to dorsal midline; cranially to last rib; caudally to tuber ischii
Hip	Tarsus to 2 clipper-widths past dorsal midline; cranially to last rib; caudally to tail head
Pelvis	Depends on area of pelvis to have surgery (ilium vs. pubis, vs. ischium); consult surgeon

adequate prepping of the neurologic surgical patient. Particularly in the event of a cervical vertebral surgery, be sure to ascertain if the surgeon will make a ventral or dorsal incision. If multiple intervertebral spaces are affected, clipping should extend from the most cranial and the most caudal space affected. Table 1-7 provides clipping guidelines for neurologic surgical cases.

Some surgeries may fall into either the soft tissue category or the orthopedic category, depending on the reason for the surgery. For example, aural surgeries are generally considered soft tissue, but if a bulla osteotomy is done, it is more of an orthopedic case. Likewise, facial surgery is soft tissue if it is a tumor removal or nasal procedure, but if there is maxillary or mandibular involvement, it is considered orthopedic. Table 1-8 provides guidelines for clipping these types of surgical patients.

After clipping, the patient and the area need to be thoroughly vacuumed (Figure 1-45). The hair removed from the animal must be cleared from the surgical site as well as from the work area. Loose hair can be a source of contamination in the OR, so it is important to avoid transporting any hair into the surgical suite. Brushing away loose hair from the clipped site with a hand is not as effective as vacuuming (Figure 1-46).

Urination

The urinary bladder should be emptied independently by the animal or manually by the technician before the surgical prep. Caution should be used if the abdomen has been traumatized or if the surgery will involve the urinary bladder. Expression of the bladder may be contraindicated, and more damage may be done to the bladder in these situations.

TABLE 1-7	Clipping Guidelines for Selected Neurologic Surgeries
VERTEBRAE	**GUIDELINES**
Cervical: ventral approach	Midventral mandible to mid-sternum; laterally to halfway between dorsal and ventral midline
Cervical: dorsal approach	Mid-skull to two vertebral spaces caudal to affected space; laterally to halfway between dorsal and ventral midline
Thoracic	Two vertebral spaces cranial and caudal to affected space; laterally to edge of transverse process
Lumbar	Two vertebral spaces cranial and caudal to affected space; laterally to edge of transverse process

TABLE 1-8	Clipping Guidelines for Miscellaneous Surgical Cases
PROCEDURE/AREA	**GUIDELINES**
Aural	Lateral canthus of eye; dorsal midline on head and neck; ventrally to ventral midline
Ophthalmic: intraocular	Trimming of eyelashes; limited skin clip because of potential irritation
Ophthalmic: extraocular	*Entropion, ectropion:* one clipper-width past lateral canthus, lower lid, and medial canthus
	Enucleation: midline of muzzle to cranial edge of ear pinna; dorsally to midline; ventrally to commissure of lip
Facial	Procedures vary widely among nasal, maxillary, and mandibular; best to consult surgeon
Perineal	Dorsally to tail head; laterally to tuber ischii (bilaterally); ventrally to mid-thigh (caudal aspect)

The technician may contact the surgeon either to request permission to attempt manual expression or to state that the bladder was not expressed. Nonabdominal surgical patients must also have the bladder emptied if possible. The patient may urinate during the surgical procedure, soaking the table linens as well as the patient's hair coat and skin. Lying in urine for any period of time exposes the patient to the risk of "urine scald" (the moist, irritating effect of urine in contact with the skin). Even if the animal does not urinate during the surgery, it will probably urinate during recovery. The patient soaked in urine is at increased risk of not only urine scald, but also contamination of the surgical wound with urine. Patients that will require critical care nursing postoperatively may have a urinary catheter placed to help prevent these problems.

The bladder can be expressed with the patient either in dorsal or in lateral recumbency. Some type of receptacle should be used to collect the expressed urine to avoid saturating the fur with urine or having the urine pool under the animal. When expressing the bladder, care is taken to use gentle, constant pressure rather than a pulsating action.

Surgical Site Preparation

The skin of a patient cannot be "sterilized," in the true definition of the word, but reducing the contaminants on the skin can greatly reduce the risk of wound infection. Multiple options exist for the products used to prep the patient, as well as the applicators used to apply these products. The use of the particular cleansing products, in a particular fashion and in a particular order, is done to render the skin as clean as possible by eliminating or decreasing as many of the skin flora as possible.

Antiseptics

The first product used in the preparation of the patient is a "scrub" product. This solution has a soap or detergent base and therefore creates a sudsy appearance when used. There are some properties of the scrub product that are desired for maximum effect. Although no available scrub product has all the desired qualities to achieve maximum effect, the choice of product should contain as many of these qualities as possible.

One product available for use as a patient scrub is *povidone-iodine*. This scrub is an iodine-based product that has a detergent and a wide spectrum of antimicrobial activity. Povidone-iodine is bactericidal, virucidal, fungistatic, and fungicidal. Its toxicity to tissues is relatively low, and it is inexpensive and readily available. Because of the iodine base, it does stain clothing and discolor the white hair of animals. Povidone-iodine has a better residual activity level than hexachlorophene but is not as effective as chlorhexidine. The povidone-iodine scrub is generally diluted 50:50 with tap water when used.

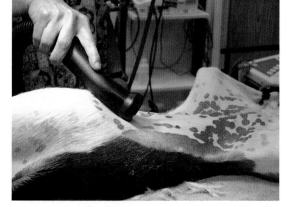

Figure 1-45 Thoroughly vacuum the area after clipping.

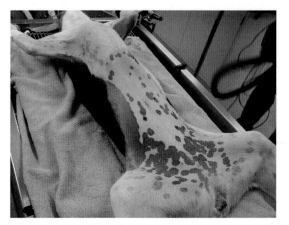

Figure 1-46 Clipped abdomen ready to be prepped.

Chlorhexidine gluconate is another scrub product available. Its residual effect is the best of any available product, and it works well in the presence of organic material. Chlorhexidine has shown bactericidal action against 30 bacterial genera, including *Escherichia coli* and *Pseudomonas* species. It also has demonstrated virucidal and fungicidal properties. Chlorhexidine scrub has relatively low tissue toxicity, except for mucous membranes. Although it is more expensive than other products, it does have the advantage of not staining. Chlorhexidine is generally used as a 60:40 dilution.

Rinsing Agents

After the application of a scrub product, a rinsing agent is needed to remove the detergent. A common rinsing product is *70% isopropyl alcohol.* Isopropyl alcohol at the 70% concentration is effective against most gram-negative bacteria. Alcohol coagulates protein, which contraindicates its use on open wounds and mucous membranes. Isopropyl alcohol is generally well tolerated by patients, and it is inexpensive and readily available. Alcohol can be used with either povidone-iodine or chlorhexidine scrub. Residual properties of the chlorhexidine seem to be enhanced when used with 70% isopropyl alcohol, whereas povidone-iodine does not show any increase in residual activity.

The property of alcohol to evaporate rapidly is both an advantage and a disadvantage. The advantage of rapid evaporation is the ability to move quickly through the prepping process without diluting subsequent products. The extreme cooling effect that results from rapid evaporation is a disadvantage. Excessive amounts of alcohol used to prepare the patient can significantly contribute to the hypothermia experienced by the anesthetized patient. Alcohol that is allowed to pool under an animal or saturate the fur can contribute to the risk of thermal burn if electrocautery is used. Therefore, alcohol should not be used as a rinsing agent if electrocautery will be used intraoperatively.

Another rinsing agent available is bottled *sterile water* or *sterile saline.* Sterile water or saline is effective at removing the detergent product, although it has no antimicrobial properties itself. When prepping open wounds, compound fractures, or mucous membranes, this is the rinsing agent used. Because 70% isopropyl alcohol is not appropriate in certain situations, sterile water or sterile saline is a practical and reasonable alternative.

Applicators

Regardless of the prepping products used, applicators used can vary widely depending on the site being prepared. The most common applicator used is a *gauze sponge.* Sponges can be used individually as needed and saturated with the product, by squirting the liquid from a bottle onto a dry sponge, or sponges can be mass-produced and stored in jars or plastic containers. If mass-produced, the prep sponges and the containers need to be dumped and cleaned weekly to inhibit the growth of contaminants. It is best to place the sponges needed in a separate, smaller container (e.g., "weigh boat") to avoid reaching into the large storage container with dirty hands.

As an applicator, *cotton balls* usually are practical only when prepping small areas, so their use is limited. Cotton balls would be indicated for IV catheter sites and perhaps ophthalmic surgeries.

Similarly, a *cotton-tipped applicator* is usually chosen only for intraocular procedures. The limited amount of preparation needed for the eye can be best accomplished with the delicate control provided by a cotton-tipped applicator.

A *spray bottle* is an appropriate "applicator" only for application of the final "paint" solution (e.g., povidone-iodine). This is an efficient method of application but can be messy. The mist from the spray bottle can easily be deposited on the patient's skin as well as other areas. Monitoring devices, table linens, and even the rest of the animal may be covered with a mist of paint solution (see Chapter 5).

Special Male Dog Preparation

If preparing the abdomen of a male dog, one task must be done before beginning the surgical site prep. After all the hair has been removed from the prepuce, the sheath must be flushed to remove potential contaminants. Combine 1 ml of povidone-iodine solution with 9 ml of tap water. Insert the syringe tip into the prepuce and inject 5 ml of solution (Figure 1-47). Pinch the prepuce around the syringe tip before removing the syringe. While still pinching the prepuce closed, gently massage the solution in the prepuce. Place a towel over the end of the prepuce to absorb the solution. Release the pinch hold on the prepuce. Repeat the process with the remaining 5 ml of solution. This step is required only for intra-abdominal cases when the prepuce will be in the draped surgical field.

Patterns for Scrubbing

Depending on the area of the body that is having surgery, one of three patterns of action should be used to prepare the site: target, orthopedic, or perineal.

Target Pattern

The most common pattern is the target pattern, which resembles a target or bull's-eye. This pattern is primarily used to prepare surgical sites for abdominal, thoracic, and neurologic cases. The prep begins after the hair has been removed by the clipper and vacuumed from the area. The first step is to take one of the rinsing sponges and wipe around the periphery of the clipped margin. This moistens the hair and flattens it down, which helps prevent the hair from flying onto the clipped area once the prep begins.

To begin preparation of the surgical site, pick up one scrub sponge and fold it in half and then in half again, or bring all four corners to the center and hold the sponge by the corners. Either method will produce a smaller contact surface that will be easier to control. Starting at the proposed incision site, move the sponge back and forth for approximately 15 seconds (Figure 1-48). Excessive pressure is not encouraged because it may abrade the skin; the wound may be more prone to healing complications if the dermal layer is compromised. After scrubbing the intended incision site, move the sponge in a progressively outward circle until the hair is reached (Figure 1-49). It is important to continue the scrubbing action with the wrist as the sponge is moved outward.

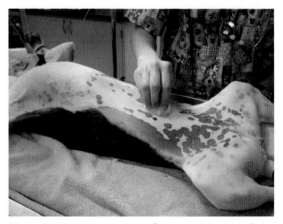

Figure 1-48   Target pattern for preparing surgical site begins at proposed incision site.

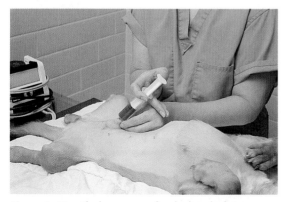

Figure 1-47   Flush prepuce of male dogs before preparing surgical site for abdominal cases. (From Fossum TW: *Small animal surgery,* ed 2, St Louis, 2003, Mosby.)

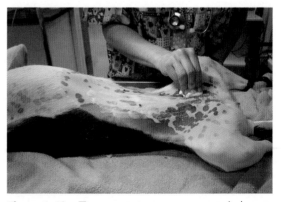

Figure 1-49   Target pattern moves progressively outward from proposed incision site.

This should not be a wiping action, but rather a scrubbing movement. Once the hair or any other dirty or contaminated area has been touched with the sponge, the sponge must *never* return to the incision site.

If using povidone-iodine, the scrub should be repeated at least two more times before rinsing off the chemical. Ensure the proper *contact time* (length determined by manufacturer) to reach the desired efficacy level with povidone-iodine. Alternating the povidone-iodine scrub and the alcohol rinse for the patient prep may decrease the efficacy. After three scrubs with the povidone-iodine, the surgical site should be rinsed with 70% isopropyl alcohol. The same target pattern should be used with the alcohol rinsing sponges as with the scrub sponges (Figure 1-50). Once all of the scrub material has been removed from the surgical site, as evidenced by alcohol sponges that have little to no scrub product, the patient should be positioned appropriately on the surgery table. Final sterile scrub and prep can then be performed (see Chapter 5).

If chlorhexidine is the product used to prepare the surgical site, the contact time is not as critical because chlorhexidine binds with keratin, and the residual effect is better than that of povidone-iodine. Chlorhexidine scrub should be applied using the same target pattern. The rinsing agent can be 70% isopropyl alcohol or sterile saline or water.

Orthopedic Pattern

The second prep pattern is that used with orthopedic surgeries. After the hair has been removed from the surgical site (Figure 1-51), any hair remaining on the foot needs to be covered. An inverted examination glove is placed over the foot (Figure 1-52) and secured with tape (Figure 1-53). To avoid a tourniquet effect, be sure the tape is not applied too tightly. The glove should be covered

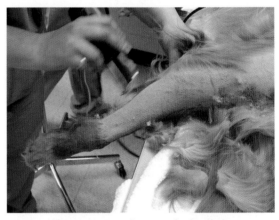

Figure 1-51   Clipping of a forelimb.

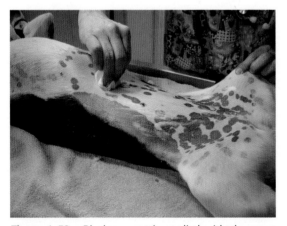

Figure 1-50   Rinsing agent is applied with the same target pattern.

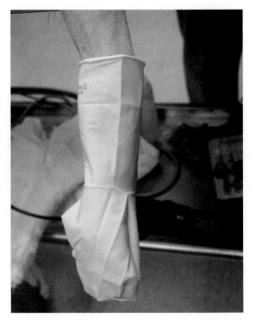

Figure 1-52   Inverted glove placed over unshaven foot.

with tape (or Vetrap), again not too tightly. A stirrup also needs to be made to allow suspension of the limb for prepping and draping. A stirrup is made by taking a long piece of white tape (~2-3 feet), leaving 2 to 3 inches at either end, then folding the remainder of the tape on itself to make it ½ inch wide. Place the ends of the stirrup on either the medial and lateral or anterior and posterior sides of the gloved foot. Secure the stirrup to the foot with tape (Figure 1-54). The limb should be suspended for the preparation to allow access to all surfaces of the limb. Place the stirrup over the hook of an IV pole and then fully extend the pole to elevate the limb (Figure 1-55). In the event of a fracture, it is imperative that the limb and bones be supported as the pole is extended. With fractures the extension of the limb may

actually provide some distraction and traction to fatigue the muscles, which will aid in reduction of the fracture. Once suspended, clipping can be completed (Figure 1-56), and the scrub prep can begin.

With a scrub sponge in hand, begin the prep at the tape edge of the suspended limb. Scrub the limb from distal to proximal, moving circumferentially

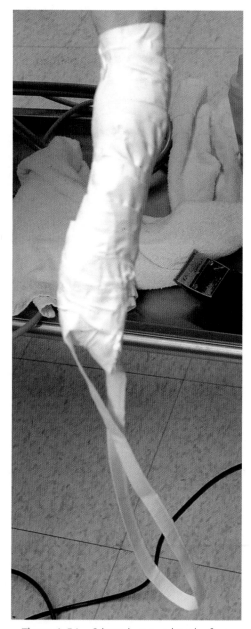

Figure 1-54   Stirrup is secured to the foot.

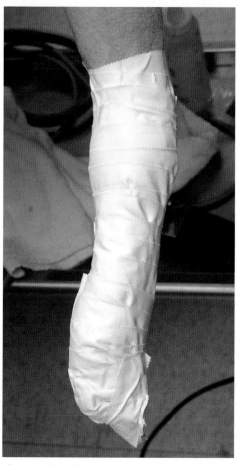

Figure 1-53   Tape covering examination glove.

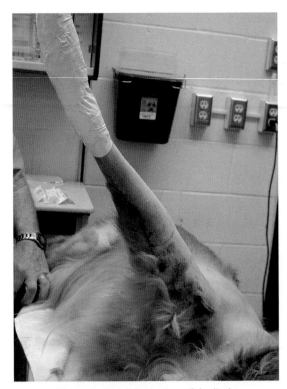

Figure 1-55   Suspension of the limb.

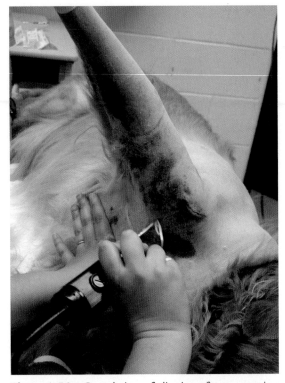

Figure 1-56   Completion of clipping after suspension of the limb.

around the limb. As the sponge dries out, discard the sponge and continue with a new sponge. As with the target pattern, the wrist must be kept moving to provide the scrubbing action. Repeat the scrub a minimum of three times before rinsing to achieve the best antimicrobial efficacy. The rinsing agent is applied in the same pattern, starting at the taped foot and moving proximally to the dorsal midline (Figure 1-57). Generally a final solution is not applied as another prep will be done once the patient is positioned on the surgery table. (See Chapter 5 for the sterile prep discussion.)

After the final rinse, place a clean towel over the medial surface of the down limb. This provides a clean surface on which the prepped limb can lie. The final prep is performed in the OR, so the towel only needs to be clean, not sterile. Carefully lower the limb, supporting any broken bones, to the towel (Figure 1-58). The patient is now ready to be transported to the surgical suite.

Perineal Pattern

The third pattern that can be used is that for perineal surgeries. It is important that a purse-string suture be placed in the anus before beginning the preparation. Placement of the purse-string suture prevents the evacuation of fecal material onto the surgical site during the procedure. The purse-string suture needs to be placed carefully to avoid puncturing the anal glands. It is the technician's responsibility to ensure that the suture is removed after the surgery; a reminder note on the anesthetic monitoring sheet will help the technician to remember this task.

The perineal pattern is basically three separate target patterns performed in a particular sequence. The first step is to do a target pattern on the clipped area to the right of the anus. The second step is to perform another to the left of the anus, and the third pattern is done on the anus itself. The "dirty" area should always be prepared

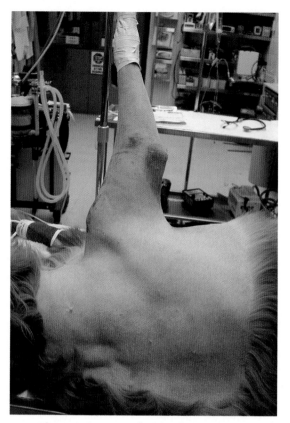

Figure 1-57   Completed orthopedic prep.

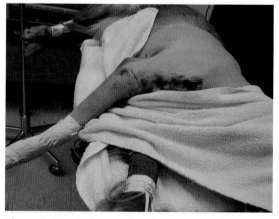

Figure 1-58   Patient ready to be transported to surgery room.

last to minimize contamination. As with other patterns, the scrub is followed by a rinsing agent.

Potential Reactions

Clipper-Related Reactions

If dull clipper blades are used or technique is harsh, clipper burn can occur. Clipper blades should be checked before use for chipped or missing teeth, rust, and other inhibitors of performance. Such inhibitors will pull on the skin and can cause clipper burn. Using excessive pressure with the clippers can also cause clipper burn. Irritation of the skin can inhibit wound healing if the irritation is over the proposed incision site. Irritation can also promote bacterial growth, which could cause an infection. Clipper burns on the peri-incisional skin can be an irritation to the animal, promoting excessive licking. This too can compromise the healing process.

Chemical-Related Reactions

Reactions to prepping products generally present as plaques or wheals. Certain breeds (Labradors, shar-peis) seem more prone to these reactions, although any breed may be affected. Povidone-iodine tends to cause more reactions than chlorhexidine. If a patient has a chemical-related reaction, a notation should be made in the medical record so that an alternative product can be used the next time.

KEY POINTS

1. Taking an accurate history and recording it in a concise, chronologic order create the foundation for the treatment plan for each surgical patient.
2. During the interview of the history taking, the technician needs to confirm the patient's signalment (age, gender, breed) and chief complaint (reason for the visit to the surgical hospital).
3. While interviewing the client, the patient should be allowed to explore the examination room at will, and the technician should make a mental note of the patient's overall condition and mentation (mental status, attitude).
4. The physical examination needs to be thorough and systematic and performed on the day of the scheduled surgery with the owner present.

5. Any abnormalities found on the physical examination need to be brought to the attention of the attending veterinarian and recorded in the medical record.

6. The consent form should identify the patient, the procedures to be performed on the patient, the potential risks involved with those procedures, the name of the veterinarian who will perform the procedures, and a place for the owner to sign indicating consent.

7. The consent form should provide confirmation that the patient was fasted appropriately before admission, that the owner was given an estimate for the costs of the procedures, and that the owner's phone number is readily available to contact the owner during the procedure if necessary.

8. Selection of preanesthetic diagnostic tests depends on the patient's age and health status, type of surgery, and results of initial diagnostic screening tests.

9. Preoperative medications should provide preemptive analgesia and tranquilization and allow for easier anesthesia induction and smoother recovery from anesthesia.

10. To provide the most effective pain prevention and relief, different types of analgesics with different mechanisms of action (multimodal analgesia) need to be administered to surgical patients.

11. The benefits of placing an intravenous (IV) catheter for every anesthetic procedure outweigh any risks.

12. The five factors that should be considered when choosing a catheter are site of placement, length of time the catheter will be needed, reason for placement, diameter of vessel, and length of vessel.

13. Catheter sites must be aseptically prepared to avoid complications.

14. Having all supplies readily available will aid in the success of the procedure.

15. Some surgical patients may require intensive care after surgery and may be better served by placement of a jugular catheter.

16. Successful endotracheal (ET) tube placement depends on using the appropriate equipment and minimizing irritation to the patient.

17. Most patients can be intubated using the one-person technique, although the two-person technique is generally the more common practice.

18. Multiple options are available for checking the ET tube for proper placement in the trachea.

19. Clean, neat, symmetric clipping is an important skill to master for the patient's well-being as well as good client relations.

20. Appropriate hair removal helps to prevent contamination of the surgical site.

21. Rather than pressure, contact time is the important consideration when using skin preparation materials.

22. When preparing a surgical site, always move the applicator from clean to dirty surfaces to avoid introducing contaminants to the proposed incision site.

REVIEW QUESTIONS

1. What information is included in the patient's signalment?
   a. Age, gender, breed.
   b. "Proceed with caution" signals (e.g., "will bite").
   c. Previous surgeries.
   d. All of the above.
   e. None of the above.

2. Why is it important to review all medications and supplements that a patient is taking before beginning the surgery?
   a. To avoid possible drug interactions.
   b. To know if other diagnostic tests are indicated.
   c. To make any necessary adjustments to the anesthesia protocol.
   d. All of the above.
   e. None of the above.

3. Why are leading questions inappropriate to ask during the history taking?
   a. They make the owner feel compelled to answer a certain way.
   b. They may encourage the owner to answer inaccurately.
   c. They are appropriate and should be asked.
   d. Both a and b.
   e. None of the above.

4. Which of the following should be assessed during the history taking?

a. Patient's attitude and mental status.
b. Patient's previous medical problems and treatments.
c. Patient's ability to see and hear.
d. Patient's gait and body condition.
e. All of the above.

5. Why should taking the patient's temperature be saved for the end of the physical examination (PE)?
   a. It is the least important part of the PE.
   b. Most animals dislike having their temperature taken, and it is easier to do a PE on a cooperative patient; taking the temp early during the PE may make the patient uncooperative for the rest of the examination.
   c. By the end of the PE, the examiner should have already ascertained whether the patient is febrile, and only then will the temperature need to be taken.
   d. None of the above.
   e. All of the above.

6. Which of the following should be performed on the day of the surgery?
   a. Thorough physical examination.
   b. Review of the patient's medical history with the owner.
   c. Verbal review of the consent form and obtaining the owner's signed consent for anesthesia and surgery.
   d. All of the above.
   e. None of the above.

7. Which tactic(s) may stop a cat from purring during thoracic auscultation?
   a. Gently squeezing the thorax with one hand while the other holds the stethoscope on the chest wall.
   b. Massaging under the cat's chin.
   c. Holding the cat near a sink or faucet, with or without the water running.
   d. All of the above.
   e. None of the above.

8. The minimum database (MDB) for a young, healthy feline patient having elective surgery would most likely include which of the following diagnostic tests?
   a. CBC, parvo test, electrolytes, and blood typing.
   b. CBC, serum chemistry panel, FeLV/FIV test, intestinal parasite test, and urinalysis.

c. FeLV/FIV test, abdominal radiographs, and ECG.
d. PCV/TS, estimate of BUN, and blood glucose.
e. PCV/TS, thyroid panel, and FeLV/FIV test.

9. What is the purpose of premedicating a patient before inducing anesthesia for surgery?
   a. To provide a smooth transition to anesthesia.
   b. To provide preemptive analgesia.
   c. To facilitate a smooth recovery from anesthesia.
   d. All of the above.
   e. None of the above.

10. *True* or *False:* Anesthesia (as provided by gas anesthetics) provides multimodal analgesia.

11. Which of the following provide multimodal analgesia?
    a. Gas anesthetics, morphine, butorphanol, and fentanyl.
    b. Nonsteroidal anti-inflammatory drugs (NSAIDs), carprofen, and meloxicam.
    c. Xylazine and medetomidine.
    d. Opioids, NSAIDs, local anesthetic agents, and alpha$_2$-adrenergic agonists.
    e. None of the above.

12. *True* or *False:* Anticholinergics, such as glycopyrrolate and atropine, increase the heart rate and provide purely beneficial effects for the patient.

13. *True* or *False:* Peripheral catheters generally suffice for short-term use, and central lines are more appropriate for long-term vascular access (days).

14. *True* or *False:* Central venous pressure measurements require that a central line be placed.

15. How can the patient's correct identity be verified?

16. Why should the patient's identity be verified before anesthetizing the animal for surgery?
    a. To avoid anesthetizing the wrong patient.
    b. To avoid performing surgery on the wrong patient.
    c. It is not necessary to cross-check the patient's correct identity because any good technician should be able to distinguish all black cats in the hospital on any given day based on physical appearance alone.
    d. Both a and b.
    e. None of the above.

17. Why does an orthopedic "clip and prep" of an extremity need to include a circumferential clip around the entire limb?

a. If the incision goes all the way through the limb and out the other side, the other side will already be prepared for this scenario.

b. If the surgeon mistakenly incises the wrong side of the limb with the first incision, and if the leg is clipped circumferentially, the mistake is easily corrected.

c. For patient comfort.

d. All of the above.

e. None of the above.

18. What needs to be done to the patient after the hair clip and before moving the patient into the OR?

a. Vacuum the clipped hair and clipped area of skin.

b. Check to see if bladder needs expressing

c. Perform initial skin scrub.

d. All of the above.

e. None of the above.

19. *True* or *False:* It is accepted practice to scrub a patient initially with a povidone-iodine product.

ANSWERS

1. a
2. d
3. d
4. e
5. b
6. d
7. c
8. d
9. d
10. False
11. d
12. False
13. True
14. True
15. Cross-check the signalment and description in the medical record, cross-check the neck ID band or cage card, and ask a co-worker (e.g., surgeon) to confirm the patient's identity.
16. d
17. e (The entire circumference of the extremity needs to be clipped and prepped so that the surgeon can move and manipulate the leg without contaminating the sterile field.)
18. d
19. True

BIBLIOGRAPHY

Cunningham JG: *Textbook of veterinary physiology,* ed 2, Philadelphia, 1997, Saunders.

Fossum TW: *Small animal surgery,* ed 2, St Louis, 2002, Mosby.

McCurnin DM, Bassert JM: *Clinical textbook for veterinary technicians,* ed 5, St Louis, 2002, Saunders.

McKelvey D, Hollingshead KW: *Veterinary anesthesia and analgesia,* ed 3, St Louis, 2003, Mosby.

Stoeberl TA: Preparing the small animal patient for surgery, *AHT* 4(5):271, 1983.

Romich JA: *An illustrated guide to veterinary medical terminology,* Albany, NY, 2000, Delmar.

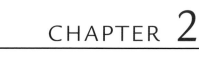

CHAPTER 2

Scrubbed Personnel

Mary Scherer

LEARNING OBJECTIVES

After studying this chapter, the reader should be able to do the following:

- Know what is considered proper attire in the surgical area.
- Understand the general guidelines for personal hygiene of veterinary surgical personnel.
- Define and perform a surgical hand "scrub."
- Define and perform a surgical hand "rub."
- Describe the different types of surgical hand prep solutions.
- Aseptically dry hands and arms after performing a surgical hand scrub or rub.
- Don a surgical gown.
- Perform open and closed gloving.
- Define and perform assisted surgical gloving.

PROPER ATTIRE IN SURGICAL AREA

The surgical area should be a restricted clean area, separate from the rest of the hospital. This restricted surgical environment should be kept as free of microorganisms as possible. Proper operating room (OR) attire reduces microbial shedding, which occurs when microorganisms are released into the environment from the body of the surgical personnel. These microorganisms are present in sebaceous and sweat glands around the hair follicles of the entire body.

The physical and emotional stress associated with surgery can compromise the immune system during surgery and during the convalescent period and make surgical patients vulnerable to infections and disease. Proper surgical attire of OR personnel helps to decrease the risk of infection for the patient by providing barriers against microorganisms. In the OR, proper surgical attire

should include freshly laundered scrub suits, head covers, masks, and possibly shoe covers. A dress code should be written and posted so that it can be easily followed and enforced. This dress code should include the definition of areas where surgical attire must be worn, appropriate attire within those defined areas, and the choice of cover apparel outside the surgical suite. Cover apparel must be removed when entering the surgical area. In addition, guidelines should be provided for general cleanliness, including care of fingernails and the wearing of jewelry. The scrub suit should be covered with a clean laboratory coat at all times when outside the surgical area. A dress code for use in the surgical preparation area should also be written and posted to avoid contamination of the scrub suit while working in this area. A laboratory coat, a plastic apron, or some other adequate covering should be considered when restraining and clipping the animal.

Scrub Suit

Street clothes should never be worn in surgery because they carry dirt, debris, and microorganisms. Instead, a clean, freshly laundered scrub suit ("scrubs") should be donned at the veterinary hospital. Ideally, all scrubs should be laundered in the hospital laundry. Scrubs should not be worn from home to the hospital, nor should they be worn home from the hospital. These scrub suits could bring microorganisms into the hospital and home to infect the surgery personnel's own pets. Clean scrub suits should be worn only in the surgical area. Scrubs should be changed if they become visibly dirty or wet.

The scrub top should fit the body snugly and be tucked into the scrub pants (Figure 2-1). This prevents body scurf (epidermal scales) from being shed as a result of friction produced by the body rubbing against the scrub top. The scrub top should be short sleeved so personnel can scrub their hands and arms for surgery. It is recommended that all nonscrubbed personnel wear long-sleeved, snug-fitting scrub jackets (not loose-fitting laboratory coats) in the OR to prevent any scurf from the arms falling onto the sterile field. Personnel should not wear the OR attire outside the surgical area because microorganisms could be transferred onto the scrub suit. Therefore, when leaving the surgical area, the scrub suit should be covered by a clean laboratory coat, which is removed when reentering the restricted area.

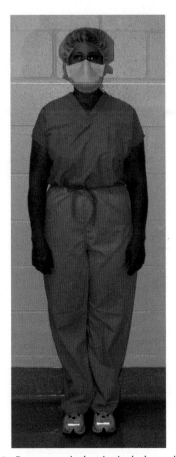

Figure 2-1 Proper surgical attire includes a clean scrub suit. The scrub top is tucked into the pants. All jewelry and name tags are removed. A head cover, mask, and clean shoes are worn.

Head Covers

Everyone in the surgical area should wear head covers. All hair on the head and facial hair should be covered; hair collects bacteria when left uncovered. The head cover prevents bacteria, dandruff, and other contaminants from falling either onto the scrub suits or into the surgical environment. Several types of head covers are available, including the bouffant, the hood, and the skullcap. The head cover chosen should fit well and should cover all hair. The bouffant covers the hair on the head adequately and is preferred over the skullcap (Figure 2-2). The hood should be worn if there is facial hair that is not covered by the mask.

Skullcaps should be worn only if the hair is very short and there is no hair outside the cap at the side or the nape of the neck. Figure 2-3 is an example of a poor choice of head covering; this person should not wear a skullcap.

Masks

The mask should be worn in the OR when open sterile supplies or scrubbed personnel are present. The mask should be worn over the mouth and nose. Because the mask functions to filter droplets containing microorganisms that come from the mouth and nose, it should be changed frequently. The strings should be tied tightly, and

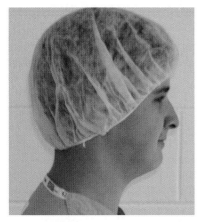

Figure 2-2   A bouffant head cover effectively covers all hair on the head and prevents hair from falling into the surgical site.

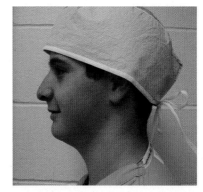

Figure 2-3   This skullcap does not effectively contain all hair on the head and should not be worn; it cannot effectively prevent hair from falling into the surgical site and contaminating the site.

the mask should conform to the face so that no air escapes without being filtered by the mask. If a sneeze or cough is imminent, without turning the head, the person should step back from the sterile field. If the mask is secured properly, the cough or sneeze should be filtered. If the mask is not secured properly, or if the head is turned, the cough or sneeze will be vented out of the side of the mask, directly onto the sterile field.

Shoes and Shoe Covers

Shoes worn in the OR should be comfortable and cleaned frequently (whether or not shoe covers are worn). Shoes should have enclosed toes and heels to protect personnel from dropping heavy or sharp objects onto their feet and injuring them. Shoe covers are optional. If worn, shoe covers should be changed if they become torn, wet, or soiled and when personnel reenter the surgical area. Foot attire has no proven significance in reducing the incidence of postoperative wound infections, and the primary reason for its use is to decrease floor contamination.

Jewelry

It is recommended that all jewelry and watches be removed, although some hospitals will allow jewelry if it is confined within the scrub suit or bouffant.

Rings, bracelets, and watches must be removed for scrubbed personnel and should be removed by all surgical personnel. Jewelry may harbor microorganisms that routine handwashing cannot remove, and earrings, necklaces, and body-piercing objects could fall into the surgical field.

GENERAL GUIDELINES FOR PERSONAL HYGIENE

All personnel should practice proper body hygiene. Everyone who works in the OR should bathe daily with an antimicrobial soap. Deodorant should be worn to prevent excessive sweating and body odor. Body odor is caused by the presence of microorganisms in the hair-bearing areas of the body. This can become unpleasant when confined to an OR.

Fingernails

Fingernails should be well manicured. They should be short, clean, and healthy. Healthy nails are desired because any small cuts or torn cuticles can harbor microorganisms. Fingernails should not extend past the fingertips because they could cause tears in the surgical gloves, which could be a source of infection to the patient. Artificial nails are unacceptable because they harbor microorganisms, especially fungi. Nail polish should not be worn because polished nails, if chipped, harbor more microorganisms than unpolished nails. In addition, personnel may not be thorough in handwashing and cleaning to avoid damaging their nail polish.

SURGICAL HAND SCRUB AND HAND RUB

The surgical hand scrub is defined as the process of removing as many microorganisms as possible from nails, hands, and arms by mechanical washing and chemical antisepsis before participating in a surgical procedure. The surgical hand scrub is also designed to maintain the lowest possible microbial counts throughout the surgical procedure.

The surgical hand scrub should always begin with a brief, general hand and arm wash to loosen surface debris and "transient" microorganisms (organisms that are loosely attached to the skin surface.)

When performing the surgical hand scrub, it is important to remember that the skin is never made "sterile." Skin becomes *surgically clean;* if there are any holes (detected or undetected) in the surgical gloves or gown, the probability of introducing microbes into the surgical field is reduced. Even though prophylactic antibiotics may be used, this should never be considered a substitute for a proper hand scrub.

The scrub procedure consists of a mechanical and a chemical part. The *mechanical* part is the removal of bacteria and debris by producing friction when rubbing or brushing. This removes dirt, oil, and transient organisms that are loosely attached to the skin. During the *chemical* part of the scrub, the antiseptic, antimicrobial skin-cleansing agents are used. These agents inactivate or inhibit the growth of microorganisms found on the surface of the skin and in hair follicles, sebaceous glands, and sweat glands.

The antimicrobial scrub agent or an alcohol-based hand rub should be chosen from the U.S. Food and Drug Administration's (FDA) product category defined as "hand scrubs" or "alcohol-based rubs." Avagard (3M) is an example of a scrubless, brushless, waterless antiseptic hand preparation product referred to as a "rub." The agent selected should be nonirritating and fast acting and should provide a prolonged depressant effect on residual bacteria. It should cover a broad spectrum of bacteria. The length of scrub time varies according to the manufacturer's recommendations and written directions for use. Scrubbing usually is performed for 5 minutes. A nail-cleaning pick should always be used to remove debris from the subungual area of each finger. Stiff brushes are not recommended on the skin because they can cause skin abrasions and may release more resident microbes from the deep layers of the skin, which is counterproductive. Many scrub agents come with disposable, antiseptic-impregnated scrub brushes that have soft brushes, sponge, and nail-cleaning pick included. The new brushless technique (alcohol rub), with or without water, consists of rubbing an antimicrobial agent on the hands and arms. Brushless rubbing agents typically are alcohol based, with the addition of moisturizing emollients and surfactants that help clean the skin. Some agents are combinations of alcohol and other antimicrobial agents, such as chlorhexidine gluconate or alcohol with preservatives.

Whichever FDA-approved antimicrobial scrub agent or alcohol-based rub is chosen, a standardized protocol should be established and written for each surgical hand procedure according to the manufacturer's recommendations for the particular scrub or rub agent used. A copy should be posted in the scrub room. Every person scrubbing for a surgery should be familiar with these instructions.

Before performing the surgical hand scrub (or rub), the animal should be properly clipped, prepped, moved into the surgery room, and positioned on the table correctly for the surgical procedure. The OR should be set up with the proper pack and instrumentation (Figure 2-4). The major special equipment necessary for the procedure should be sterile and ready.

Prescrubbing Guidelines

1. Remove all rings, watches, and jewelry. Remove pens, name tag, and other items from scrub top pockets.

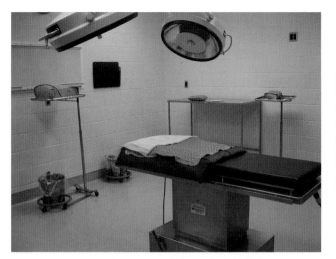

Figure 2-4   The operating room is arranged with the appropriate surgical packs before performing the surgical hand preparation. Note the circulating warm water pad on the surgical table and the kick buckets with plastic liners. Also note that the surgical room is free of clutter. Only those items needed for the specific surgery to be performed are in the OR.

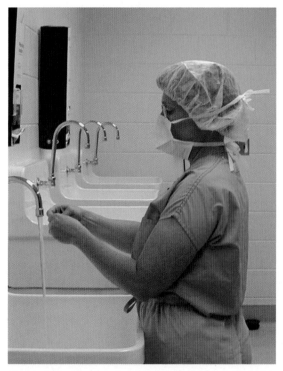

Figure 2-5   The hands and forearms are washed with soap and water before beginning the official surgical hand preparation. Note that the head cover and mask are already on before the hand prep begins. The gown and glove pack should be opened before starting the hand prep.

2. Fingernails need to be well maintained and should not be longer than the fingertips. Do not wear artificial nails or nail polish.
3. Clean and thoroughly dry eyeglasses, if worn. Elastic bands are recommended to hold eyeglasses in place, thus preventing them from falling into the surgical field.
4. Apply cap and mask. Make sure all hair is covered by headgear and that the mask is snug and comfortable. To prevent eyeglasses from fogging up because of the mask, tape can be put over the upper edge of the mask, or specially designed masks can be purchased.
5. Hands should be thoroughly washed with an antimicrobial soap and water and towel-dried.
6. Open sterile gown and gloves in the surgery area, as well as any other sterile equipment that needs to be opened, if the circulating nurse is not available.

Surgical Hand Scrub Using Antimicrobial Scrub Agent

A traditional, standardized, surgical hand antisepsis scrub procedure should include, but may not be limited to, the following steps:

1. Wash hands and forearms with soap and running water immediately before beginning the surgical scrub (Figure 2-5).

2. Clean the subungual areas of both hands under running water using a disposable nail-cleaning pick (Figure 2-6).
3. Rinse hands and forearms under running water.
4. Hold hands higher than elbows and away from surgical attire.
5. Dispense the approved antimicrobial scrub agent according to the manufacturer's written directions.
6. Apply the antimicrobial agent to wet hands and forearms. Some manufacturers may recommend using a soft, nonabrasive sponge (Figure 2-7).
7. Visualize each finger, hand, and arm as having four sides. Wash all four sides effectively. Repeat this process for opposite fingers, hand, and arm.
8. Repeat this process if directed to do so by the manufacturer's written directions for use.
9. Avoid splashing surgical attire.
10. For water conservation, turn water off when it is not directly in use, if possible.
11. Discard used sponges in appropriate containers, without contaminating hands.
12. In the OR, dry hands and arms with a sterile towel before donning a sterile surgical gown and gloves. Make sure not to touch scrub suit with the sterile towel.

The scrub should always start with the fingers, proceed to the hands, and continue up the arms to 2 inches above the elbow. Most manufacturers' directions recommend using one brush. Two methods typically are used when scrubbing; either the timed method or the counted brush stroke method is acceptable. With the *timed method* the hands, fingers, and arms are scrubbed for a prescribed period of time, as indicated in the manufacturer's directions for the particular scrub agent. The directions may also specify how long the scrub should be done on each specified surface. The number of strokes and time may both be incorporated into a scrub policy. The *counted brush stroke method*, or *anatomic scrub*, involves a prescribed number of brush strokes applied lengthwise with the brush or sponge and used for each surface of the fingers, hands, and arms. Whichever method is used, always continue to hold your hands higher than your elbows so that the water can run from the hands (cleanest area) to the elbows (area less likely to have direct contact with the sterile field).

Surgical Hand Rub Using Antimicrobial Rub Agent

A standardized protocol for alcohol-based surgical hand rubs should follow manufacturers' written instructions and should include, but may not be

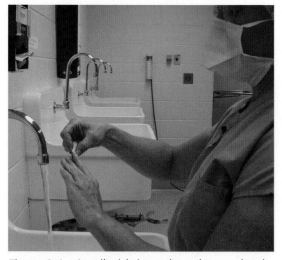

Figure 2-6   A nail pick is used to clean under the fingernails as part of the surgical hand prep.

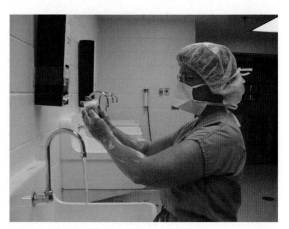

Figure 2-7   In this surgical hand prep, a soft sponge is used. Note that the hands are held above the elbows throughout the scrub.

limited to, the following steps:

1. Wash hands and forearms with soap and running water immediately before beginning the surgical hand antisepsis procedure.
2. Clean the subungual areas of both hands under running water using a nail-cleaning pick.
3. Rinse hands and forearms under running water.
4. Dry hands and forearms thoroughly with a paper towel.
5. Dispense the manufacturer-recommended amount of surgical hand rub product.
6. Apply the product to the hands and forearms, following the manufacturer's written directions. Some manufacturers may require the use of water as part of the process.
7. Rub thoroughly until dry.
8. Repeat the product application process as indicated in the manufacturer's written directions.
9. In the OR, don sterile surgical gown and gloves.

The rub should always start with the fingers, proceed to the hands, and continue up the arms to 2 inches above the elbow.

TYPES OF SCRUB SOLUTIONS

When choosing an antimicrobial (antiseptic) detergent, several desirable characteristics are recommended for the surgical scrub product: (1) FDA compliant, (2) broad spectrum of activity, (3) fast acting and effective, (4) nonirritating, and (5) persistent effects and cumulative activity. Whatever type of scrub agent is chosen, it is important to follow the manufacturer's written directions for use. These include the scrub time, whether the use of a brush is recommended, and whether it is a brushless, alcohol-based surgical rub.

Several types of antimicrobial skin-cleansing agents are available. The following agents are discussed: chlorhexidine gluconate, iodophors, triclosan, alcohol, hexa-chlorophene, parachlorametaxylenol (Table 2-1), and the brushless rub.

Chlorhexidine gluconate (4%) is a broad-spectrum antimicrobial agent. It is more effective against gram-positive bacteria than gram-negative organisms. Chlorhexidine gluconate is a fair inhibitor of fungi. It is active against enveloped viruses and has minimal action against tubercle bacillus. Organic matter minimally affects it. Most importantly, chlorhexidine gluconate 4% is persistent (the ability to stop microbial regrowth with repeated use). The residual effect is maintained for more than 6 days.

Iodophors (7.5%) are complexes consisting of iodine and a carrier. Iodophors have a wide range of activity against gram-positive and gram-negative bacteria, tubercle bacilli, fungi, viruses, and some spores. Iodophors are neutralized rapidly in the presence of organic materials. These agents have minimal residual effect and can cause skin irritation and damage.

Triclosan is a broad-spectrum agent with good activity against gram-positive and most gram-negative bacteria, but it does not work well against fungi. Little is known about its activity against viruses. It has an intermediate speed of action, has excellent persistence on the skin, and is affected minimally by organic matter. Triclosan is less effective than chlorhexidine gluconate and iodophors.

Alcohol (60%-90%) is an agent with rapid antimicrobial properties against organisms, but it does not have residual activity. It has excellent bactericidal activity against gram-positive and gram-negative bacteria and good activity against tubercle bacillus as well as many fungi and viruses. It is not sporicidal. It aids in removing oils from the skin. The disadvantages of alcohol are its drying effect on the skin and its flammability, so it needs to be stored carefully.

Hexachlorophene (3%) is bacteriostatic for gram-positive bacteria but has little activity against gram-negative bacteria, fungi, tubercle bacilli, or viruses. It is persistent and is most effective after a buildup of cumulative suppressive action. A major disadvantage is that hexachlorophene has a known neurotoxicity and can produce neurologic effects. Therefore it is rarely used.

Parachlormetaxylenol (PCMX) has good activity against gram-positive bacteria and less activity

TABLE 2-1   Characteristics of Selected Antimicrobials Used in Surgical Scrub Solutions

ANTIMICROBIAL	SPECTRUM OF ACTIVITY*	FUNGI	VIRUSES	TUBERCLE BACILLI	AFFECTED BY ORGANIC MATTER	SPEED OF ACTION	DISADVANTAGES	ADVANTAGES
Chlorhexidine gluconate 4%	Broad spectrum (more effective against gram+ than gram−)	Fair	Enveloped viruses	Minimal	Minimal	Intermediate Significant immediate antimicrobial effect	Eye irritant	Persistent; ability to stop microbial growth with repeated use Residual effect maintained for more than 6 days
Iodophors 7.5% (complexes that consist of iodine and carrier)	Broad spectrum (some spores)	Yes	Yes	Yes	Neutralized rapidly	Significant immediate antimicrobial effect	Odor, staining, tissue irritation	Persistent for 4-6 hours
Triclosan	Broad spectrum	Poor	Little known	—	Minimal	Intermediate	—	Excellent persistence
Alcohol	Broad spectrum (not sporicidal)	Many	Many	Yes	Conflicting evidence	Rapid No residual activity	Drying effect Volatile and flammable	Lacks persistence
Hexachlorophene	Gram+ (very little activity against gram−)	Poor	Poor	Poor	—	Slow; most effective after buildup of cumulative suppressive action	Known neurotoxicity and neurologic effects	Persistent
Parachlormeta-xylenol (PCMX)	Broad spectrum (good activity against gram+, less activity against gram−)	Some	Some	Yes	Minimal	Intermediate	Highly formula dependent; does not sustain residual activity	Persistence limited to a few hours Skin sensitivity low

*Including against gram-positive (*gram+*) and gram-negative (*gram−*) bacteria.

against gram-negative bacteria. It has fair activity against some fungi, viruses, and tubercle bacilli. PCMX has a persistent effect of a few hours and is minimally affected by organic matter. Its antimicrobial effect can be altered by the composition of the antiseptic product. Efficacy data should be reviewed before these products are used for surgical scrubs.

A *brushless rub* (with or without water) is now available (e.g., Avagard). This brushless technique has an alcohol base with an antimicrobial ingredient such as chlorhexidine gluconate or triclosan. These agents reduce bacterial counts on hands more rapidly than antimicrobial soaps or detergents. Combining alcohol (for rapid reduction of microbial growth) and chlorhexidine (for persistent and cumulative effect) prevents microbial regrowth. The advantage of the brushless rub is that the scrub time is shorter compared with other agents and techniques, and damage to the skin from brushes is avoided.

GOWNING AND GLOVING

The purpose of gowning and gloving is to create a barrier between the sterile and nonsterile areas. Gowns and gloves cover the surgical team members' skin to prevent it from being a possible contaminant.

Gowns and gloves should be opened on a surface away from other sterile supplies so that dripping water from the scrub person's arms will not contaminate them.

Drying the Hands

After completing the surgical hand scrub, the hands and arms need to be thoroughly dried with a sterile towel. From the sterile gown and towel pack, pick up the towel by the corner (Figure 2-8). Be careful not to drip water on the gown pack. Step back from the sterile table, always being aware of the sterile items in the environment to prevent contamination. Open the towel full length, using one end of the towel to gently rub the fingers, hand, and arms (in that order) of the first hand and arm (Figure 2-9). Do not rub back and forth; instead, rub circumferentially. Bend at the waist slightly so that the towel does not brush against the scrub suit. When ready to dry the second hand and arm, bring the first dry hand to the opposite end of the towel and repeat (Figure 2-10). When completed, drop the towel onto the floor with the hand that is currently

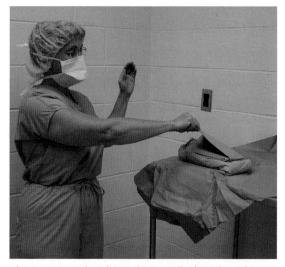

Figure 2-8   A hand towel is usually found on the top of a sterilized gown pack. Note the distance between the nonsterile scrub top and the sterile, open gown pack.

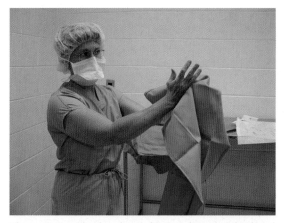

Figure 2-9   The hand towel is used to dry the hand first, then the wrist, then the forearm. Once the towel leaves the hand, it cannot go back up to the hand. Note the bend at the waist and the extended arms required to prevent the sterile towel from touching the nonsterile scrub top.

holding it, without allowing either hand to fall below waist level.

Gowning

The gowns are folded inside out in the packs. Lift the folded gown out of the package, then step away from the table, making sure there is adequate space to gown without contaminating anything (Figure 2-11). After locating the neckline and armholes, the gown is held by the neckline (Figure 2-12). The inside front of the gown is unfolded (do not shake it), keeping the inside toward the body and the hands in the armholes. Both arms are slid inside the gown by reaching and extending both arms at the same time (Figure 2-13). The "circulator" (the nonsterile assistant) will continue to pull the gown on the scrubbed-in personnel, carefully bringing the gown over the shoulders, fastening the neck of the gown, and tying the waistline, all while standing behind the person gowning and touching only the hem of the collar and back of the gown. The cuffs of the sleeves must be extended over the hands. (The hands must not be exposed in the closed-gloving technique.)

If the surgical gowns used are the "wraparound style," the front tie should not be touched until sterile gloves have been donned. On reusable gowns the wraparound ties are tied in the front of the gown by a single bow-tie knot. Another sterile team member must assist in this process to properly finish the donning of the gown. On disposable gowns a disposable paper tag covers the end of the ties. This gown can be properly donned with the help of a nonsterile circulator. Both these gowns cover the back of the body, thereby reducing the chance of contamination because most of the body is covered. The back of the gown or the

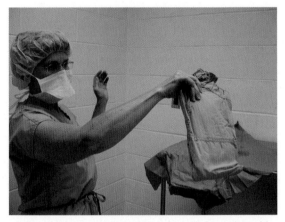

Figure 2-11   As the gown is removed from the table, the person steps back away from the table to prevent the gown from touching any nonsterile items as it unfolds.

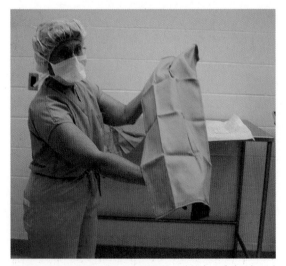

Figure 2-10   Use the opposite end/side of the hand towel to dry the second hand/arm.

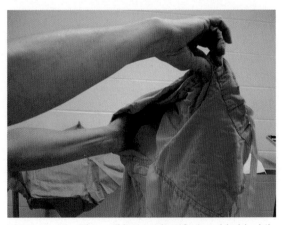

Figure 2-12   The neckline is identified and held while the armholes are found, and the gown is allowed to open.

body is never considered sterile. If either tie drops on the reusable gown or the disposable gown, the circulator retrieves both ties and fastens them behind the scrubbed person's back.

Gloving

There are three methods of gloving: (1) closed gloving, (2) open gloving, and (3) assisted gloving. Both open and closed gloving enable the scrubbed personnel to glove themselves. Assisted gloving requires the assistance of another scrubbed-in team member.

Closed Gloving
Closed gloving provides assurance against contamination because no bare skin is exposed in the process.
Technique
1. Keep the hands within the cuffs of the gown. With the left hand, pick up the right glove from the inner wrapper of the glove package by the folded cuff (Figure 2-14).
2. Extend the right hand (still within the cuff) with the palm facing upward. Place the palm of the glove palm down against the palm of the hand with the thumb and fingers of the glove facing the body. (The thumb side should be underneath on the same side

as the thumb of the right hand facing upward.) When performing closed gloving, remember the saying, "Palm to palm, thumb to thumb, fingers of glove facing the elbow."
3. Through the gown cuff, grasp the back of the glove cuff with the right hand (Figure 2-15). With the left hand, pull and lift the cuff up and over the gown cuff and the right hand (Figure 2-16). The hand is still inside the sleeve.
4. With the left hand, grasp both the top of the right glove cuff and the gown cuff, and pull toward the elbow while pushing the hand through the gown cuff and into the glove. Be sure the cuff of the glove completely covers the cuff of the gown (Figure 2-17).
5. Glove the left hand using the same technique (Figures 2-18 to 2-20).

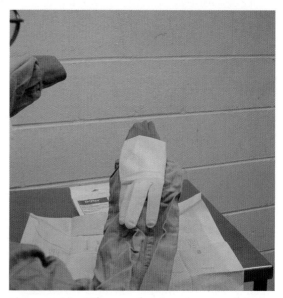

Figure 2-14 When performing the closed-gloving technique, "palm to palm, thumb to thumb, and fingers face the elbows" means that the palm of the hand covered by the cuff of the gown is facing up, and the palm side of the glove is facing down toward the palm of the hand. The thumb of the hand covered by the cuff of the gown is directly beneath the thumb of the glove. The fingers of the glove are lying over the wrist of the gown-covered hand, facing toward the elbow of the gown-covered arm.

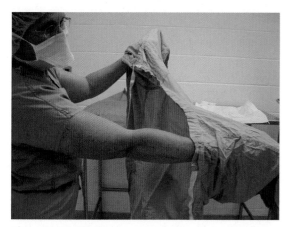

Figure 2-13 Both arms are advanced into the sleeves simultaneously, but the hands are not allowed to pass all the way through the cuffs in order to allow for closed gloving.

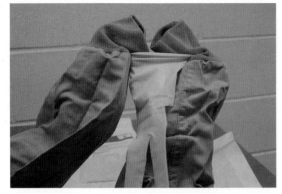

Figure 2-15   During closed gloving the hands remain within the cuffs of the gown until the gloves are secured over the cuffs of the gown, and then the hand can be extended out of the gown and into the glove. This requires manipulating the gloves through the material of the gown.

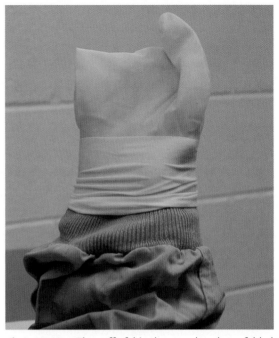

Figure 2-17   The cuff of this glove needs to be unfolded and pulled down to cover the entire cuff of the gown; this will assist placement of the fingers and thumb into the glove.

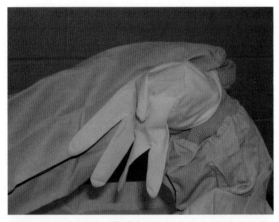

Figure 2-16   The cuff of the glove is extended over the cuff of the gown to perform closed gloving.

Open Gloving

Open gloving is another method that enables the scrubbed personnel to glove themselves. The open-gloving method should not be used routinely for surgical gowning and gloving. The closed or assisted technique is preferred, but the open method is used if one glove becomes contaminated in surgery and an assistant is not available to perform assisted gloving. Open gloving is also used when only the hands need to be sterile and no gown is needed, such as for minor surgical

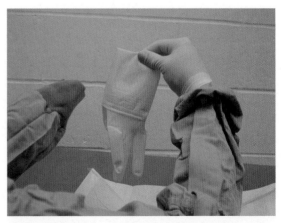

Figure 2-18   Once the first hand is gloved, use that hand to place the second glove palm down onto the extended left hand covered by the cuff of the gown. Note that the palm of the left hand covered by the cuff of the gown is facing up.

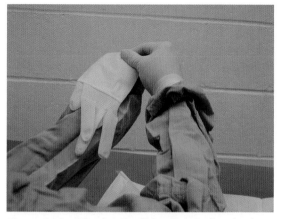

Figure 2-19   The thumb of the glove is directly above the thumb of the left hand covered by the cuff of the gown, and the fingers of the glove are facing the elbow of the left arm. "Palm to palm, thumb to thumb, and fingers facing the elbow."

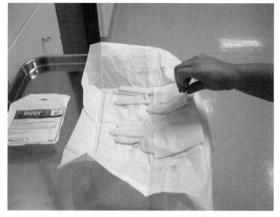

Figure 2-21   Only the "skin surface" of the glove being put on during open gloving can be touched. This means that only the folded cuff of the first glove can be touched.

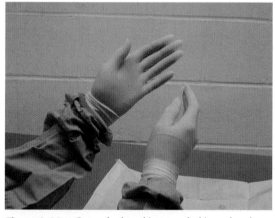

Figure 2-20   Once the hand is extended into the glove, the cuff of the glove needs to be unfolded and to cover the entire cuff of the gown.

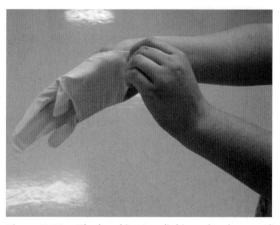

Figure 2-22   The hand is extended into the glove, and the cuff is pulled up the wrist.

procedures, bone marrow biopsies, or catheterizations. For open gloving in surgery, instead of leaving the hands in the sleeves of the surgical gown, the hands are extended all the way through the cuff and the sleeves. The hands are entirely exposed.

Technique

1. With the left hand, pick up the right glove by grasping the cuff on the "future" inside surface ("nonsterile" surface) of the fold only (Figure 2-21).

2. Gently guide your fingers into the glove, leaving the cuff well turned over the hand. Keep the thumb in the palm of the hand until it is well inside the glove. Do not adjust the cuff (Figures 2-22 and 2-23).

3. Place the gloved fingers of the right hand under the everted left glove cuff, on the sterile side of the left glove (Figure 2-24).

4. Slide the fingers of the left hand into the glove, keeping the thumb inside the palm of

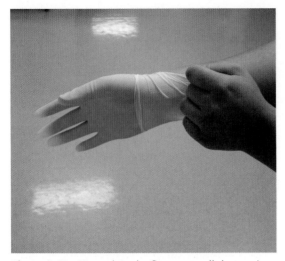

Figure 2-23   Even when the fingers are all the way into the glove, the cuff is *not* unfolded yet.

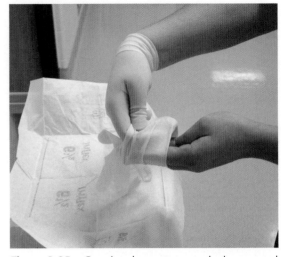

Figure 2-25   Care is taken *not* to touch the exposed skin of the hand being gloved with the sterile glove already donned. This would contaminate the first glove.

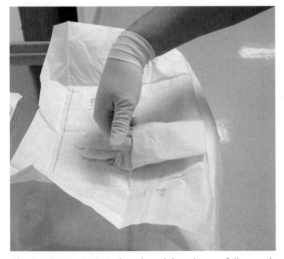

Figure 2-24   Using the gloved hand, carefully reach under the folded cuff of the second glove to pick it up. The second glove is put on before the cuff of the first glove is unfolded up the wrist.

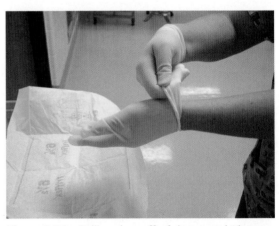

Figure 2-26   Pulling the cuff of the second glove up the arm and away from the wrist prevents the gloved hand from touching the exposed skin and assists in finishing the step of pulling on the second glove.

the hand, until inside the glove. Pull the glove on all the way (Figures 2-25 and 2-26).

5. With the left hand, slide your fingers under the outside edge of the right cuff and unfold it by stretching it up the wrist. Avoid touching any bare, exposed skin (Figure 2-27).

Assisted Gloving

Assisted gloving is used when a sterile team member assists in gloving another scrubbed-in team member. The hands are extended all the way through the cuffs and sleeves as in open gloving.

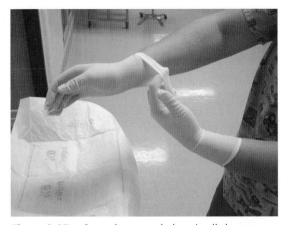

Figure 2-27 Once the second glove is all the way on, the cuff of the first glove can be unfolded and extended up the arm. Only the fingers (not the thumb) of the second hand to be gloved are used to unfold the cuff. This prevents the thumb from touching the exposed skin on the arm.

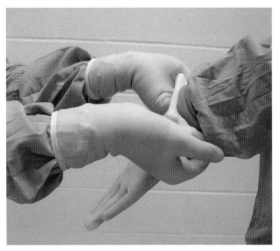

Figure 2-29 The cuff of the glove is stretched wide, and the thumbs of the assistant are not used to hold the glove. This prevents the assistant from accidentally touching the exposed hand of the person needing the glove.

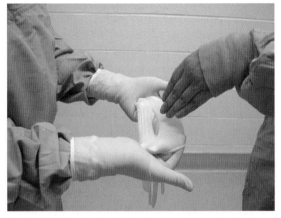

Figure 2-28 Assisted gloving requires the help of another scrubbed-in and gloved person. The palm of the glove being placed is held toward the person needing the glove.

Technique

1. The already-gloved, sterile team member picks up the sterile glove, then places fingers from both hands under the cuff on the sterile sides of the glove. The palm of the glove is held toward the person being gloved (Figure 2-28).
2. The cuff of the glove should be stretched widely open so that the hand can be placed in the glove without touching the sterile assistant. The sterile assistant can avoid touching the hand to be gloved by holding the thumbs out (Figure 2-29).
3. As the person slips into the glove, pull up on the glove (Figure 2-30).
4. When pulling up on the glove, bring the cuff of the glove over the cuff of the sleeve.
5. Repeat for the other hand. The person being gloved can assist by using the one gloved hand to hold open the cuff of the other sterile glove being donned, while the assistant's thumbs are kept under the glove's cuff until the glove is donned.

Contaminated Gown

If a gown becomes contaminated during surgery, it must be removed. The contaminated person steps away from the sterile field. The circulating nurse opens new sterile gloves and gown. The circulator unfastens the gown and pulls it off inside out. The contaminated person then removes the gloves by grabbing the cuff of the glove (not the gown) and pulling the glove off inside out.

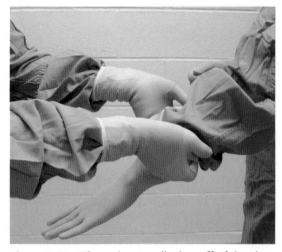

Figure 2-30   The assistant pulls the cuff of the glove over the cuff of the gown as the hand is pushed into the glove. Note that the thumbs are still held away from the glove.

Rescrubbing is not required to regown and reglove. If only a sleeve has been contaminated, sterile sleeves may be used to cover the contaminated area.

If a glove is contaminated during surgery, it needs to be changed. The contaminated person should step away, or at least keep the contaminated hand away from the sterile field. The circulating nurse grasps the outside of the glove cuff, but below the top of the glove, to ensure the sterile gown is not touched. The glove is pulled off inside out. Assisted gloving is the best method to use to reglove. If this is not possible, open gloving away from the sterile field is necessary. Closed gloving is inappropriate; the cuff of the gown should not be pulled over the hand because the cuff is contaminated with skin cells and scurf.

3. The scrub suit should be covered with a clean laboratory coat at all times when outside the surgical area.
4. Personnel are not allowed to wear laboratory coats in the OR.
5. Scrub suits worn in the OR should not be worn home from the hospital.
6. Clean, freshly laundered scrub suits should be donned just before going into the OR and should not be worn from home into the hospital.
7. Proper surgical attire includes wearing a head cover that completely covers all head and facial hair, surgical masks that effectively cover the mouth and nose, and clean shoes with or without shoe covers.
8. Proper surgical attire requires the removal of *all* jewelry; this includes wedding bands, body-piercing objects, and watches.
9. Fingernails need to be well manicured and cannot extend beyond the tips of the fingers. Fingernails cannot be covered with nail polish.
10. The purpose of the surgical hand scrub or hand rub is to remove as many microorganisms as possible from the nails, hands, and arms.
11. All jewelry, name tags, and pens need to be removed before beginning the surgical hand scrub or hand rub.
12. Head covers and masks need to be donned before beginning the surgical hand scrub or rub.
13. Sterilized gown and glove packs need to be opened before beginning the surgical hand scrub or rub.
14. When using an antimicrobial detergent, it is important to follow the manufacturer's directions regarding the scrub time and whether or not a scrub brush should be used.
15. Closed gloving is the best gloving technique to guard against contamination because no bare skin is exposed in the process.

KEY POINTS

1. A surgical dress code should be written and posted so that it can be easily followed and enforced.
2. The dress code should include the defined areas where surgical attire must be worn, appropriate attire within those defined areas, and the acceptable options for cover apparel outside the surgical area.

REVIEW QUESTIONS

1. Which of the following is *true?*
   a. Proper surgical attire includes wearing freshly laundered scrub top and pants, head cover, and mask.
   b. Each surgical facility should have its own posted surgery dress code.

c. Proper surgical attire decreases the risk of infection associated with surgery.

d. All of the above.

e. None of the above.

2. What should the surgical nurse don on leaving the surgery suite?

a. Street clothes.

b. Laboratory coat.

c. Shoe covers.

d. Cap and mask.

e. None of the above.

3. Why should scrub suits *not* be worn from home to the hospital?

4. Why should scrub suits *not* be worn home from the hospital?

5. *True* or *False:* The surgical nurse's scrub top should be tucked into the scrub pants.

6. Why should scrub tops be short sleeve?

7. *True* or *False:* It is recommended that all non-scrubbed personnel wear long-sleeve laboratory coats in the OR.

8. *True* or *False:* Jewelry and long fingernails are protected by the sterile gloves worn by scrubbed-in surgical personnel and therefore do not need to be removed (jewelry) or cut (nails).

9. Which of the following is *false* regarding the surgical hand preparation?

a. The preparation should begin with a quick, general hand and arm wash.

b. The purpose of the prep is to sterilize the skin on the surgeon's hands and arms.

c. Stiff scrub brushes should not be used to scrub the hands and arms.

d. The product manufacturer determines the recommended length of time the product should be scrubbed on the hands and arms during the surgical hand prep.

10. Which of the following is the correct order of events associated with performing the surgical hand prep and donning the surgical gown and gloves?

a. Confirm removal of or remove all jewelry → open gown and glove packs → don cap and mask → perform hand prep → dry hands using sterile hand towel → gown → perform closed gloving.

b. Perform hand prep → open gown and glove packs → don cap and mask → don gown and perform open gloving.

c. Remove all jewelry → do short hand wash → perform hand prep → open gown and glove packs → don cap and mask → don gown and gloves.

d. Remove all jewelry → gown and glove → perform hand prep.

e. None of the above.

ANSWERS

1. d
2. b
3. Scrub suits can carry microorganisms into the hospital
4. Scrub suits can bring microorganisms home and infect the personnel's own pets
5. True
6. To allow for scrubbing above the elbows
7. False
8. False
9. b
10. a

BIBLIOGRAPHY

Association of periOperative Registered Nurses (AORN): *Standards, recommended practices, and guidelines,* Denver, 2004, AORN.

Fairchild S: *Perioperative nursing principles and practice,* ed 2, Philadelphia, 1996, Lippincott.

Fossum T: *Small animal surgery,* ed 2, St Louis, 2002, Mosby.

Gruendemann BJ, Bjerke N: Is it time for brushless scrubbing with an alcohol based agent? *AORN J* 74:859, 2001.

Paulson D: Comparative evaluation of five surgical hand scrub preparations, *AORN J* 60:246, 1994.

Phillips N: *Berry & Kohn's operating room technique,* ed 10, St Louis, 2004, Mosby.

Slatter D: *Textbook of small animal surgery,* ed 3, Philadelphia, 2003, Saunders.

Spry C: *Essentials of perioperative nursing,* ed 2, Boston, 2004, Jones & Bartlett.

CHAPTER 3

The Operating Room and Asepsis

Mary Scherer

LEARNING OBJECTIVES

After studying this chapter, the reader should be able to do the following:

- Understand the terms and principles of cleaning, disinfecting, asepsis, sterile field, and surgical conscience.
- Perform routine and terminal cleaning of the operating room.

- Maintain asepsis.
- Maintain a sterile field.
- Open sterile packs without contaminating their contents or the sterile field.

CLEANING THE SURGICAL AREA

The surgical environment should be kept as free from bacterial contamination as possible to minimize the chance of the patient being infected from an exogenous source. Routine cleaning and disinfection accomplish this goal. *Cleaning* is the process by which any type of soil, including organic material, is removed by using detergent, water, and scrubbing action. *Disinfection* is the process of destroying some forms of microorganisms by using a disinfecting agent on inanimate surfaces. The disinfectant selected should be hospital grade (virucidal, bactericidal, nonstaining, and noncorrosive).

The surgery rooms should have a thorough, once-daily cleaning at the completion of the daily surgical schedule (once in a 24-hour period, which could be in the evening or first in the morning) in addition to the routine cleaning between patients to provide the optimal surgical environment.

To facilitate cleaning, the surgery room should be simple and uncluttered, and it should not be used as a storage room for equipment or supplies.

Daily Terminal Cleaning

The daily thorough cleaning, or terminal cleaning, includes cleaning and disinfecting the floors, all horizontal surfaces (that collect dust), the surgical lights, surgical tables (e.g., Mayo stands), the patient surgery table, and any other items (e.g., monitoring devices, electrocautery machines, suction, anesthesia machines) in the operating room (OR) according to the manufacturer's directions. The cleaning and disinfecting should begin at the ceiling and end with the floor, always starting at the high point of the room and working down.

All horizontal surfaces should be damp-dusted with a lint-free cloth and a hospital-grade disinfectant. Countertops and instrument tables should have smooth surfaces and should be able to withstand frequent disinfecting. The best surface is stainless steel.

Surgical lights should be damp-dusted and cleaned according to the manufacturer's directions. The kick buckets should also be disinfected and the wheels cleaned. The scrub sinks should be scrubbed and disinfected daily. The scrub sinks should not be used for any tasks other than scrubbing hands.

The floors should be wet-vacuumed or damp-mopped. Although wet vacuuming is preferred, it is not always available. If a damp mop is used, the mop should be laundered and dried daily, rinsed between uses, and soaked in disinfectant.

Routine Cleaning after Each Surgical Case

At the end of each surgical procedure, the surgical instruments are removed and brought to the instrument-cleaning station. Waste should be separated according to the requirements of the Office of Radiation, Chemical and Biohazard Safety (ORCBS). The waste materials are collected, separated, and placed in the proper containers. Separate, properly labeled biohazard containers should include those for bloody saturated waste, tissues, and sharp instruments ("sharps"). All sharps (blades, needles) are discarded in designated puncture-resistant containers that have a biohazard label. In the OR the surgery tables, water blankets, and V-troughs or positioning bags should be cleaned and disinfected. Instrument tables and Mayo stands should be cleaned and then wiped with a disinfectant. Any visibly soiled areas on the floor should be spot-cleaned and disinfected. The gurney or cart for transportation of the patient to and from the surgery room should be thoroughly cleaned and disinfected after each use.

Cleaning Protocols

Detailed tasks should be written to avoid confusion among the individuals responsible for cleaning the OR. A written protocol should be readily available for proper daily cleaning instructions as well as terminal cleaning instructions. A written protocol should be posted for appropriate separation of all waste. For more information regarding the cleaning of the surgery room, see Chapter 9.

ASEPSIS

The surgical area is a restricted area because it needs to be as free of microorganisms as possible. A surgical wound could easily become infected if the proper techniques are not used. These acquired infections can be serious and even fatal. Asepsis (absence of pathogenic microorganisms that cause infection) makes the environment surgically clean, but not sterile (absence of all living microorganisms, including spores). Keeping the surgical area as aseptic as possible, by properly cleaning and disinfecting it, adhering to the written dress code, preparing the patient correctly, and performing proper handwashing and hand scrubbing, helps to prevent pathogenic microorganisms from contaminating the environment and entering the surgical wound. Aseptic techniques, along with sterile techniques, are the most important practices to prevent infection in the patient.

Surgical Conscience

Surgical conscience is the commitment of the surgical personnel to adhere strictly to aseptic technique, because anything less could increase the potential risk of infection, resulting in harm to the patient. Any break in aseptic technique is immediately reported and addressed or corrected, whether or not anyone else is present to observe the violation.

Maintaining Asepsis

Maintaining asepsis in the surgical area is accomplished by practicing aseptic and sterile techniques. The Association of periOperative Registered Nurses (AORN) has listed several "Recommended Practices for Maintaining a Sterile Field," as follows:

1. Scrubbed personnel function within a sterile field.
   a. The scrubbed personnel's gowns are sterile in front from the chest, to the level of the sterile field.

b. The sleeves are sterile from 2 inches above the elbow to the top of the edge of the cuff.

c. The neckline, shoulders, and cuffed portion of the sleeves may become contaminated by perspiration and therefore are not considered sterile.

d. The back of the gown is never considered sterile because a member of the surgical team cannot observe it constantly.

e. The cuffs of the gown are considered contaminated because hands have passed through them.

2. Sterile drapes should be used to establish a sterile field.

Drapes are barriers that help to prevent microorganisms from passing between sterile and nonsterile areas. The drapes should cover the entire animal, the furniture, and the equipment that is part of the sterile field. The circulating nurse, or any other nonscrubbed personnel, should never reach over the draped, sterile areas. Also, if any drapes become wet, they are considered contaminated because strike-through will occur. *Strike-through* occurs when liquids soak through a drape from a sterile area to an unsterile area, and vice versa.

3. All items used within a sterile field should be sterile.

Before opening any sterile items for the surgeon to be placed on the sterile field, make sure the packages are inspected for sterility.

a. Make sure there are no tears or holes in the outer package.

b. Make sure the items have gone through the proper sterilization by checking the sterile indicators. These are located on the outside of the package, or there may be indicator tape on the front of the package (Figure 3-1).

c. Check the seal of the package to make sure it is secure and not broken at any point.

d. Check the package itself. If it looks worn by being handled too much, it should be considered contaminated.

e. The larger surgical packs should have a sterile indicator inside to ensure that the

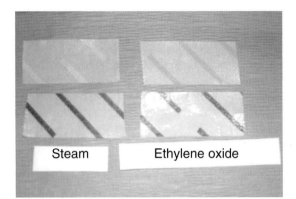

Figure 3-1 Sterilization indicator tape. *Top left,* Steam sterilization indicator tape before being exposed to steam. *Below,* Steam sterilization indicator tape after it has been exposed to steam. The color change from yellow to black indicates the tape was exposed to steam. *Top right,* Ethylene oxide gas sterilization indicator tape before being exposed to ethylene oxide gas. *Below,* Ethylene oxide gas sterilization tape after it has been exposed to ethylene oxide. The color change from green to red indicates the tape was exposed to ethylene oxide gas.

sterilizing agent has penetrated the entire thick pack (to the center).

f. The expiration date should be checked, although AORN maintains that the sterility of the item is *event* related and not time related (see Chapter 10). This means that if all the above (*a* through *e*) have been checked on the package, the time and expiration date of sterilization are not significant.

4. All items introduced onto a sterile field should be opened, dispensed, and transferred by methods that maintain sterility and integrity.

a. Edges of all sterile wrappers and packages are considered nonsterile. Therefore, when opening an item, be sure all edges are secured so that they do not contaminate the field or the sterile packaged item.

b. Sterile supplies are opened by unwrapping the flap farthest away first, the sides next, and the nearest flap last.

c. Irrigation fluids should be poured carefully to prevent any spills onto the

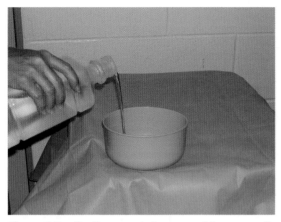

Figure 3-2   Sterile water being poured into a sterile bowl. Care is taken to avoid splash-back. Note that the bowl is set in the corner of an empty table to avoid possible contamination should splashing occur.

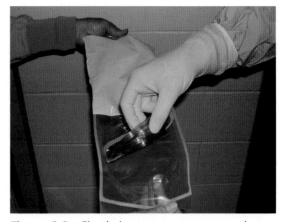

Figure 3-3   Circulating nurse opens a peel-away pouch. Fingers of the circulating nurse touch only the outer edges of the pouch and carefully peel away the sides to open the pouch and expose the contents for easy, sterile removal by scrubbed-in personnel.

sterile field and to avoid splash-back. Therefore, it is best to have the scrubbed-in person hold the basin away from the field or to place it at the edge of the sterile table. Once the fluids have been opened, the cap is considered contaminated and cannot be replaced unto the bottle, so the remaining fluids must be discarded (Figure 3-2).

d. If the sterile item cannot be carefully flipped or placed on the sterile field, a scrubbed-in person must lift the item straight out of the package, without touching any of the edges of the package (Figure 3-3).

e. Heavy, sharp, or large items should not be tossed onto the sterile field because they could damage other instruments on the table, cause a perforation in the sterile barrier drape of the table, roll off the table, or displace other items on the table.

f. Flash-autoclaved items (items needed for immediate use are placed in "flash pan" with handle) are given to the scrub nurse so that the sterile items can be transferred to the sterile field without contamination.

5. A sterile field should be maintained and monitored continuously. The sterile field should never be left unattended.

6. All personnel moving within or around a sterile field should do so in a manner to maintain the integrity of the sterile field. The surgical team must be aware of the sterile and nonsterile areas in the surgery room *at all times.*

a. Movement creates air currents, which can be a source of contamination in the OR. Minimal movement is required.

b. Scrubbed personnel should not walk away from the sterile field by wandering around the room or leaving the room.

c. When scrubbed-in personnel must change positions around the sterile field, they should be a safe distance apart so as not to touch. When they pass each other, they should pass face to face (sterile to sterile) or back to back (unsterile to unsterile).

d. Unscrubbed personnel should *always* face the surgical field.

e. Unscrubbed persons should not walk between two sterile fields. For example, unscrubbed personnel should not walk between the sterile, draped patient and the sterile equipment table.

f. The surgical scrub team should not change levels of position during a procedure. *Levels of position* are from sitting to standing, and vice versa. The lower portion of the gown is considered contaminated, and when the scrubbed person sits, this portion of the gown is closer to the hands, arms, and the sterile field and therefore could cause contamination.

g. The surgical conscience is followed to report any breaks in aseptic or sterile technique.

h. There should be minimal talking in the OR.

i. OR doors should remain closed as much as possible.

j. All non–scrubbed-in persons should be a safe distance from the sterile field.

k. A limited number of non–scrubbed-in observers should be allowed in the OR at one time. The more congested the OR, the more difficult it is to monitor the sterile field, and the sterile team has less room to move adequately around the sterile field.

OPENING STERILE PACKS

Proper opening of sterile packs is important to maintain a sterile field. All packages have to be checked thoroughly, as discussed in practice 3 above. Speed should *not* be a top priority. Although opening items in a timely way is necessary, rushing can cause unnecessary mistakes. Timing is also a factor. If the scrubbed-in person is not ready to receive the item, or if the equipment table is not properly prepared, the circulating nurse should consider delaying opening the item until a later, more convenient time.

Wraps and packages can be sterilized at the hospital or by the manufacturer. Wraps and packages sterilized by the manufacturer are usually disposable items. Packages sterilized at the hospital often do not come with directions how to open them. This skill comes with knowledge and practice. The manufacturer often will have directions explaining which end to open first.

Opening Peel-Away Pouches

Many paper or plastic pouches for packaging individual sterile instruments have a side sealed with an arrow (↑) indicating which end to open.

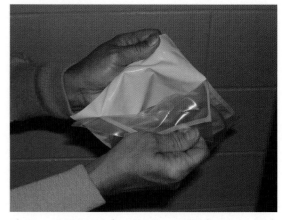

Figure 3-4 Properly opening a peel-away pouch requires holding and touching only the outer edge of the separated ends, then carefully pulling them apart by adducting the thumbs.

Holding the packet at the end with the arrow allows easy opening of this type of seal; with both hands, grasp the package with the thumbs and slowly peel the package open by adducting the thumbs (Figure 3-4). While peeling the package open, hold the item firmly so that the item is stabilized and does not slide across the nonsterile edges of the package.

The plastic or paper tubing or pouches with a straight seal are opened similarly, except that a constant pull must be maintained on both sides. Instruments and sutures can be either handed to the surgeon or unwrapped to make them available for the surgical team. Small, sterile items can be gently tossed onto the sterile table by opening the package as described. Lift the paper side, with the sterile item still on it, without reaching over the sterile field, then give the item a lifting toss onto the sterile table, still holding on to the package and making sure the item does not slide over the edge of the package, to avoid contamination. These items can also be opened in the same manner on a clean, dry, flat, nonsterile surface. Place the item, paper side down, and hold on to the top sealed edge with a thumb and finger of one hand, and pull the plastic side with the other hand. The scrubbed-in assistant can carefully pick the item off the sterile paper and transfer it to the sterile table. Suture can be aseptically provided by

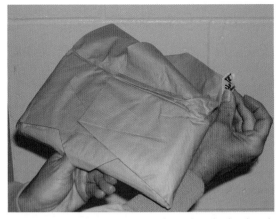

Figure 3-5   Opening a pack with one hand. The thumb of one hand is slid under the tab of the taped edge, and the pack is held between that thumb and the fingers of that hand while the other hand unwraps the pack.

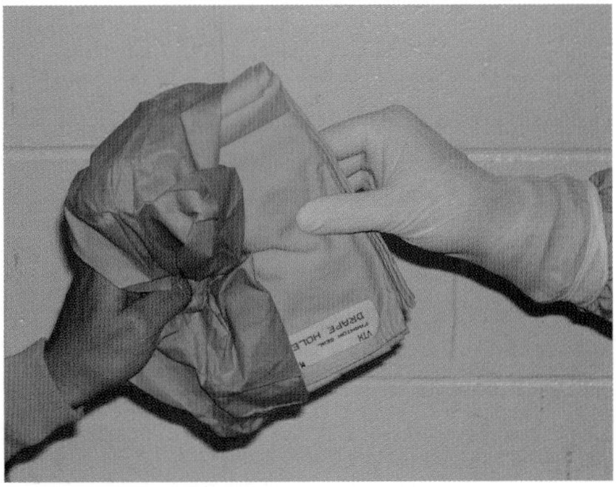

Figure 3-6   Circulating nurse holds the outer wrap of an opened pack in an extended hand to allow the scrubbed-in person to reach in to remove the pack's contents without breaking sterility.

"flipping" the inner suture packet onto the table. Suture can also be given directly to the scrubbed-in personnel by opening the package and allowing the scrubbed-in person to retrieve the inner suture package.

Opening Wrapped Packs with One Hand

Some wrapped items are small enough to be opened with one hand by the circulating nurse. Opening a pack correctly with one hand allows the circulating nurse to hand the item to the scrubbed-in team member for its removal from the wrap, without contaminating the scrubbed-in person. To open a sterile pack with one hand, follow these steps:

1. Hold the pack in one hand (hand A), then insert thumb of hand A under the taped fold (Figure 3-5).
2. Using hand B, remove the tape.
3. Using hand B, lift the top fold back, and tuck the top flap into the grasp of hand A by folding the top flap under the pack.
4. Using hand B, unwrap the two side folds, one at a time, tucking each one into the grasp of hand A underneath the pack.

5. Using hand B, grasp the last corner tab, and pull it back to be held by hand A, as the item is carefully removed from the wrap by the scrubbed-in personnel (Figure 3-6).

Opening Large Packs

Wrapped sterile packs are opened on a clean, flat surface in the OR, as follows:

1. Stand back from the surface on which the pack is to be opened.
2. Place the sterile pack on a flat surface so that the wrapped edges are uppermost.
3. After confirming that the steps for maintaining a sterile field have been met (as listed in practice 3 earlier), remove the indicator tape.
4. Open the distant flap first, taking care not to reach over the sterile contents of the pack.
5. Open the side flaps one at a time, taking care to touch *only* the exposed tabbed corners and no other part of the wrap.
6. Open the nearest flap last. For especially large packs, the circulating nurse may need to walk around the table to avoid reaching over the sterile field. If the wrap is double wrapped, the scrubbed-in team member can open the inner wrap.

KEY POINTS

1. Terminal cleaning of the OR is performed daily.
2. Terminal cleaning includes disinfecting all surfaces of the room and objects contained in the room.
3. The OR floor should be wet-vacuumed daily.
4. The surgical environment needs to be thoroughly cleaned on a daily basis to prevent contamination of the surgical site and to prevent hospital-acquired patient infection.
5. Aseptic technique is used to maintain the absence of disease-causing organisms in the surgical environment.
6. Asepsis does not guarantee sterility.
7. Sterile items are used in surgery and are free of all microorganisms, including spores.
8. A surgical conscience requires acknowledging when a breach in asepsis or sterility has occurred and taking the necessary steps to address and correct it, even if no one else witnesses the breach.
9. The *space* above and surrounding an open sterile pack is considered part of the sterile field.
10. The sterile field cannot be entered or touched by non–scrubbed-in personnel.
11. If non–scrubbed-in personnel enter or touch the sterile field, it is no longer sterile and is considered contaminated.

REVIEW QUESTIONS

1. *True* or *False:* The surgery room does not need to be spot-cleaned between patients because the thorough cleaning performed at the completion of the day's surgery should sufficiently disinfect any soiling that occurs through normal use.
2. Why is stainless steel considered the best surface for surgical tables?
   a. It is not considered the best; in fact, it is the worst because it gets cold and promotes hypothermia.
   b. Its durability provides for long usefulness.
   c. Its smooth surface allows for easy cleaning and discourages harboring of microorganisms.
   d. Both b and c.
   e. All of the above.
3. *True* or *False:* Wet vacuuming of the surgery room floor should not be done because it introduces more microorganisms than wet mopping.
4. Why is it important to restrict traffic through the surgical area?
   a. To keep microbial counts as low as possible.
   b. To promote elitism in the OR.
   c. To minimize distractions.
   d. Both a and b.
   e. None of the above.
5. *True* or *False:* The words "aseptic" and "sterile" are synonyms and can be used interchangeably.
6. What are the two most important practices used to prevent surgical infections?
   a. Aseptic and septic technique.
   b. Sterile and septic technique.
   c. Septic and antiseptic technique.
   d. Aseptic and sterile technique.
   e. Sterile and antiseptic technique.
7. What areas of the scrubbed-in personnel's gown are part of the sterile field?
   a. Back of the gown.
   b. Front from chest to the level of sterile field.
   c. Cuffs of the sleeves.
   d. All of the above if the gown was autoclaved.
   e. None of the above.
8. *True* or *False:* "Strike-through" renders surgical drapes "sterile proof," and therefore drapes affected by strike-through cannot become contaminated under any circumstance.
9. *True* or *False:* The edges of all sterile packages are considered nonsterile.
10. *True* or *False:* It is acceptable practice for the circulating nurse to reach over the sterile field if required to assist the surgeon or surgical assistant.
11. Which of the following is *true* regarding the sterile field?
    a. Only scrubbed-in personnel need to know what is sterile and nonsterile.
    b. Only the circulating nurse needs to keep track of what is sterile and nonsterile.
    c. Excessive talking and movement among scrubbed-in personnel are acceptable, but not among non–scrubbed-in personnel.
    d. All of the above.
    e. None of the above.

12. Which of the following is *false* regarding the sterile field?
    a. Unscrubbed personnel should not walk between two sterile fields.
    b. Unscrubbed personnel should never face the sterile field.
    c. All unscrubbed personnel should keep a safe distance from the sterile field.
    d. Only sterile items should be in the sterile field.
    e. The sterile field should never be left unattended.
13. *True* or *False:* If unscrubbed personnel enters *or* touches the sterile field, it is no longer considered sterile.
14. *True* or *False:* The space above and surrounding an open sterile pack is considered part of the sterile field.

ANSWERS

1. False
2. d
3. False
4. a
5. False
6. d
7. b
8. False
9. True
10. False
11. e
12. b
13. True
14. True

BIBLIOGRAPHY

Association of periOperative Registered Nurses (AORN): *Standards, recommended practices, and guidelines: recommended practices for maintaining a sterile field,* Denver, 2004, AORN.

Fairchild S: *Perioperative nursing: principles and practice,* ed 2, Philadelphia, 1996, Lippincott.

Spry C: *Essentials of perioperative nursing,* ed 2, Boston, 2004, Jones & Bartlett.

CHAPTER 4

Surgical Supplies and Equipment

Teri Raffel

LEARNING OBJECTIVES

After studying this chapter, the reader should be able to do the following:

- Describe the steps used to manufacture surgical instruments.
- List the common surgical instruments used in general, orthopedic, and ophthalmic surgery in veterinary medicine.
- Describe the function of an anesthesia machine.
- List the individual components of the anesthesia machine.
- Describe the method for performing a leak check of an anesthesia machine.
- Describe the difference between rebreathing and non-rebreathing circuits and the indications for their use.

- Describe how to calculate the size of rebreathing bag to be used.
- Describe the use of different oxygen flow rates and the indications for their use.
- Describe the different styles of suture needles.
- Describe the characteristics of suture material.
- List examples of suture material and their main properties.
- List examples of equipment used perioperatively in veterinary surgery.
- List examples of anesthesia monitoring devices.
- Describe the functions of anesthesia monitoring devices.

SURGICAL INSTRUMENTS

Surgical instruments are a major investment for the veterinary hospital. It is important that instruments be used for their designed purpose. Improper use can damage or destroy instruments.

Manufacturing

Instruments are generally made of stainless steel, although some disposable models may be made from plastic. The stainless steel used is composed of iron, chromium, and carbon. *Martensitic* stainless steel has a higher carbon content and is generally used for cutting instruments because the potential for hardness during the tempering stage is greater. *Austenitic* stainless steel has a higher chromium content and a lower carbon content. This metal is used for hemostats and needle holders. Austenitic steel is not as hard as martensitic steel, and as a result, tungsten carbide inserts are often added to the austenitic needle holders to increase their durability.

There are five steps involved in the production of surgical instruments, as follows:

1. Forging: forming or shaping of an instrument by heating and hammering.
2. Milling: cutting a forged piece to produce a final product.
3. Tempering: hardening the instrument by slowly heating in a salt bath and then immersing in oil, or "quenching."
4. Passivation: using a chemical bath to remove the particles created from grinding and other foreign materials, strengthen the steel, and aid in rust protection.
5. Polishing: refining the surface to produce a shiny or matted finish.

Components

Veterinary surgery personnel must know the basic parts of surgical instruments to use, clean, and inspect them appropriately (Figure 4-1).

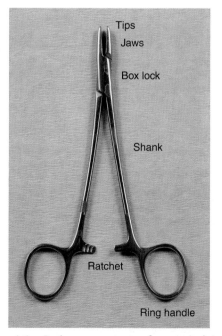

Figure 4-1 Basic components of a surgical instrument. (From McCurnin DM, Bassert JM: *Clinical textbook for veterinary technicians*, ed 5, Philadelphia, 2002, Saunders.)

The first part of the instrument to identify is the *jaw* or *tip*. This area can be traumatic or atraumatic in design, depending on the intended use, and can be straight or curved. The jaw or tip can have serrations, teeth, or flat surfaces. Serrations can be horizontal, vertical, or a combination (e.g., Rochester Carmalt hemostatic forceps). The arrangement of the teeth can be 1×2, 2×3, and so on. Tips with a 1×2 configuration have one tooth on one side of the tip and two teeth on the opposite side. The teeth can also be arranged in rows (e.g., Adson Brown thumb tissue forceps). The tips or jaws can easily become damaged. Teeth and serrations of the tips or jaws should be thoroughly evaluated after each use to observe any defects that may have resulted from use. Blades are available on most types of scissors as curved or straight. Some types of scissors also have the option of blades with sharp or blunt tips. When describing or identifying instruments, the blades or tips can provide important information. For example, identifying an instrument as a "curved Metzenbaum dissecting scissors" defines the shape and type of scissors. Identifying an operating scissors as a "curved, sharp/blunt [s/b] operating scissors" reveals even more about the instrument.

The second important part of the instrument, the *box lock,* is present only on instruments with ring handles. The box lock is the joint or hinge of the instrument. This area absorbs great stress when the instrument is in use, and therefore the box lock must be inspected carefully to detect any cracks or evidence of degradation.

The third part of the instrument to identify is the *shank* (also referred to as the "shaft") or *body* of the instrument. This part is usually the longest area and determines the instrument's overall length. Instruments may range from 3 to 12 inches in total length depending on the length of the shank.

The *ratchet* is the next important part of the instrument, but it is found only on some instruments with ring handles. The ratchet is a device with interlocking teeth that will lock an instrument jaw in a closed position. Degradation of this part of the instrument is usually seen as the inability of the ratchet to remain locked.

Some instruments also have *ring handles,* which serve as the means for using and controlling the instrument. Proper handling of an instrument with ring handles is achieved by placing the thumb and ring finger in the rings. The thumb ring should not advance beyond the first knuckle of the thumb, and the ring on the ring finger should not advance beyond the second knuckle. The index finger can rest on the shank to help stabilize the instrument (Figure 4-2).

General Surgery Instruments

Scissors

Many types of scissors are available to the veterinary surgeon (Figure 4-3). As with all instruments, it is important that scissors be used only for their intended function.

Operating Scissors

The intended use of operating scissors is to cut only inanimate objects (e.g., suture, paper drapes, sponges). Its design can be straight or curved, and the blades can be sharp tipped or blunt tipped.

Mayo Dissecting Scissors

The Mayo dissecting scissors is used when cutting large muscle masses, cartilage, or any other nondelicate tissue. The blades are thick and approximately one-third the instrument's length. The blades can be straight or curved.

Metzenbaum Dissecting Scissors

The Metzenbaum dissecting scissors is used for delicate surgical dissection. The blades are thin, delicate, and approximately one-fourth the

instrument's overall length. The shaft is long and thin, and the blades can be straight or curved.

Suture Removal Scissors

Sometimes called a "suture scissor," the suture removal scissors usually is not found in the surgery pack but rather is stored in the treatment area or examination room. The suture scissors has one blade in the shape of a hook that cradles the suture to be cut (Figure 4-4). This instrument is designed to remove external sutures from the skin.

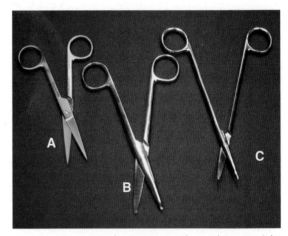

Figure 4-3   Surgical scissors: **A,** Sharp/sharp straight operating scissors; **B,** straight Mayo dissecting scissors; **C,** curved Metzenbaum dissecting scissors. (Photo by John T. Miller.)

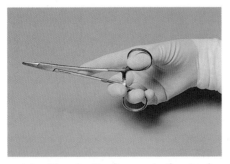

Figure 4-2   Thumb–ring finger grip for ring-handled instruments. (From Fossum TW: *Small animal surgery,* ed 2, St Louis, 2002, Mosby.)

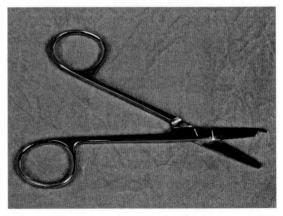

Figure 4-4   Suture removal scissors.

Hemostats

Although there are many types of hemostats, only five styles are typically used in veterinary surgery (Figure 4-5). As their name implies, hemostats are used to aid in controlling hemostasis in the surgical field. Hemostats can have jaws that are straight or curved and serrations that are horizontal, vertical, or a combination. Serrations also may be partial or may extend the full length of the jaw.

Halstead Mosquito Hemostatic Forceps

This instrument has small jaws with fine horizontal serrations that extend the entire length of the tip. The Halstead hemostat is generally used to clamp small vessels (e.g., "skin bleeders").

Kelly Hemostatic Forceps

This instrument is larger than the mosquito hemostat. The horizontal serrations are wider and only extend half the length of the jaw. The Kelly hemostat can be used for medium sized vessels or small tissue masses.

Crile Hemostatic Forceps

The Crile hemostat is similar to the Kelly hemostat, with the difference being how far the serrations extend along the jaws. The Crile hemostatic forceps has serrations that extend the entire length of the jaw.

Ferguson Angiotribe

Although not a true "hemostat," the Ferguson angiotribe is an extremely strong forceps that is quite traumatic, with a crushing jaw design that has one raised jaw and one recessed jaw. This clamp can be used on vessels of almost any size and on any tissue that will not need to be viable in the body (e.g., uterine stump).

Rochester Carmalt Hemostatic Forceps

This hemostat is quite different from other hemostats. The Rochester Carmalt hemostat has both horizontal and vertical serrations on the jaw near the tip. The result is a checkerboard appearance at the tip of the jaw. This hemostatic forceps is usually about 8 inches long, making it a large instrument, and the jaw is approximately $3\frac{1}{2}$ inches of the total length. It can be used to clamp large vessels or large tissue masses.

Needle Holders

Needle holders have very short jaws that have a roughened platform in the tips to allow for a secure grip of the suture needle (Figure 4-6). As previously mentioned, tungsten inserts may be used in the jaws of needle holders to increase instrument longevity. Needle holders are the only surgical instruments designed with the specific intent of holding metal. Therefore the needle holder is the *only* instrument that should be used to hold needles or to place scalpel blades onto scalpel handles.

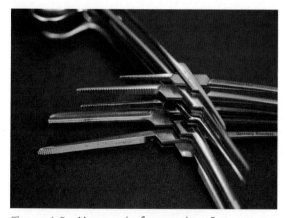

Figure 4-5 Hemostatic forceps tips. *Bottom to top,* Straight Rochester Carmalt hemostatic forceps, straight Ferguson angiotribe, straight Kelly hemostatic forceps, straight Crile hemostatic forceps, and straight Halstead Mosquito hemostatic forceps. (Photo by John T. Miller.)

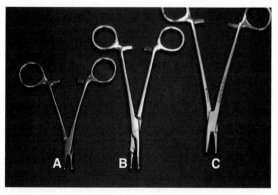

Figure 4-6 Needle holders: **A,** Derf; **B,** Olsen-Hegar; **C,** Mayo-Hegar. (Photo by John T. Miller.)

Derf

The Derf needle holder is small in length and is used with small animals, with special species, and in extraocular ophthalmic procedures (considered too large for intraocular surgery).

Olsen-Hegar

The Olsen-Hegar instrument is different from other needle holders in that it has scissors built into the jaws. This added feature is a time-saving device that allows suture to be cut without having to reach for another instrument. The main disadvantage to having the scissors as part of this needle holder is that an inexperienced user may inadvertently cut suture material when trying to grasp the needle.

Mayo-Hegar

The Mayo-Hegar is a commonly used needle holder available in a variety of lengths, depending on the surgical procedure and the surgeon's preference.

Crile-Wood

Although similar to the Mayo-Hegar, the Crile-Wood needle holder has a finer, more delicate jaw.

Scalpels

Scalpel Blade Handles

Scalpel blade handles are designed to hold the scalpel blade for easier and safer use. Scalpel blades numbered 10 through 19 fit on the No. 3 scalpel handle (Figure 4-7). Blades numbered 20 through 29 fit on the No. 4 handle (Figure 4-8). Handles often have units of measurement on them to be used as needed. One such use may be as a reference marker for cases requiring photographic documentation (e.g., mass removal, foreign body removal). Scalpel handles should be held in a pencil grip with the index finger on the noncutting edge of the blade to stabilize the scalpel (Figure 4-9).

Scalpel Blades

The most common scalpel blade used in small animal surgery is the No. 10 (Figure 4-10). This blade is used primarily for skin incisions. A No. 11

blade is tapered to a pointed shape and is generally used to create a "stab" incision. The No. 12 blade resembles a hook, with the cutting edge on the inside curve, and is frequently used when declawing a cat. A No. 15 blade has the appearance of a No. 10 blade, but with only half the No. 10's length. The larger scalpel blades (Nos. 20-29) are generally reserved for use in large animal surgery.

Thumb Tissue Forceps

A thumb tissue forceps (casually referred to as a "pick-up") is an instrument used to grasp and retract tissue on a short-term basis (Figure 4-11). Instruments in this category resemble a tweezer, but thumb tissue forceps should never be referred to as "tweezers." A pencil grip is used to hold this instrument in the nondominant hand (Figure 4-12). The best control of pressure is achieved when holding the forceps as if it were a pencil. The shaft of a thumb tissue forceps is generally straight, but some

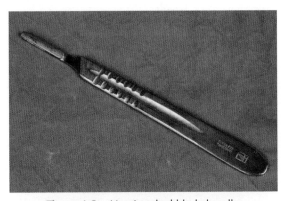

Figure 4-8   No. 4 scalpel blade handle.

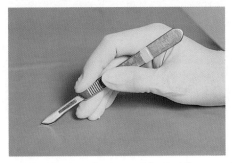

Figure 4-9   The pencil grip used for holding a scalpel. (From Fossum TW: *Small animal surgery,* ed 2, St Louis, 2002, Mosby.)

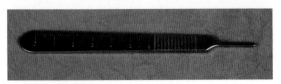

Figure 4-7   No. 3 scalpel blade handle.

designs have unique shapes to the shaft that help distinguish them from others (e.g., Adson, Bayonet). The tips can be toothed, smooth (atraumatic), or fairly traumatic in design.

Debakey Thoracic Thumb Tissue Forceps

Originally designed as a cardiovascular thumb tissue forceps, the Debakey thoracic forceps is an excellent example of an atraumatic forceps that should be used only on delicate tissue. The tips have no teeth but rather a ridge or groove design.

Tissue Thumb Forceps

This instrument has a straight shaft and can range in length from 5 to 12 inches. The tips can have 1 × 2 teeth or 3 × 4 teeth.

Russian Thumb Tissue Forceps

This instrument has a very traumatic, bulky tip. The Russian thumb tissue forceps is generally reserved for use on skin or tissue that is being removed from the animal.

Adson Thumb Tissue Forceps

The Adson thumb tissue forceps has a very narrow tip that broadens to a ½-inch-wide shaft.

The tips can be of various designs and are described as follows:

- *Adson dressing.* The tip has no teeth but does have flat, atraumatic serrations. This Adson style is generally used as an aid in placing or removing dressings on wounds.
- *Adson-Brown.* The tip of this instrument has two parallel rows of nine shallow teeth on both tips. A common general surgery tissue forceps, the Adson-Brown can be found in most general instrument packs.
- *Adson 1 × 2.* The tip of this style has one tooth on one tip and two teeth on the opposite side. The teeth interdigitate to grasp tissue firmly. It can be fairly traumatic if used on delicate tissue or used too aggressively.

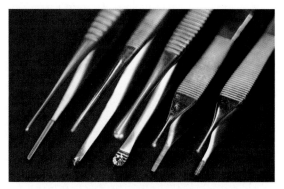

Figure 4-11 Thumb tissue forceps. *Left to right,* Debakey, 1 × 2, Russian, Adson dressing, and Adson-Brown. (Photo by John T. Miller.)

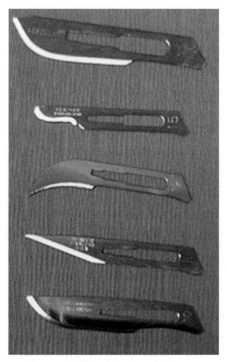

Figure 4-10 Scalpel blades. *Top to bottom,* Nos. 20, 15, 12, 11, and 10.

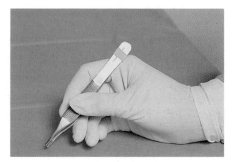

Figure 4-12 The pencil grip used for holding thumb tissue forceps. (From Fossum TW: *Small animal surgery,* ed 2, St Louis, 2002, Mosby.)

Allis Tissue Forceps

The Allis tissue forceps is neither a hemostat nor a thumb tissue forceps. Its intended use of grasping tissue in a fairly traumatic way makes it a unique instrument. This ring-handled instrument has tips that may have teeth configured in a 3 × 4 or 4 × 5 style (Figure 4-13). Because of its traumatic nature, the Allis tissue forceps is generally used to grasp tough tissue (e.g., linea alba) or tissue being removed from the animal (e.g., tumor, skin).

Retractors

Retractors are instruments used to deflect or retract tissue or other structures away from the surgical field where the surgeon is working. Retractors can be *handheld* (Figure 4-14), which require at least two sterile members of the surgical team, or *self-retaining* (Figure 4-15).

Handheld Retractors

U.S. Army This handheld retractor is a double-ended retractor with different lengths of blades on either end. It has no teeth on the blades and therefore causes little tissue trauma, other than

pressure damage if applied too forcefully to the tissue.

Senn The Senn retractor is also a double-ended handheld retractor. One end is a narrow, blunt blade, and the other end is a toothed, traumatic end. The teeth can be sharp or blunt, which may affect where it is used.

Self-Retaining Retractors

Gelpi With its single, sharp-pointed tips, the Gelpi self-retaining retractor is a fairly traumatic instrument. It has limited use in soft tissue surgery but is extremely useful in orthopedic and neurologic surgery.

Weitlaner This self-retaining retractor has teeth in the jaw that can be blunt or sharp. Although used more often in orthopedic surgery, the blunt-toothed style of the Weitlaner retractor can be used in some soft tissue surgical cases.

Balfour The Balfour retractor is one of the few self-retaining retractors frequently used in soft tissue surgery (Figure 4-16). Available in adult and pediatric sizes, it is extremely useful for abdominal procedures. While keeping the abdominal walls in lateral retraction, it also has a third blade for cranial retraction as well. This widespread retraction provides excellent visualization of the abdominal cavity for the surgeon.

Towel Clamps

Towel clamps are instruments used to secure the sterile drapes to the patient during surgery or to

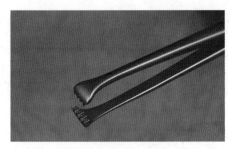

Figure 4-13   Allis tissue forceps: tips. (Photo by John T. Miller.)

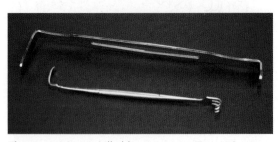

Figure 4-14   Handheld retractors. *Top,* U.S. Army retractor. *Bottom,* Senn double-ended retractor. (Photo by John T. Miller.)

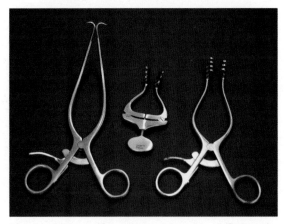

Figure 4-15   Self-retaining retractors. *Left to right,* Gelpi, Jansen, and Weitlaner. (Photo by John T. Miller.)

secure the sterile drapes to one another (Figure 4-17). Towel clamps may have a *penetrating* design, which means the tips are sharp and pointed and are intended to pierce the patient's skin to hold the sterile drape in place. They also may have a *nonpenetrating* style, which is more likely to be used to secure one drape to another.

Backhaus

The most common style of towel clamp, the Backhaus has penetrating tips and is available in 3½- or 5½-inch sizes.

Roeder

The Roeder style is unique in that it has balls on the tips. The balls prevent the towel clamp from being placed too deeply into the tissue.

Jones

This penetrating towel clamp is more delicate and lightweight than the other styles. Instead of the usual ratchet and ring handle, the Jones towel clamp has a squeeze-handle mechanism, which makes it convenient to use on smaller patients.

Lorna

Also known as the Edna nonpenetrating towel clamp, the Lorna, like the Backhaus, is available in 3½- and 5½-inch sizes. The feature of nonpenetrating tips makes this an ideal clamp for securing second-layer drapes, whether cloth or paper, to the ground drapes.

Miscellaneous Instruments

A few miscellaneous instruments are found in most veterinary surgical packs.

Snook Spay Hook

Some surgeons use this hooklike instrument to find and exteriorize the uterine horns when performing an ovariohysterectomy on dogs and cats.

Needle Rack

The needle rack is a spring mounted on a metal base designed to store "eyed" free needles during the autoclaving process.

Groove Director

This instrument is designed to aid the surgeon in making incisions on the linea alba. The groove director provides a "channel" that the scalpel can follow, to avoid accidental incising of abdominal viscera (Figure 4-18).

Bowls

Every instrument pack should have at least one bowl. The bowls can be used for holding saline for lavage or for storing sharps during the procedure to help keep the instrument table safe and clean (Figure 4-19).

Orthopedic Surgery Instruments

Many types of orthopedic instruments are available. The instruments described here are the

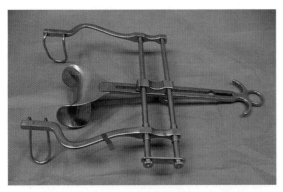

Figure 4-16   Balfour abdominal retractor.

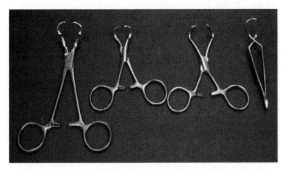

Figure 4-17   Towel clamps. *Left to right,* Roeder, Backhaus, Lorna, and Jones. (Photo by John T. Miller.)

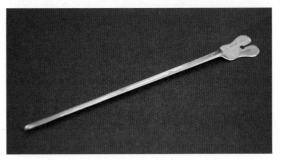

Figure 4-18   Groove director. (Photo by John T. Miller.)

basics needed for orthopedic surgery and provide a starting point for building an orthopedic surgical instrument inventory.

Bone Holders

Bone-holding clamps are designed to hold bone fragments together until permanent fixation can be achieved. Bone holders can have pointed tips, toothed tips, or serrated tips (Figure 4-20). Bone holders are available in a variety of sizes and styles (Figure 4-21). Depending on the bone that is fractured and the type of fracture, certain styles of bone holders may be better suited than others.

Periosteal Elevators

The periosteal elevator is used to prepare the fractured bone for permanent fixation. As the name implies, the intended use is to elevate the periosteum from the bone so that the implants can be placed. Periosteal elevators are available in many shapes and sizes, with the most popular styles being the Freer elevator (Figure 4-22), ASIF (Synthes) elevator (Figure 4-23), and Adson elevator.

Bone Rongeurs

Rongeurs have cupped tips with sharp edges and work with a squeezing action of the handles (Figure 4-24). Rongeurs are used to break up bits and pieces of bone for grafting purposes. Pieces of bone too small to reattach to the animal are broken down into small pieces and packed around the fracture lines to encourage new osteoblast formation and promote healing. Rongeurs can also be used to remove pieces of unnecessary bone.

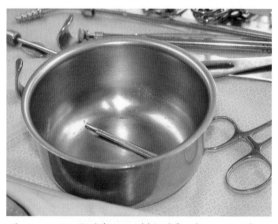

Figure 4-19   Stainless steel bowl for sharps or saline.

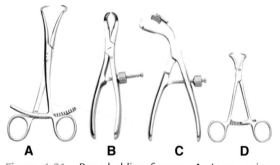

Figure 4-21   Bone-holding forceps. **A,** Large point-to-point bone reduction forceps. **B,** Bone reduction forceps with speed lock. **C,** Verbrugge bone-holding forceps with speed lock. **D,** Small, sharp, bone reduction forceps. (Courtesy Synthes, West Chester, Pa.)

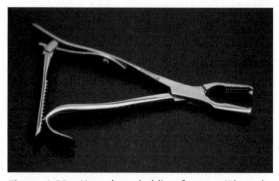

Figure 4-20   Kerns bone-holding forceps. (Photo by John T. Miller.)

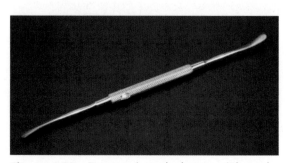

Figure 4-22   Freer periosteal elevator. (Photo by John T. Miller.)

Bone Cutters

Bone cutters have handles with squeezing and spring action, similar to the rongeurs. Bone cutters have cutting-edged tips designed to cut through bone and to remove small pieces of bone.

Bone Curettes

Bone curettes are single-handled instruments that have a cupped tip surrounded by sharp edges. Bone curettes are used to collect ("harvest") bone graft material or to shape and scrape bony surfaces.

Hand Chuck (Jacob's Chuck)

A hand chuck is designed to hold and drive intramedullary pins for repair of a fracture or for other orthopedic surgeries requiring the use of pins (Figure 4-25). The hand chuck is a manual drill. It can hold wires with sizes from 0.035 inch and up to $^{3}/_{16}$-inch pins. The pins are held securely in the hand chuck when the key is used to tighten the chuck. An extension piece is available to protect the surgeon from the pin, which may extend beyond the end of the chuck.

Internal Fixation Implants

Implants can be used for internal fixation of bone fractures, as curative measures for traumatic situations (e.g., tibial plateau leveling osteotomy, cranial cruciate ligament repair), and to correct congenital limb deformities. Many types of implants are available, from pins and orthopedic wire to standard dynamic compression plates (DCP) and specially designed bone plates. This section describes the basic types of implants and the equipment necessary to use them.

Intramedullary Pins

These implants are made of metal and range in size from $^{1}/_{16}$ to $^{1}/_{2}$ inch (Figure 4-26). Intramedullary (IM) pins are used to stabilize certain types of fractures or soft tissue in specific orthopedic situations.

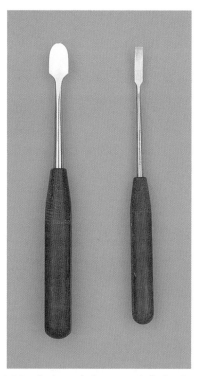

Figure 4-23   Periosteal elevators. *Left,* Synthes round edge. *Right,* Synthes curved blade, straight edge. (From Fossum TW: *Small animal surgery,* ed 2, St Louis, 2002, Mosby.)

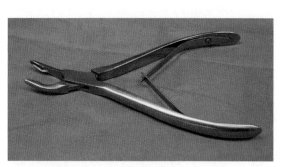

Figure 4-24   Single-action rongeur.

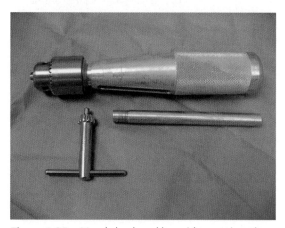

Figure 4-25   Hand chuck and key with extension piece.

These pins can be smooth tipped or can have threaded ends. IM pins can be used alone or in conjunction with wire, plates, and screws. Pins can be placed using a hand chuck or a nitrogen air drill or electric drill.

Pin Cutter

A pin cutter is used to cut pins once they have been placed in the animal (Figure 4-27). Depending on the size of the pin, a squeeze-handle cutter or a bolt cutter may be needed.

Orthopedic Wire

Orthopedic wire is stainless steel wire designed for long-term implantation in a patient (Figure 4-28). This wire is sized from 16 to 30 gauge; the smaller the number, the larger (thicker) the wire. The most common sizes used in veterinary surgery are 18, 20, and 22 gauge, but the choice depends on the size of the patient, the procedure performed, and the expected stress level of the wound (and therefore its ability to heal). Wire can be used in conjunction with pins, plates, or screws. Wire twisters are used to secure the wire and are available in many styles (Figure 4-29). Previously used needle holders are often reserved for the purpose of securing wires as well.

Bone Plates

Bone plates are stainless steel (except for vertebral plates, made of plastic) and are designed to aid in the reduction of fractures and the repair of bone fragments. Plates are available in a wide variety of sizes (Figure 4-30). The size chosen by the

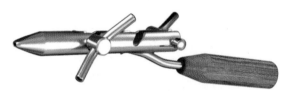

Figure 4-28   Orthopedic wire. (Photo by John T. Miller.)

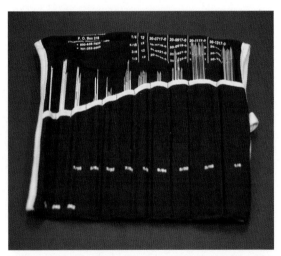

Figure 4-26   Intramedullary pin set. (Photo by John T. Miller.)

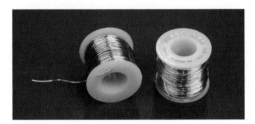

Figure 4-29   Wire twister. (Courtesy Synthes, West Chester, Pa.)

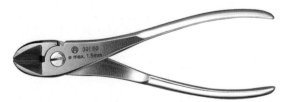

Figure 4-27   Pin cutter. (Courtesy Synthes, West Chester, Pa.)

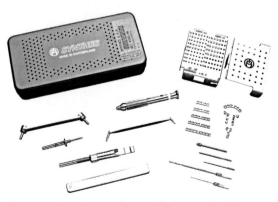

Figure 4-30   Bone plates (plating set). (Courtesy Synthes, West Chester, Pa.)

surgeon primarily depends on the size of the patient, the particular bone being repaired, and the size of the bone to be repaired. Plates can have different shapes (e.g., straight, T-plates, L-plates), widths (e.g., 2.0, 2.7, and 3.5 mm), and lengths (e.g., four, five, or six hole). The *width number* indicates the size of screw that should also be used to secure the plate, and the *length* is defined by the number of holes available to be filled with screws. Accordingly, the larger the implant, the more expensive is the piece.

Implant Specialty Instrumentation

Each type of implant has accompanying specialty instrumentation that must be used to place the implant properly. For example, IM pins are generally placed with a hand chuck or power drill. The drill can be an electric drill or powered by nitrogen. Plates and screws require an entire set of specialized instruments for proper use of the implants (Figures 4-31 and 4-32). Even orthopedic wire should be used with dedicated instruments such as wire cutters and wire twisters.

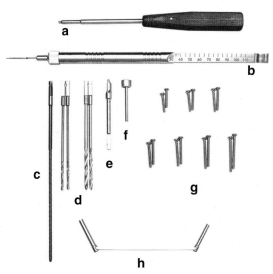

Figure 4-31   Specialty instrumentation for implant (plate and screw) placement: *a,* screwdriver; *b,* depth gauge; *c,* tap; *d,* drill bits; *e,* countersink; *f,* insert drill sleeve; *g,* screws; *h,* tap sleeve. (Courtesy Synthes, West Chester, Pa.)

Ophthalmic Surgery Instruments

Every veterinary surgical area should have a basic set of ophthalmic instruments available for use. These instruments are extremely delicate and expensive and should be handled with great care. Because of the nature of the tissue for which these instruments are routinely used, the tips are very fine, the shafts tend to be short, and the mechanism of use may be box lock or squeeze handle.

Beaver Blade Handle

This handle is used to hold Beaver scalpel blades (Figure 4-33, *F*). Although some ophthalmic procedures can be performed using a No. 15 scalpel blade on a No. 3 handle, some intraocular procedures may require the use of a beaver blade.

Lid Speculum

An eyelid speculum may or may not be used, depending on the procedure performed. For intraocular procedures, a Barraquer wire speculum is often used to retract the eyelids away from the surgical site (Figure 4-33, *A*). For lid procedures, a chalazion lid speculum may be used (Figure 4-33, *D*). This instrument is most helpful in the removal of an eyelid tumor.

Lacrimal Cannulas

Both straight and curved lacrimal cannulas are available. These stainless steel cannulas can be used to flush lacrimal ducts. One end of the cannula is adapted to accept a syringe to allow for

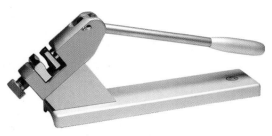

Figure 4-32   Tabletop plate bender used to bend and conform implant (plate) to bone surface. (Courtesy Synthes, West Chester, Pa.)

infusion of solution. The other end is blunt to permit easy passage into the lacrimal duct.

Thumb Tissue Forceps

Thumb tissue forceps are extremely delicate in design. Their function in ophthalmic surgery is the same as in general surgery. Gentle holding of tissue is imperative because the tips of these instruments are extremely delicate. It is crucial to handle the tissue of the eye and its associated structures in an atraumatic manner to avoid damaging the tissues. Examples of thumb tissue forceps include the iris 1 × 2 (Figure 4-33, *B*), Bishop-Harmon, and Colibri.

Scissors

The scissors used in ophthalmic surgery may be miniature versions of general surgery instruments, such as the baby Metzenbaum dissecting scissors (Figure 4-33, *H*). Others are specially designed and crafted for delicate eye surgery, such as the Castroviejo scissors. Many of the specialty scissors have a squeeze-action operation instead of the more traditional ring-handled mechanism. Two general-purpose utility scissors are typically used in ophthalmology: the Stevens tenotomy scissors (Figure 4-33, *G*) and the iris scissors (Figure 4-33, *C*). Compared with the Stevens tenotomy scissors, the iris scissors has a slightly longer blade, which tapers at a more constant rate from box lock to tip, as well as

sharper points. Both these scissors can be used to cut the extrafine suture material used in ophthalmic surgery as well as tissue.

Needle Holders

The type of needle holder used depends on whether the surgical procedure is intraocular or extraocular. Extraocular procedures may be managed with a small (4-inch) Mayo-Hegar or a Derf needle holder. Intraocular procedures may require a more delicate instrument, such as a Castroviejo needle holder (Figure 4-33, *E*). As with the scissors, the specialty needle holders may have a squeeze-handle mechanism instead of the usual, bulkier ring-handle style.

Miscellaneous Ophthalmic Equipment

Hemostasis for ophthalmic surgery involves different concerns than in general or orthopedic surgery. The delicate nature of the tissue surrounding the eye requires that materials other than sponges be used to perform hemostasis. For extraocular procedures (e.g., lid tumor, enucleation), regular, radiopaque surgical sponges are appropriate. For intraocular procedures (e.g., corneal laceration, lens luxation), a more delicate device is needed. Cotton-tipped applicators can be sterilized and used, or surgical spears (e.g., Weck-Cel) are available commercially (Figure 4-34). The spears have an arrow shape and permit pinpoint control of hemorrhages in a small working area.

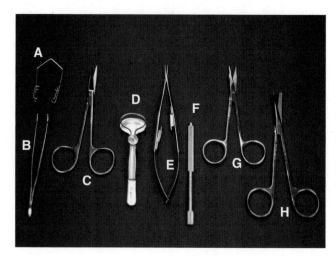

Figure 4-33   Ophthalmic surgery instruments. **A,** Barraquer wire lid speculum. **B,** Curved 1 × 2 iris thumb tissue forceps. **C,** Straight iris scissors. **D,** Chalazion lid speculum. **E,** Castroviejo locking needle holder. **F,** Beaver blade handle. **G,** Stevens tenotomy scissors. **H,** Curved baby Metzenbaum scissors. (Photo by John T. Miller.)

ANESTHESIA MACHINE

One purpose of an anesthesia machine is to deliver inhalation anesthesia to the patient and then remove the unneeded gases from the patient and the surgery suite. Generally this is accomplished with the use of a corrugated tubing system. The inhalation anesthetic gas is delivered to the patient through oxygen molecules (i.e., oxygen is the carrier gas for the anesthetic gas). Another purpose of an anesthesia machine is to deliver oxygen (O_2) as the sole gas, as in cardiopulmonary resuscitation (CPR). For the anesthesia machine to perform as intended, it must do the following:

1. Deliver O_2 at a controlled rate.
2. Vaporize (turn a liquid into a gas) a designated concentration of liquid anesthetic, mix the anesthetic with oxygen, and deliver the mixture to the patient.
3. Remove exhaled gases from the patient, then dispose of the gases through a scavenging system or recirculate them (after removing the carbon dioxide) to the patient.

The ability of the anesthesia machine to function properly depends on the equipment being in good repair and properly maintained.

Anesthesia machines are configured in many forms, depending on the manufacturer. Well-known producers of anesthesia machines include North American Matrix (Figure 4-35), Drager (Figures 4-36 and 4-37), and Ohmeda Medical. Some machines are designed with the simplest intent of delivering inhalation anesthesia (see Figures 4-35 and 4-36). Others have accessories

and the ability to provide automatic ventilation, multiple inhalation gas choices (e.g., nitrous oxide, isoflurane, sevoflurane), and space for placement and storage of monitoring devices (see Figure 4-37). Regardless of the machine's appearance, the basic function remains the same.

Components

The anesthesia machine has many components working together to perform its intended function properly. To best understand how the machine works, it is necessary to identify and understand each component. This basic information not only provides a working knowledge of the machine, but also assists the technician with troubleshooting problems in the event of a malfunction. Tracing the oxygen flow through

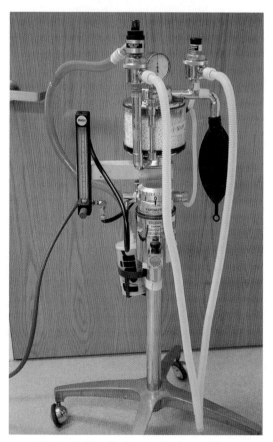

Figure 4-35   Basic anesthesia machine.

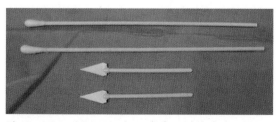

Figure 4-34   Hemostatic tools for ophthalmic surgery. *Top,* Cotton-tipped applicators. *Bottom,* Weck-Cel surgical spears.

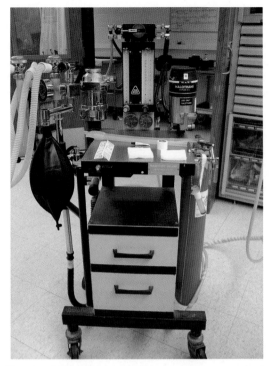

Figure 4-36   Basic double-vaporizer anesthetic machine.

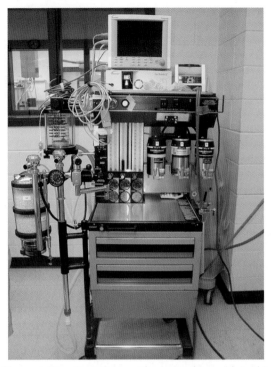

Figure 4-37   Complex anesthesia machine with multiple vaporizers, storage for monitoring devices, and a ventilator.

the machine allows a view of all the components of the machine.

Oxygen Source

The oxygen source can be a localized cylinder or a large, centrally located source (Figure 4-38). Cylinders are available in different sizes; the two most common sizes are the "E" and "H" tanks. The "E" tanks are smaller and generally attached to the machine, whereas the "H" tanks are larger and generally stand alone away from the anesthesia machine, often chained against a wall. Tanks are color-coded for easy recognition (green in the United States, white in Canada) and have a pressure reading of 2200 pounds per square inch (psi) when full. When opening a tank, personnel should remember the rule of "righty tighty, lefty loosey." When turning the valve clockwise (to the right), the tank is being closed; turning the valve counterclockwise (to the left) opens the tank. Using 100% O_2 from an oxygen source is justified

because (1) the O_2 acts as a carrier for the vaporized anesthetic gas and delivers it to the patient, and (2) anesthetized patients have a decreased tidal volume, so an increased O_2 concentration will compensate for the decrease in tidal volume.

Pressure-Reducing Valve

The first pressure-reducing valve in the system should be found near the oxygen source tank. This valve reduces the pressure leaving the tank and entering the machine to 40 to 45 psi. The lower pressure gas is carried through the source lines to the anesthesia machine.

Flowmeter

Next in the flow of O_2 is the oxygen flowmeter (Figure 4-39). The flowmeter further reduces the pressure of the gas to 15 psi. This is very close to atmospheric pressure and is well tolerated by patients. The flowmeter regulates how much O_2 is entering the system and being delivered to

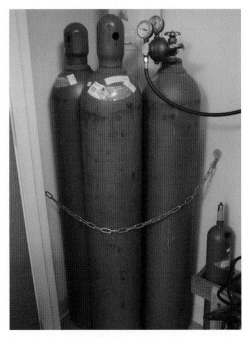

Figure 4-38 Large "H" tanks as an oxygen source.

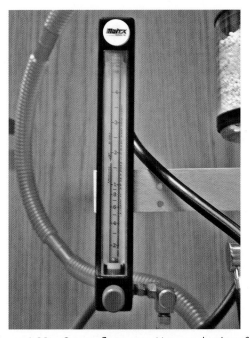

Figure 4-39 Oxygen flowmeter. Note graduations for measuring oxygen flow. Float is seen at bottom of flowmeter. Fast flush valve is to right of regulating knob.

the patient. O_2 flow is measured in liters per minute (L/min) or milliliters per minute (ml/min). The O_2 flow is regulated by a knob at the bottom of the flowmeter. Personnel must take care to avoid excessive tightening of the knob when turning off the flow. When reading the flowmeter, the "float" needs to be properly read. Ball floats are read on the scale where the middle of the ball sits on the graduations. Floats with a point are read at the top of the float. Graduations on the flowmeter may be in 100-ml increments until the 1-L level, then in 500-ml increments thereafter.

Fast Flush Valve

Next in the order of O_2 flow through the machine is the fast flush valve. On many anesthesia machines the oxygen flush valve is found near the oxygen flowmeter. The fast flush valve allows quick infusion of only O_2 into the breathing circuit. This infusion can occur because, with a vaporizer "out of the circle," the vaporizer is bypassed with the tubing arrangement of the machine. The fast flush valve should never be used with a non-rebreathing system for two reasons. First, the pressure of O_2 coming out of the system is too high and may harm the patient. Second, the non-rebreathing systems use such a high O_2 flow that the valve's purpose becomes moot; the high flows result in O_2 levels similar to those achieved with the fast flush valve. During the recovery phase, the fast flush valve is frequently employed to dilute residual anesthetic gases that remain in the system. Flushing the system of residual gases will hasten the patient's recovery because less anesthetic gas is present.

Vaporizer

The vaporizer is usually found next when tracing O_2 flow. The vaporizer *inlet* is the point where the O_2 enters the vaporizer to carry anesthetic gas molecules to the patient. The vaporizer *outlet* is the point at which the O_2 and anesthetic gas leave the vaporizer to enter the circuit. (Up to this point, the O_2 flow has been "out of the circle," assuming the anesthesia machine being used has the vaporizer out of the circle. The "circle," or circuit, is the loop that the gases travel to cycle in and out of the patient when a rebreathing ["recycling"] system is used.) The primary function of the vaporizer is to house or hold liquid anesthetic and to vaporize that liquid into a gas form that can be delivered to the patient in a controlled manner. The vaporizer is likely the most expensive component of the anesthesia machine and therefore must be used appropriately.

Vaporizers are calibrated internally for a specific type of inhalation anesthetic. Only the type of anesthetic for which the machine has been calibrated should be used in the vaporizer. All designs of vaporizers have some style of indicator window at the base of the unit. This window allows determination of the amount of liquid anesthetic remaining in the machine. Once the level reaches half to one-quarter remaining, liquid anesthetic should be added to avoid running out during a procedure. If the vaporizer does need to be filled while the machine is in use, personnel must be sure to turn off the vaporizer before filling it, to prevent the anesthetic from bubbling out and contaminating the environment with noxious, anesthetic fumes. Some vaporizers have two indicator windows, one to show how full it is and one to show when to refill. Vaporizers have

some type of device to determine the amount of anesthetic being delivered to the system. Depending on the type of vaporizer, this amount will be determined as a percentage or just a setting on the dial.

Vaporizers should be serviced annually to ensure a properly functioning mechanism. In the event that a vaporizer needs to be shipped for servicing, drain the vaporizer of any liquid anesthetic to avoid any accidental spill or leaks during shipping.

Both precision and nonprecision vaporizers are available (Table 4-1). However, nonprecision vaporizers are infrequently used now.

Precision Vaporizer

The precision vaporizer has many advantages over the nonprecision style (Figure 4-40). Precision vaporizers are used with high-vapor-pressure anesthetics and are always found out of the circle. The liquid phase of a high-pressure anesthetic vaporizes easily and quickly and must be delivered in a controlled state. If uncontrolled delivery occurs, the concentration of the drug in the carrier gas could easily become excessive and dangerous. Three factors affect vaporizer function and are

TABLE 4-1   Comparison of Precision and Nonprecision Vaporizers

PARAMETER	PRECISION VAPORIZER	NONPRECISION VAPORIZER
Temperature compensation	Output not affected by ambient temperature in most models	Output affected by ambient temperature
Flow compensation	Output not affected over a wide range of oxygen flow rates	Output affected by oxygen flow rate
Back pressure compensation	Changes in back pressure do not affect output	Changes in back pressure affect output
Maintenance requirements	Requires periodic factory recalibration and cleaning	Minimal; can be done by hospital staff
Cost	High	Minimal
Anesthetics commonly used	Isoflurane, sevoflurane, halothane (i.e., those with high vapor pressure)	Methoxyflurane (i.e., those with low vapor pressure); isoflurane and halothane with low-flow techniques
Control over anesthetic concentration	Precise; given as a percentage	Not precise; given as a control lever setting (1-10)
Position relative to anesthetic circuit	Out of circle (VOC)	In circle (VIC)

From McKelvey D, Hollingshead KW: *Veterinary anesthesia and analgesia*, ed 3, St Louis, 2003, Mosby.

compensated for in the precision vaporizer: (1) temperature, (2) gas flow rate, and (3) back pressure. First, if the room temperature is cold, the amount of volatile anesthetic vaporized may be less than the amount indicated on the dial. In a warm room, however, the amount of anesthetic vaporized may be much higher, and therefore a higher level will be delivered to the patient than indicated on the dial setting. The precision vaporizer is constructed with insulation to the liquid anesthetic chamber, so the problems with temperature are eliminated.

The second factor that the precision vaporizer compensates for is the carrier gas flow rate. The O_2 flow rate can affect the amount of vaporized anesthetic delivered to the patient. Extremely high flows (>10 L/min) or extremely low flows (<500 ml/min) are difficult to compensate for, and therefore they should not be used routinely. In a vaporizer that is compensated, the amount of vaporized gas will match the amount indicated on the dial. As the O_2 flow rate is reduced from 300 to 200 to 100 ml/min, the reliability of the dial setting becomes more questionable. Because the flow is reduced, less fresh gas is being delivered. Even though the amount of vaporized gas being sent to the circuit is constant, the amount of gas delivered to the patient is reduced. Vaporizer settings for lower O_2 flow rates need to be adjusted to deliver the amount of anesthetic gas that is actually desired.

The third factor affecting vaporizer function and compensation is back pressure. Vaporizers that have gas under pressure passing through them may release additional anesthetic, increasing the concentration to the circuit, unless the vaporizer compensated for this situation. This occurs when an animal is "bagged." Modern precision vaporizers are designed to adjust for any increase in pressure so that the amount of anesthetic released is not affected.

Precision vaporizers are designed to eliminate or reduce the effect of these three factors on the liquid anesthetic and its vaporization. Precision vaporizers have a dial that shows, in a percent unit, the amount of anesthetic that is being delivered to the circuit.

Nonprecision Vaporizer

Nonprecision vaporizers are seen less and less in veterinary medicine with the development of safer inhalant anesthetics that need to be used in precision vaporizers. A nonprecision vaporizer is basically a glass canister that allows liquid anesthetic to vaporize at an uncontrolled rate (Figure 4-41). This uncontrolled vaporization is the main reason that only anesthetics with low vapor pressure should be used in this type of vaporizer. Low-vapor-pressure liquid anesthetics are those that vaporize slowly. This slow vaporization means that a level of approximately 4% concentration is the maximum that will be reached in the carrier gas. This level of anesthetic is relatively safe for most patients because of the high blood-gas solubility and the drug's slow onset of action. The construction of the nonprecision vaporizer does not permit compensation for the three factors that affect anesthetic vaporization. Due to the lack of compensation, less accurate delivery of the anesthetic occurs, increasing the risk to the patient.

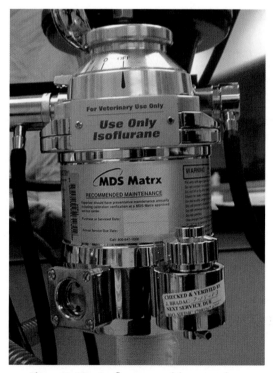

Figure 4-40 Isoflurane precision vaporizer.

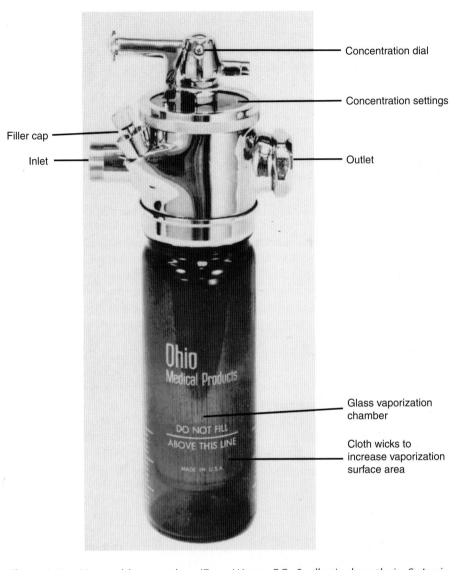

Concentration dial

Concentration settings

Filler cap

Inlet

Outlet

Glass vaporization chamber

Cloth wicks to increase vaporization surface area

Ohio
Medical Products

DO NOT FILL
ABOVE THIS LINE

MADE IN U.S.A.

Figure 4-41   Nonprecision vaporizer. (From Warren RG: *Small animal anesthesia,* St Louis, 1983, Mosby.)

Unidirectional Inspiratory Valve

The unidirectional inspiratory valve, also called the *inspiration valve* or *flutter valve,* is a component of anesthesia machines designed to allow movement of gases in only one direction (Figure 4-42, *a*). There is a thin, plastic circular piece (wafer) that moves (flutters) each time the patient inspires. As the patient inspires, the gases are moved through this valve, through corrugated tubing, and delivered via the endotracheal tube to the patient.

Negative-Pressure Relief Valve

The next part in many anesthesia machines is the negative-pressure relief valve (Figure 4-42, *b*). This valve is primarily intended as a safety device. If a negative pressure is detected in the system, this valve will allow room air to enter the system.

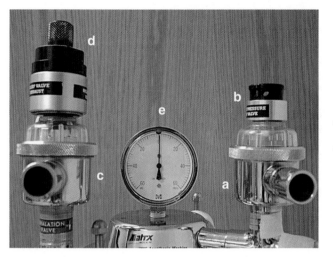

Figure 4-42   Anesthesia machine components: *a*, unidirectional inspiratory valve; *b*, negative-pressure relief valve; *c*, unidirectional expiratory valve; *d*, pop-off valve; *e*, manometer.

Negative pressure may occur, for example, if the oxygen source is empty. Without this safety device, the patient would be without oxygen. The negative-pressure relief valve allows room air into the system, thereby providing 21% O_2 rather than no O_2. Negative pressure may also result if an active scavenger has the vacuum set too high or if the O_2 flow rate is too low.

Corrugated Tubing and Y-Piece

Gases pass through the tubing as the patient inspires and expires. This corrugated tubing is available in a variety of materials, lengths, and diameters. Although there is no formula to determine the size of tubing to use, shorter tubing with a smaller diameter generally is used for smaller patients (7-20 kg). Larger tubing is used with patients weighing more than 20 kg. It is important to remember that this tubing is not unidirectional; therefore, tube ends can be placed on either the inspiratory valve or the expiratory valve. The valves determine gas flow direction.

Unidirectional Expiratory Valve

The unidirectional expiratory valve functions on the same premise as the inspiratory ("inhalation") valve, except it works with expired gases (Figure 4-42, *c*). As the patient exhales, the gases travel though the corrugated tubing to the unidirectional expiratory valve. As with the inspiratory valve, a wafer of plastic moves or "flutters" as the expired gases pass through the valve. The movement of these two valves is also a good indicator of the patient's respiration for the anesthetist.

Adjustable Pressure Relief Valve ("Pop-off" Valve)

The adjustable pressure relief valve is generally located close to the unidirectional expiratory valve (Fig. 4-42, *d*). The pop-off valve has several functions in the anesthesia machine. First, it can act as a vent. When in the completely open position, the pop-off valve prevents buildup of pressure in the system. This is important because if pressure builds up in the system, the alveoli of the lungs expand and may rupture. Second, the pop-off valve can be used to determine flow rate techniques (e.g., low flow). When varying degrees of "open" are used (i.e., pop-off valve is partially opened), different O_2 flow rates can be used. Higher flows need to be used with a wide-open pop-off valve, and a lower flow rate can be used with the valve partially closed or "closed," meaning mostly closed. (The *only* time the pop-off valve should be completely closed is when "bagging" the patient, and even then it is only temporarily closed because the patient cannot breathe against a closed pop-off valve.) Any level of being closed is dangerous because, as just mentioned, pressure may build in the system and cause alveolar damage. In the hands of a novice anesthetist, it is wise to have the pop-off completely open.

Manometer

The manometer is the pressure gauge of the anesthesia machine (Figure 4-42, *e*). This component only measures the pressure in the system; the manometer does not regulate the pressure. The pressure reading of the system, as indicated by the manometer, is useful information because it gives the anesthetist a good indication of the pressure in the patient's lungs. The unit of measure for the manometer is in centimeters of water (cm H_2O). Some manometers may have a double scale, one in cm H_2O and the other in millimeters of mercury (mm Hg). Personnel must be careful to read the correct scale because the graduations between the units are not the same and therefore display different information. For example, 20 mm Hg of pressure is approximately at the same graduation as 33 cm of water pressure, but a reading of 33 cm H_2O is a dangerous pressure for a patient. The pressure reading on the manometer should never exceed 20 cm H_2O, even when "bagging" the patient. Normal resting pressure, with the pop-off open, should read 0 cm H_2O. The manometer and the pop-off valve have a direct relationship; the more closed the pop-off valve, the higher the pressure reading on the manometer. More pressure builds up in the system as the pop-off valve is closed more.

Rebreathing Bag (Reservoir Bag)

The rebreathing bag is a rubber bag that may serve different purposes depending on the circuit with which it is being used. One purpose, when being used with a rebreathing system, is to allow the patient to rebreathe some of the exhaled gases stored in the rebreathing bag. The level of fullness of the bag adjusts as the gases enter and leave the circuit. The reservoir bag will deflate as the patient inspires and will inflate as the patient expires. This movement is a good indication of respiratory rate that the anesthetist can monitor. An indirect level of respiratory quality can also be assessed based on how much of the bag is deflated with each breath (i.e., shallow breaths will be evident as barely moving the bag).

Another purpose of the rebreathing bag, regardless of the circuit, is to allow manual ventilation of the patient ("bagging"). Whether as an alveolar expanding "sigh" or as a resuscitative measure, being able to provide manual ventilation to the animal is essential. When providing artificial ventilation, the first step is to close the pop-off valve. Then, squeeze the rebreathing bag to a pressure of no greater than 20 cm H_2O (on the manometer), and immediately open the pop-off valve. It is important to ventilate the patient with as normal a respiratory character as possible. For example, a pattern of longer inspiration and then quick expiration best simulates a "normal" breath.

With the rebreathing bag storing excess gases and providing backup quantities of gases to be inspired, it is important that the proper size of bag is used. One formula to calculate bag sizes is simple and relies on the tidal volume of the patient (Box 4-1). Tidal volume is calculated as 10 ml/kg of body weight and is the volume of air inhaled during a normal breath at rest. That volume is then multiplied by a factor of 5 to ensure that enough gas will be available for the patient in the event of a full, deep breath.

Rebreathing bags are available in several sizes, ranging from 0.25 to 5.0 L for small animals (Figure 4-43). After calculating the volume needed, the bag should be selected. When selecting the rebreathing bag based on 5 times the patient's tidal volume, rounding up to the next larger size is appropriate. It is important *not* to round down to the next smaller bag because this will not provide the minimum volume required by the patient (see Box 4-2 for examples).

Carbon Dioxide Absorber

As the patient exhales, the waste gases pass either to the carbon dioxide (CO_2) absorber or to the scavenger. The CO_2 absorber is a canister that contains a material made of either barium

---

BOX 4-1	Calculation for Size of Rebreathing Bag

$5 \times$ Tidal volume = Bag size in milliliters (ml)
Tidal volume calculated as 10 ml/kg of body weight.

hydroxide lime (Baralyme, A-M Systems) or sodium hydroxide lime (Sodasorb, WR Grace). The crystals absorb the exhaled CO_2, and the resulting chemical reaction produces heat, water, and a color change. The crystals have a pH indicator added to allow for the color change. Once the crystals have undergone the chemical reaction, they are depleted. Fresh crystals are easily crushed, but depleted crystals are very hard and may exhibit a color change from white to violet (Figure 4-44). Especially when using isoflurane, the color change may be evident only while the crystals are exposed to the anesthetic gas. Once the vaporizer is turned off, the color will disappear.

Generally, crystals are disposed of and replenished when the canister shows 50% of the crystals displaying a color change. Crystal density should also be evaluated to determine when to change the canister. The hours of use should be tracked, rather than a set time frame of every week or every 2 weeks, to determine when to replenish the crystals.

When replacing the crystals, the old material can usually be disposed of in the regular trash, but the local health department may have other guidelines or ordinances; these can be consulted if disposal options are unclear. New crystals should be added to the canister in increments, shaking the canister to settle the crystals. About $1/2$ inch of air space is left at the top of the canister to allow proper gas flow over the crystals.

Scavenging System

It is important to use some type of system to evacuate waste gases from the anesthesia machine and out of the surgery suite to the outside of

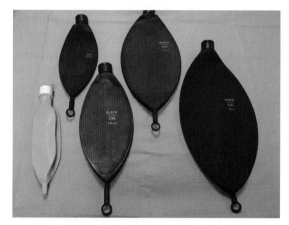

Figure 4-43 Various rebreathing bags.

BOX 4-2 Examples of Rebreathing Bag Calculations

1. 40-kg patient
   $5 \times (40\ kg \times 10\ ml/kg)$ = Volume (ml)
   $5 \times 400\ ml$ = Volume (ml)
   2000 ml, or 2 L
   Use a 3.0-L rebreathing bag because volume needed is equal to bag size.
2. 16-kg patient
   $5 \times (16\ kg \times 10\ ml/kg)$ = Volume (ml)
   $5 \times 160\ ml$ = Volume (ml)
   800 ml
   Use a 1-L rebreathing bag because 800 ml is less than 1000 ml (1 L).

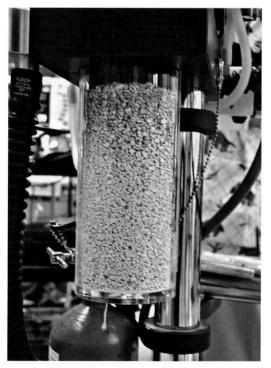

Figure 4-44 Carbon dioxide (CO_2) canister. Machine is in use with a patient attached. Partially depleted crystals are evident by color change at top of canister.

the building. There are two types of scavenging systems available: active and passive. *Active* scavenging systems are mechanical devices attached to the anesthesia machine and then connected to a general building source that produces a vacuum to remove the gases. These systems are generally incorporated into the building plans for a new facility. The centrally located vacuum in this system removes the gases from the anesthesia machine and then evacuates the waste out of the building. Anesthesia machines require a local vacuum control on the machine as well as hosing to connect to the central source, similar to the oxygen hose used to connect with the general oxygen source.

Passive scavenging systems rely on gravity to remove the gases from the system. Anesthetic gases are the heaviest of the expired gases and will naturally gravitate to the lowest point. Tubing attached to the pop-off valve can carry the anesthetic waste gas either to an activated-charcoal canister attached to the base or stand of the machine or to an outside wall vent (Figure 4-45).

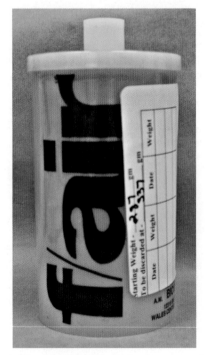

Figure 4-45   Activated-charcoal scavenger canister for waste anesthetic gas.

Wherever the canisters are attached, it is important that they be suspended so that air can circulate through the vents found on the bottom of the canisters. If the canisters are placed on the floor, these vents are effectively plugged. To ensure that the canister is effectively scavenging the waste gases, its use needs to be monitored and documented. The canister should be weighed with a gram scale before its first use and before being suspended on the machine. After each use the canister should be reweighed and the weight recorded on the canister. Once the unit has gained 50 grams from the initial weight, it should be disposed of because it will no longer adequately absorb the waste gas. Canisters can be disposed of in the regular trash. Hoses from the pop-off valve that attach to an outside wall vent should be no longer than 20 feet; hoses longer than 20 feet will compromise the system's function. Scavenging to a vent will limit the mobility of the anesthesia machine, but this is appropriate if the machine remains in the same area all the time. Scavenging waste gas to the floor without any type of collection or evacuation is inappropriate and should not be done.

Leak Testing

Properly functioning equipment is extremely important in anesthesia. Technicians are responsible for maintaining equipment and should take this responsibility seriously. In addition to using a scavenging system, leak checking the machine will aid in reducing and eliminating any gas that may be inappropriately leaving the system. Before every use, the anesthesia machine should be checked for a system leak. If the machine was cleaned or replenished or if hoses or bags were changed, the potential exists for a leak in the system. Box 4-3 outlines the steps for performing a machine leak check.

Any area on the machine has the potential for leaking, but some sites are more likely than others to develop leaks. One of the first places to check is the pop-off valve. Check that it is completely closed when doing the leak check. If the pop-off valve is left open, there is no way for pressure to build up in the system. Even if the pop-off valve is only partially closed, a leak will result, so complete closure of this valve is critical. Another common place for leaks is the rebreathing bag or the corrugated hosing. Many of these products are intended as single-use items, but the economics of veterinary medicine often dictate their reuse. Anesthetic gas can degrade the integrity of the rubber in these items, and areas of thinning or microscopic holes can develop. If the leak is isolated to the bag or hoses, these items should be discarded and replaced with new equipment. Another place for a leak is the occluding of the Y-piece. If the Y-piece is not fully occluded with a finger or the palm of the hand, a leak may persist.

Other, more subtle areas of the anesthesia machine that may leak include the metal rings on the inspiratory and expiratory valves. If removed or loosened for cleaning purposes, the rings may not have been securely replaced and fully tightened. Another "hidden" place for a leak is the CO_2 absorber. When removing the canister to replenish the crystals, it is easy to leave the tightening mechanism a little loose. Finally, all the tubing on the machine is continually exposed to the detrimental effects of anesthetic gas, which may lead to small, barely detectable holes in the tubing.

Regardless of the location of the leak, it needs to be corrected before the machine is used.

Breathing Circuits

The size of the patient will determine the breathing circuit that should be used to deliver anesthetic gases. There are two types of circuits: rebreathing and non-rebreathing.

Rebreathing Circuit

The rebreathing circuit is useful because it allows the recirculation of some expired anesthetic gases and permits a lower flow of oxygen because some of the gases are rebreathed. This circuit is used with patients that have a body weight greater than 7 kg. The traditional circuit is two corrugated hoses connected at one end by a Y-piece (Figure 4-46). The hosing can be plastic or rubber, and the Y-piece can be plastic or metal. The open end of the tubing is placed on the inspiratory and expiratory valve openings on the anesthesia machine.

An alternative to the traditional rebreathing circuit is the Universal F circuit (Surgivet, Waukesha, Wis) (Figure 4-47). This circuit is used with patients weighing more than 7 kg and offers

---

BOX 4-3   Steps in Performing Anesthetic Machine Leak Check

1. Connect oxygen hose to oxygen source, or turn on local oxygen source.
2. Attach appropriate bag and tubing to be used.
3. Check vaporizer for adequate level of liquid anesthetic.
4. Securely occlude Y-piece with thumb or palm of hand.
5. Completely close pop-off valve.
6. Adjust oxygen flowmeter to 2 L/min.
7. As the rebreathing bag fills with oxygen, the needle gauge on pressure manometer will rise. When the needle reaches 20 cm H_2O, readjust oxygen flow to 200 ml/min.
8. If the system is leak free, the pressure manometer should maintain a reading of 20 cm H_2O for 20 seconds (time with second hand on watch) with the oxygen flowmeter set at 200 ml/min.
9. If the needle gauge declines, there is a leak. Consult the text (or machine manual) for possible locations of leak, and correct.
10. After 20 seconds of a steady needle at 20 cm H_2O, maintain the occlusion on the Y-piece and open the pop-off valve. The rebreathing bag should deflate.
11. Remove thumb from Y-piece.
12. Check scavenging system to ensure connections are intact.
13. Completely open the pop-off valve.

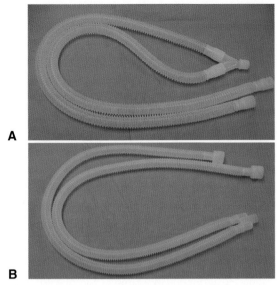

Figure 4-46   A, Large-diameter rebreathing circuit. **B,** Small-diameter rebreathing circuit.

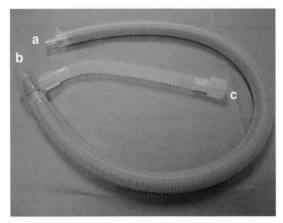

Figure 4-47 Universal F rebreathing circuit: *a,* connects to the endotracheal tube; *b,* connects to the inspiratory valve; *c,* connects to the expiratory valve.

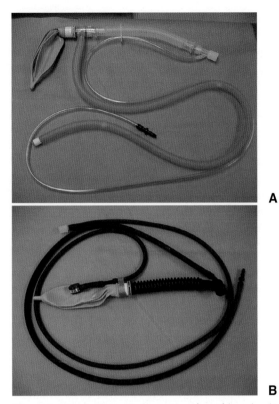

Figure 4-48   A, Ayres T-piece non-rebreathing circuit. **B,** Modified Mapleson D non-rebreathing circuit.

some distinct advantages to the traditional circuit. The design of the inspiratory tube inside the expiratory tube allows the inspired gases to be warmed by the expired gases surrounding the tube. The single-tube design is also beneficial in offering less congestion at the head and mouth. This is especially appreciated when performing a dental prophylaxis.

Non-Rebreathing Circuit

The non-rebreathing circuit is used so that none of the gases is rebreathed. Patients weighing less than 7 kg benefit the most from the use of this circuit because of the low gas resistance. The use of this circuit requires high flows of oxygen to ensure adequate levels of anesthetic. These high flows push the gases to the patient, so little effort is required by the patient to receive the gas. The disadvantage to the non-rebreathing circuit is the expense incurred because of the amount of oxygen used. Figure 4-48 shows two examples of non-rebreathing circuits.

Oxygen Flow Rates

Depending on the type of breathing circuit used, different O_2 flow rates should be employed. Providing adequate oxygen to the patient is critical, but using an excessive amount of oxygen is wasteful.

Rebreathing circuits generally use a high O_2 flow rate for induction and recovery, with large-volume delivery of gas. This perpetuates a speedy induction and assists in a quick recovery. Maintenance flows for rebreathing circuits are significantly less than the induction and recovery flow rates. Only enough oxygen to match the patient's tidal volume is needed, because in addition to the fresh gas being supplied, the patient is rebreathing some of the gases already in the system. Usually a buffer is added in calculating the flow to allow for large breaths that may be given to or taken by the patient (Box 4-4).

Non-rebreathing systems also use high O_2 flow rates (see Box 4-4), but the flows remain at a constant high flow regardless if the patient is undergoing induction, maintaining the desired depth of anesthesia, or recovering. Continuous high flow rates are necessary to provide adequate gases to the patient. Smaller patients cannot rebreathe any of the gases because of the difficulty in moving that much air with each respiration. Fresh gases need to be provided to these patients at all times. A major advantage of the non-rebreathing system is that it has low resistance for breathing for the patient. Fresh gases are constantly being provided to the patient with minimal effort required of the animal. The design and high flows of the non-rebreathing system allow the gases to be "delivered" at the endotracheal tube, and the patient merely breathes a normal respiration and takes in fresh, new gases.

Anesthesia can be a stressful time for the veterinary technician. However, a thorough understanding of the components of the machine, the flow of gas through the machine, and the options available to deliver the anesthetic gases to the patient can reduce the stress level and can even make surgery a rewarding part of the technician's day.

SURGICAL NEEDLES

Many sizes and shapes of surgical needles are available. The needle point, the needle body, and the needle eye are considered when categorizing needles (Figure 4-49).

Needle Point

The needle point helps to determine the type of tissue in which the needle should be used. A *taper-point needle* has a sharp point that pierces and penetrates tissues without leaving small cuts because the cross section is rounded. The round needle body associated with the taper point is best used in tissue when a sealed suture line is needed, such as when suturing intestine or other hollow organs. Any tissue that should not be traumatized or is not difficult to pass a needle through will tolerate a taper needle.

A *taper-cut needle* is a combination of a round, tapered body and a reverse cutting point. This type of needle is easily used with tough fibrous tissue and some cardiovascular procedures. A *reverse cutting needle* has three cutting edges on the point—the cross section is triangular, with one of the cutting edges being the outside of the curve—and it maintains that same shape in the body and is stronger than the conventional cutting needle.

A *cutting-edge needle* also has three cutting edges on the point and body, but the third cutting edge is on the inside of the curve. This style of needle may be most traumatic because the cutting edge on the inside of the curve cuts toward the edges of the wound, compromising the strength of the tissue.

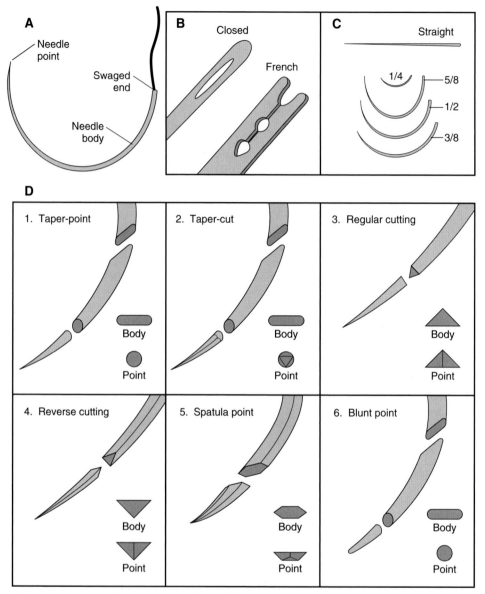

Figure 4-49   **A,** Basic components of a needle; **B,** types of eyed needles; **C,** needle body sizes; **D,** needle body shapes. (From Fossum TW: *Small animal surgery,* ed 2, St Louis, 2002, Mosby.)

Needle Body

The shape of the needle body can also vary widely. Needles can be straight, circular, or curved. Straight needles, sometimes referred to as Keith needles, are available but have limited application in veterinary medicine. One procedure made easier by the use of a Keith needle is the placement of a purse-string suture in the anus. The straight shape of the needle makes it easier to avoid the anal glands by allowing superficial placement of the suture.

Curved needles can either be full curve, half curve, or double curve. Needles that are double curved have either end of the needle curved, in opposite directions. Double-curved needles are generally reserved for use in large animal surgery, especially bovine surgical closures.

Half-curved needles are classified as such because only half the body of the needle is curved. They are rarely used in veterinary surgery.

Full-curved needles have the entire body of the needle involved in the curve. Varying degrees of curvature can be found, based on the portion of a full circle that is involved. For example, a ⅜-circle needle means that if a full circle were divided into eight equal parts, the continuous curve of three of those parts would be this shape. Likewise, a half-circle needle would mean that four continuous parts (or ½ the circle) would be the shape of the needle. Other common circular needle shapes are ¼ circle and ⅝ circle.

Suture Attachment End

The final portion of the needle is the suture attachment end. Some needles have eyes, which can be single or French style. *Single-eyed needles* must have the suture material passed through the needle eye. Suture is threaded through the eye from the inside of the curve to the outside. The threading of the needle results in a rather bulky portion of suture that must pass through the tissue, therefore creating excessive tissue drag and damage. The *French-eyed needle* has one complete eye and one split eye. The suture is passed through the complete eye and then pushed down through the split eye, which securely grips the suture.

The most atraumatic and therefore most common method of suture attachment is with the *swaged needle,* or *eyeless needle.* When the suture is manufactured, the needle and suture are attached to one another. With this type of attachment, the tissues undergo minimal damage because the point and diameter of the needle create the hole, and the suture simply follows along without causing further trauma. The ease of use and limited trauma of the eyeless needle make it the first choice of almost all veterinary surgeons.

SUTURE MATERIAL

The purpose of suture material is to hold together wound edges until the wound can withstand the stress of healing without additional support. Some examples of tissue instability that would require suture material are an intentional surgical incision, ligated vessels, and ligament, tendon, or muscle repair. Suture material is available in many forms, sizes, and colors. It is important to understand the terminology used when discussing suture to know the options available and to select the appropriate material for the procedure being performed. Although the technician will not be making the decision about which type of suture to use, it is important to have a working knowledge of the types of suture available. Veterinary technicians who can anticipate the type of suture that may be requested, based on knowledge and experience, will be an invaluable member of the surgical team.

Characteristics

Tensile Strength
Tensile strength is the amount of force in pounds per square inch (psi) that the suture can withstand (as an untied fiber) before it breaks.

Memory
Memory is the ability or tendency of the suture to return to its original packaged form.

Flexibility
Flexibility is the ease with which the suture is manipulated, either by the surgeon or in the tissue. Flexibility is somewhat determined by the size (diameter) and material used to make the suture. For example, silk has better flexibility than stainless steel.

Absorbability
Suture can be classified as either nonabsorbable or absorbable. *Nonabsorbable suture* is not broken down by the body and can remain intact in the body for at least 2 years. *Absorbable suture* can be broken down by the body through different processes. During phagocytosis, leukocytes, usually

neutrophils, are released and travel to the site of concern (incision) to ingest and destroy the microbes or, in the case of suture material, the foreign suture material. Suture is also absorbed through hydrolysis. The chemical compound in the suture is decomposed as it is exposed to water. Absorption of suture may begin as soon as 7 days after placement. Complete absorption may take 60 days to 2 years.

Capillarity

Capillarity describes the ability of the suture to allow microbes to "wick" (be carried) to the interior of the suture strand. This action can be curtailed if the manufacturer coats the suture at production to decrease the "wicking" action. Teflon, wax, paraffin, silicone, and calcium stearate are substances used to coat suture. Generally, multifilament sutures are treated more often for capillarity than monofilament sutures.

Structure

There are two basic structure types of suture: multifilament and monofilament (Figure 4-50). *Multifilament suture,* also called *braided suture,* has two or more strands braided together to form the single strand of suture. *Monofilament suture* is a single, solid strand of suture material.

Monofilament suture material tends to have less "tissue drag" or friction when it is being pulled through the tissues than multifilament suture material.

Knot Security

The ability of suture to hold the knots the surgeon has placed is imperative. Some types of suture materials hold knots better than other types. Usually, braided material has less knot slippage than monofilament suture. Once knots have been formed with the suture, they must stay secure. The slippage of a knot can result in the death of a patient if the knot was around a major vessel, slips, and the animal bleeds to death.

Color

Some sutures are dyed during the manufacturing process for easier identification after placement in the tissue. Suture material is available in dyed or undyed styles. Although not as great a concern with veterinary patients as with human patients, suture color should be considered in some cases. For example, if the patient is a black Labrador and the surgeon can use either black nylon or blue polypropylene for the skin sutures, the blue sutures will be much easier to identify at suture removal in 10 days.

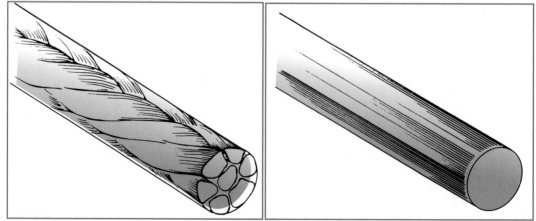

A   B

Figure 4-50   **A,** Multifilament suture. **B,** Monofilament suture. (From Meeker MH, Rothrock JC: *Alexander's care of the patient in surgery,* ed 12, St Louis, 2003, Mosby.)

Origin of Material

Suture material is also classified by the origin of the material from which it is made. *Natural* suture material is a product made from fibers found in nature. Some examples include cotton, silk, and catgut (made from sheep intestinal mucosa).

Synthetic material is other suture produced with the use of man-made products. This group includes almost all the remaining suture not previously mentioned (e.g., nylon, polyglactin 910). *Metallic* suture is a small category of sutures and is limited to surgical stainless steel suture, which includes suture wire and staples.

The ideal suture material would have no knot slippage, would have high tensile strength, would be absorbable, would cause no tissue reactivity, would be easy to handle, and would be inexpensive. Unfortunately, no one "perfect" suture material exists, so the surgeon much consider all the characteristics of the material when deciding whether to use it for a particular procedure. In addition to the physical characteristics of the suture material, the surgeon must also consider the following criteria when selecting the suture type and size:

1. Patient size
2. Area (tissue) of placement (skin vs. hollow organ)
3. Strength required
4. Healing potential of the tissue
5. Importance of cosmetic appearance
6. Cost

Sizing

Suture material is classified by size according to the *United States Pharmacopeia* (USP). The USP uses a numeric scale to denote size from fine to coarse. Hypodermic needles are classified by *gauge,* which indicates the diameter size of the needle. Intramedullary pins are classified by fractions of an inch to identify their size in diameter (e.g., $\frac{1}{8}$, $\frac{5}{32}$, $\frac{1}{4}$).

Suture is classified by the term *ought.* When sizing suture, the numeral "0" is used to represent "ought" or "zero." The more zeros in a size, the smaller is the suture. For example, "0000" (pronounced "four-ought") is the same as 4-0 (also pronounced "four-ought"). Similarly, "00" is the same as 2-0, which some refer to as "double-ought." Size 5-0 suture material is smaller in diameter (finer) than 3-0 suture. Whole numbers alone can also be used to identify the size of suture (e.g., No. 1, No. 2, No. 3). When sizing suture material, whole numbers used alone, that is, without any "oughts," increase in size with an increase in the number; the larger the number, the larger the suture. Suture is manufactured in a wide range of sizes, from 11-0 to No. 5. Smaller patients and more delicate tissue (ophthalmology or cardiovascular procedures) tend to use the small sizes, whereas the larger sizes are primarily used in large animal surgery.

Packaging

Most suture material is packaged as single-use items sterilized at the factory by the use of gamma radiation (Figures 4-51 and 4-52). Suture packaged and sterilized in this manner will have a rather long shelf life, which is indicated by an expiration date on the box. Individual suture

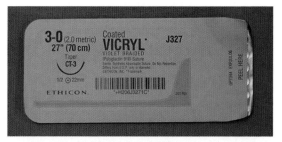

Figure 4-51 Single-use multifilament, absorbable, synthetic suture.

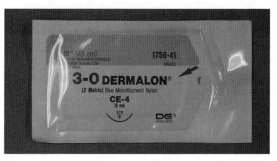

Figure 4-52 Single-use monofilament, nonabsorbable, synthetic suture.

packs are opened on an as-needed basis, aseptically, onto the surgical field. Exposed but unused suture should not be resterilized but rather saved for use in nonsterile procedures (e.g., necropsy closure). If the inner suture pack was unopened and unused on the sterile field, resterilizing the package may be possible. Under no circumstances should suture be steam-sterilized. Any sterilization should be accomplished by the use of an ethylene oxide (EtO) sterilizer.

Another packaging option is to have long lengths (50-100 meters) of suture placed on a reel or "cassette" by the manufacturer (Figure 4-53). Although economically a good idea, this method of storing suture material has a greater potential for contamination than individually packaged products. Also, a knot in the middle of the reel of suture is a common risk and can prove to be a difficult obstacle in removing suture from the cassette.

Staples

Internal and external staples are available for use in veterinary surgery and differ dramatically in cost, ease of use, and applicability.

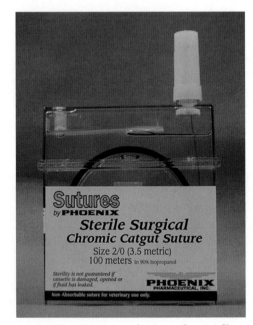

Figure 4-53   Cassette packaging of monofilament, absorbable, natural suture.

External Staples

Skin (external) staples are stainless steel staples placed perpendicularly to an incision to close a wound (Figure 4-54, *A*). If a patient has a history of postsurgical incisional licking or tissue reaction to other suture material, external staples may be a good option. Self-contained in a disposable stapling device, the staples can be placed quickly, which significantly decreases anesthesia time. Once placed in the skin, the staples take on a unique shape to inhibit accidental removal. A special staple removal device is required to remove the staples safely and comfortably from the patient at the appropriate time.

Internal Staples

Specific soft tissue cases may benefit from the use of internal stainless steel staples. Internal staples may be most advantageous in certain thoracic cases (e.g., pulmonary resection, excision of tumors in certain locations). Thoracoabdominal (TA) staples are designed to place multiple rows of staples in tissue (Figure 4-54, *C*). Special staples are also used with gastrointestinal procedures, such as gastrointestinal anastomosis (GIA; Figure 4-54, *B*) and end-to-end anastomosis (EEA). A number may follow the initials of the staple type to indicate the length of the row of staples. For example, TA 90 is a row of staples 90 mm in length with the TA design. Special staplers are required for each of the different types of staples. Although expensive, these staples can save time in critical cases. The benefit must be weighed against the cost so that these staples are used judiciously.

Table 4-2 summarizes the characteristics of common types of suture material. Remember that, in addition to suture characteristics, the surgeon must also consider other criteria (e.g., patient size, type and location of tissue being sutured) when selecting suture material.

PERIOPERATIVE EQUIPMENT

Many pieces of equipment besides surgical instruments are critical to the success of a surgical procedure. Whether related to providing patient

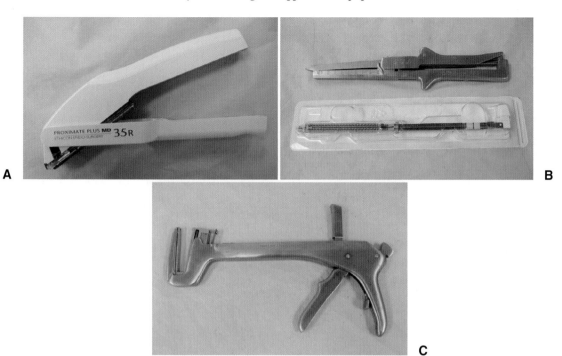

Figure 4-54 Surgical stapling equipment. **A,** Surgical skin stapler applies a single staple with each squeeze of the trigger (staple guns typically hold 25-35 staples). **B,** Gastrointestinal anastomosis (GIA) stapler. Cartridge of staples are for one-time use and are purchased in presterilized package. **C,** Thoracoabdominal (TA) stapler. Staple cartridges are purchased as for GIA. Shown here with staple cartridge in place. (From McCurnin DM, Bassert JM: *Clinical textbook for veterinary technicians,* ed 6, Philadelphia, 2006, Saunders.)

TABLE 4-2	**Summary and Comparison of Common Suture Material**					
GENERIC NAME	**BRAND NAME**	**MANU-FACTURER**	**ABSORB-ABILITY**	**MULTI/MONO-FILAMENT**	**COLOR**	**NATURAL/SYNTHETIC**
Nylon	Ethilon	Ethicon	Nonabsorbable	Mono	Black	Synthetic
Nylon	Dermalon	Davis & Geck	Nonabsorbable	Mono	Black	Synthetic
Polyester	Surgidac	USSC	Nonabsorbable	Multi	Green	Synthetic
Polyester	Ethibond	Ethicon	Nonabsorbable	Multi	Green	Synthetic
Polyglactin 910	Vicryl	Ethicon	Absorbable	Multi	Purple/ undyed	Synthetic
Polyglycolic	Dexon-Plus	Davis & Geck	Absorbable	Multi	Beige	Synthetic
Polypropylene	Surgilene	Davis & Geck	Nonabsorbable	Mono	Blue	Synthetic
Polypropylene	Prolene	Ethicon	Nonabsorbable	Mono	Blue	Synthetic
Polidioxanone	PDS	Ethicon	Absorbable	Mono	Violet/ clear	Synthetic
Silk	Silk	Davis & Geck	Nonabsorbable	Multi	Black	Natural
Chromic gut	Chromic gut	Davis & Geck	Absorbable	Mono	Beige	Natural
Chromic gut	Chromic gut	Ethicon	Absorbable	Mono	Beige	Natural
Stainless steel	Surgical steel	Ethicon	Nonabsorbable	Mono	—	Metallic

comfort, assisting the surgeon, or monitoring anesthesia, each item is an integral part of the process.

Patient Warming Devices

Circulating warm water blankets are used frequently with surgical patients and critically ill patients. The circulating warm water blanket is a good way to provide a heated surface on which the patient can lie during surgery (Figure 4-55). The heated surface helps prevent the loss of body heat to a cold metal surface, thereby diminishing the hypothermia that so often occurs during surgery. Water blankets are available in a variety of sizes, and some are considered disposable. Unless damaged by a patient, water blankets can be used repeatedly. A cat's claw, a misplaced towel clamp, or even a set of teeth can easily puncture holes in the water blanket, making it unusable. Single puncture holes or small tears can be repaired using a vinyl patch kit in some cases, but more often the best solution is disposing of the blanket.

One alternative to constantly replacing the water blanket is using a hard heated pad (Figure 4-56). This pad, made of acrylic plastic glass (Plexiglas), operates on the same principle as the disposable pad and connects to many currently available circulating water pumps. The hard heated pad also is available in a variety of sizes. The main advantage to this style of heating system is the pad itself, because the acrylic plastic glass is puncture proof.

Another option for thermoregulation of the surgical patient is the use of forced warm air (Figure 4-57). One example is the Bair Hugger. The pad is placed around the patient, then "inflated" with warm air. A variety of pads are available to best suit the size of the patient. The constant flow of warm air that envelopes the patient is very effective at maintaining body temperature. Although expensive, this pad is a viable alternative or addition to a circulating warm water blanket. The pad is not puncture proof, but there is less risk of puncture because the pad is not placed near the animal until the patient is anesthetized.

Surgical Lights

The lights used in the surgery room can make a huge difference for the surgeon. Adequate lighting is imperative. Many brands and styles of lights are available. Single-beam lights that have a mechanism for a wide lateral as well as a vertical range of motion are desirable. Ceiling or wall-mounted lights are a much better choice than the standing floor models. If installed in the ceiling, the lights are out of the way and easily manipulated. Removable light handles that can be autoclaved are a helpful feature because once wrapped and sterilized, the handles can be aseptically opened and placed on the sterile field (Figure 4-58). The surgeon or surgical assistant can then place the handles on the lights, which allows them to adjust the lights themselves (Figure 4-59).

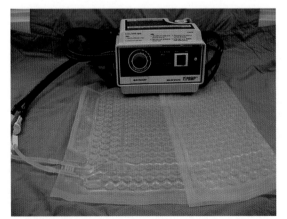

Figure 4-55   Circulating warm water blanket.

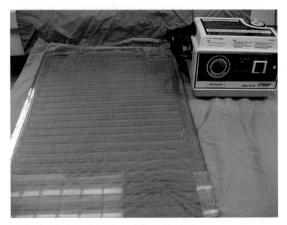

Figure 4-56   Hard pad for circulating warm water.

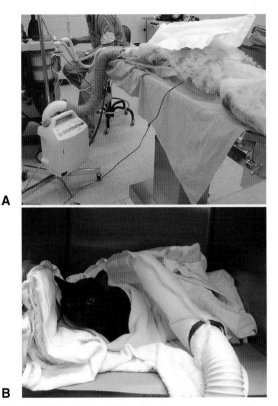

A

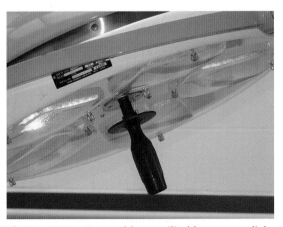

B

Figure 4-57   **A,** Forced hot-air unit on a surgery patient. **B,** Forced hot-air unit on a recovering patient.

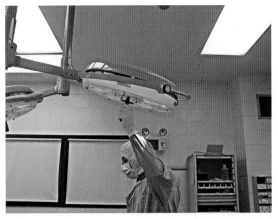

Figure 4-59   The surgeon is able to manipulate and position the lights as needed if the handles have been sterilized.

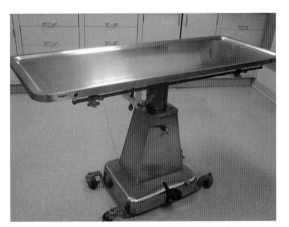

Figure 4-60   Solid-top, adjustable surgery table.

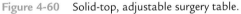

Figure 4-58   Removable, sterilizable surgery light handles.

Surgery Table

It is also important to have a quality surgery table. Many different types are available depending on the size of the surgery room and financial constraints. Tabletops can be a solid surface or can be designed in a split-surface style. The solid-top model is generally less expensive and can be more difficult to work with because fluids pool on the tabletop and can soil the patient (Figure 4-60). The split-top tables have the double advantage of (1) a tray under the space in the table to collect any fluid that may run off the surgical field and

(2) the ability to be adjusted to help maintain the patient (especially large, deep-chested dogs) in dorsal recumbency (Figure 4-61).

Another available feature in surgery tables is the incorporation of a heated tabletop. This heated surface aids in thermoregulation and eliminates the need for a circulating water blanket under the patient. Surgery tables should also have the capability to raise and lower and to tilt in one direction. Hydraulics or electric power can be employed to accomplish variation in height, whereas manual effort is generally required to tilt the table.

Electrosurgery

The use of electricity, transmitted through a special hand piece to cut or coagulate vessels, is very advantageous in surgery. Hemostasis is vital during surgery, and cautery is an important tool available to accomplish this. Both single-use and reusable cautery hand pieces are available. Hand pieces are activated by a member of the sterile team by pushing switches or buttons on the hand piece or by stepping on a foot pedal (Figures 4-62 and 4-63).

Electrosurgery can be either monopolar or bipolar. When using *monopolar* electrosurgery, a ground plate must be placed under the patient. When the hand piece is activated, the electric current passes through the patient to the ground plate and then is diverted away from the patient.

The ground plate must have sufficient contact with the patient to transmit the current properly to the ground plate. A water- or saline-saturated sponge should be placed on the ground plate between the patient and the plate. Never use alcohol to saturate the sponge because it may lead to patient burns or even fire. *Bipolar* electrosurgery utilizes a hand piece that resembles a thumb tissue forceps. As the hand piece is activated, the current passes from one tip to another, and therefore no ground plate is needed.

Monopolar electrosurgery can be used in one of two ways. First, the hand piece can be activated, and the tip of the hand piece can directly touch the

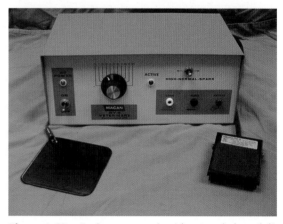

Figure 4-62   Basic cautery unit with ground plate *(left)* and foot pedal *(right)*.

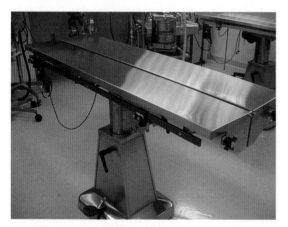

Figure 4-61   Split-top, heated surgery table.

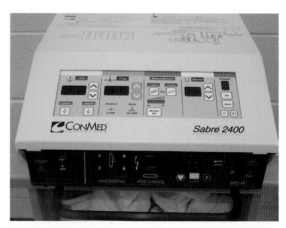

Figure 4-63   Cautery unit with option of hand or foot control.

tissue or vessel that needs cauterizing (Figure 4-64). Second, the surgeon can place a hemostat on the tissue or vessel that needs to be cauterized. The hemostat is then elevated off of the surgical field such that the only metal touching the patient is the tip of the hemostat. The cautery hand piece tip can then be touched to the hemostat as the hand piece is activated. The metal of the instrument conducts the electric current, therefore cauterizing the tissue held in the clamp (Figure 4-65).

Charred material may build up on the tip of the hand piece, causing an impeded flow of current. It may be cleaned by scraping with a scalpel blade (away from the sterile field) or by using a commercially available "scratch pad." Because it is designed as a thumb tissue forceps, bipolar electrosurgery can pick up tissue or a vessel that needs to be coagulated.

Suction

Suction can be defined as the ability to remove fluid or air from an area by using either a manual or a mechanical device. Suction can be performed with a syringe, a bulb syringe, or a mechanical pump. For application in surgery, the mechanical pump is most frequently used. Suction is an extremely important tool in surgery and if unavailable can make the surgery increasingly more difficult and frustrating for the surgeon. Whether performing an abdominal, orthopedic,

or neurologic procedure, having suction available is essential. For abdominal cases, suction can be used to remove abdominal fluid in the event of a hemoabdomen or uroabdomen. Abdominal lavage is a common practice after an exploratory surgery, and mechanical suction assists in the removal of the lavage fluid better than any other option. Lavaging a joint, flushing a septic site, and removing bone dust created while drilling screw holes for a fracture repair are examples of how suction is useful in orthopedic surgery.

There are also risks associated with suction, and veterinary personnel must understand these risks to prevent unnecessary trauma to the patient. The vacuum pressure of the suction is easy enough to control when using manual devices, but care must be taken to use appropriate levels of vacuum on mechanical devices. In abdominal cases, if the vacuum level is too high, omentum may become entrapped in the suction tip and may be damaged. A sufficiently strong vacuum that meets the needs of the surgical procedure, without being excessive, is the goal. Inappropriately low vacuum settings will not adequately suction the fluid and debris on the field and will prove to be frustrating.

Suction Machines
Many different models of suction machines are available. Some models are run on electric power; a motor is used to generate the vacuum (Figure 4-66).

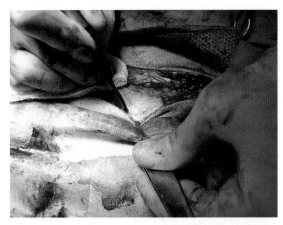

Figure 4-64   Electrocautery applied directly to the tissue to be cauterized.

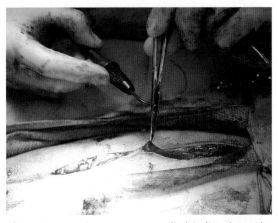

Figure 4-65   Electrocautery applied indirectly to the tissue to be cauterized through an instrument grasping the tissue.

Other models require a central vacuum system to operate (Figure 4-67). Any type of machine will require some sort of bottle or receptacle for the collected fluid. Older models may still have glass jars, which can be dangerous and easily broken.

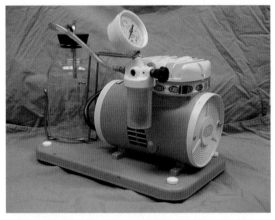

Figure 4-66   Electric, motorized suction machine.

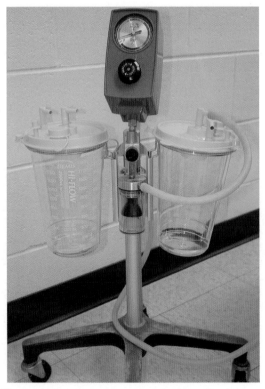

Figure 4-67   Central vacuum, double-collection suction unit.

Plastic bottles or canisters are more desirable. Usually the cover of the bottle has some type of "float" or safety device that will not allow fluid into the working mechanism of the suction machine if the bottles become too full.

In addition to the suction machine, a suction tip and tubing are needed. Suction tubing is available in 6- and 10-foot lengths (Figure 4-68). The tubing is usually prepackaged and sterilized for single-time use. After being opened onto the sterile field, one end of the tubing attaches to the suction tip (usually sterilized separately), and the other end is dropped off the field to be connected to the nonsterile suction unit. Due to the length of the tubing and the difficulty in cleaning appropriately, this is one piece of equipment that is truly disposable and should be discarded after the surgery. If for some reason the tubing is not used after being opened, it can be resterilized. Ethylene oxide sterilization must be used because this vinyl tubing will not withstand steam sterilization.

Suction Tips

Different designs of suction tips are more appropriate for some procedures than others.

Poole

A Poole suction tip is a two-piece instrument best used to remove large volumes of liquid or fluid (Figure 4-69). The inner cannula can be used alone or in conjunction with the outer basket. The basket is designed with many holes to remove the liquid quickly without entrapping any tissue.

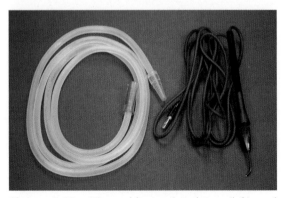

Figure 4-68   Disposable suction hose *(left)* and reusable foot-operated cautery pencil *(right)*.

Frazier/Adson

The Frazier/Adson suction tip is a single tube with a fairly small opening (Figure 4-69). Often there is a thumb hole to help control the amount of vacuum. This instrument is frequently used in orthopedic and neurologic surgeries.

Yankauer

The Yankauer suction tip is also a single-tube design, but it is bulkier than the Frazier (see Figure 4-69). The Yankauer is a general-purpose suction tip.

Plastic Tubing Connector

Some surgeons have concerns about the abrasive metal tip of the Frazier suction tip traumatizing the bone or cartilage during orthopedic procedures. A good alternative that is frequently used is an Argyle Bubble connector (Figure 4-70). This plastic tubing connector fits securely into the suction hose and is small enough to be efficient and lightweight enough to be easy to use.

Clippers

Electric clippers are a necessity when discussing perioperative equipment. In addition to removing hair for the intravenous (IV) catheter or Doppler crystal, the clippers are the only logical, practical option for removing the hair from the surgical site. Two basic options are available: an electric clipper (with a cord) or a battery-operated, rechargeable, cordless clipper. The traditional electric clipper has a proven history of efficient, dependable performance. The interference of the cord, however, can be frustrating and hazardous. The cord does allow the clipper to be hung from an IV pole or anesthesia column hook or attached to a ceiling reel cord to prevent the clipper from rolling off the table onto the floor.

Cordless clipper models have the advantage of less congestion in the induction area and may be appropriate for limited clipping situations, and they are portable. However, two main disadvantages of the cordless clipper should be considered. First, the battery in the clipper must be appropriately recharged in order for the unit to function properly. If not placed correctly (or not placed) in the recharger, the unit will not have sufficient power to perform as needed. Second, even if fully charged, certain extensive clipping procedures (e.g., stifle surgical clip on a giant-breed dog) may drain the battery before the clipping is complete. Therefore, it is wise to have a minimum of two sets of clippers available.

Clipper Blades

The clipper blade used to prepare the site is also another important consideration. IV catheter sites, any "-centesis" (e.g., abdomino, thoraco,

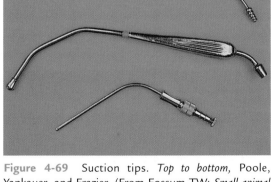

Figure 4-69 Suction tips. *Top to bottom,* Poole, Yankauer, and Frazier. (From Fossum TW: *Small animal surgery,* ed 2, St Louis, 2002, Mosby.)

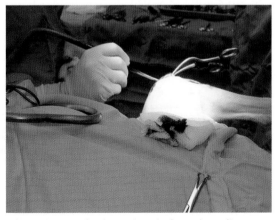

Figure 4-70 Plastic suction tip for orthopedic cases.

arthro), and surgical preparations should all be clipped with a size 40 or 50 blade. These two styles of clipper blades have a single row of close-set, fine teeth to achieve the closest shave possible. Ideally, no hair stubble should be left on the skin after the site has been clipped for surgery.

Maintenance

Clippers and their blades should have the recommended routine maintenance performed in order to extend the life of the equipment as well as achieve optimal performance. Each new blade should be cleansed in Blade Wash before use, according to the manufacturer's directions, to remove the thin, protective film applied during production. After each use the blade should be brushed clean of any hair, lubricated, and disinfected. The brush used can be the brush provided by the company, an old toothbrush, or an old scrub brush. Also, most manuals with the clipper provided by the manufacturer include instructions for basic oiling of the clipper. Careful attention to these instructions, as well as strict adherence to the procedure outlined in the manual, will enhance and lengthen the performance of the clipper.

ANESTHESIA MONITORING DEVICES

The monitoring of a patient that is under the effects of anesthetic drugs is a highly involved and critically important responsibility of the veterinary technician. The veterinary technician must be willing and prepared to anticipate and troubleshoot potential problems to provide the safest anesthetic episode for the patient. Although there is no ideal monitoring device, multiple devices used together can provide useful information on the patient's status.

A well-trained, educated, sensitive, alert technician is probably the best "device." The senses of the technician are constantly relied on while monitoring a patient. The technician's sense of sight can watch for changes in mucous membrane color or patient movement or changes in respirations; the sense of sound is applied to listen to heart rates and rhythm; the sense of smell can detect the presence of anesthetic gas; and the sense of touch can feel for changes in peripheral pulses, indicating changes in blood pressure.

Even the best technician has limitations, however, so the use of auxiliary monitoring devices is extremely helpful. Many types of monitors are available with varying capabilities and limitations. Some monitoring devices combine multiple capabilities into one unit for convenience and optimal anesthetic evaluation. Table 4-3 lists normal values for anesthetic monitoring of dogs and cats.

Pulse Oximeter

Pulse oximetry is based on the ability to evaluate the level of oxygen saturation in the blood to help assess tissue perfusion. Pulse oximeters also monitor pulse rates. Oxygen in the blood is carried by the hemoglobin in the red blood cells. The pulse oximeter measures how much (or the percentage) of the available hemoglobin is saturated with oxygen. This measurement is achieved using

TABLE 4-3	Anesthetic Monitoring: Normal Parameters		
SPECIES	SaO_2	$ETCO_2$	BLOOD PRESSURE
Canine and Feline	95%-99%	35-45 mm Hg	Systolic: 90-160 mm Hg Diastolic: 50-90 mm Hg MAP (awake): 85-120 mm Hg MAP (under anesthesia): 70-90 mm Hg

SaO_2, Arterial oxygen saturation, $ETCO_2$, end-tidal carbon dioxide level; *MAP*, mean arterial pressure.

two different wavelengths of light transmitted through tissue with a pulsatile blood flow. The sensors (or probes) emit wavelengths of both red light and infrared light. The infrared light determines oxygen saturation, and the red light determines the pulse rate. The light is transmitted through the tissue, and the photo detector (located opposite the transmitter) senses the light. The software within the unit compares the absorption ratio of the two different wavelengths. Oxygen-rich blood (arterial) absorbs less light, so more of the light wavelength is sensed by the detector; therefore a higher arterial oxygen saturation (SaO_2) reading is displayed.

Models

Some pulse oximeters are single-function units that measure only SaO_2 and pulse. Units can be small handheld versions, whereas other versions are larger and more cumbersome (Figure 4-71). Most models have the capability to set alarms for high and low limits of acceptable readings. These alarms emit an audio tone when the high or low limits of SaO_2 or pulse are reached, and they can alert the person monitoring the patient to potential problems. Other models are capable of monitoring multiple parameters, including SaO_2, heart rate, respiratory rate, and end-tidal CO_2.

Sensors

The choice of sensor depends on the placement site and species of animal being monitored (Figure 4-72). One of the most common sensors is the *lingual sensor,* which resembles a clothespin in design and is available in large and small versions. Other common sensors are the reflectance probe and universal C-clamp. The lingual sensor, as the name implies, is most frequently used on the

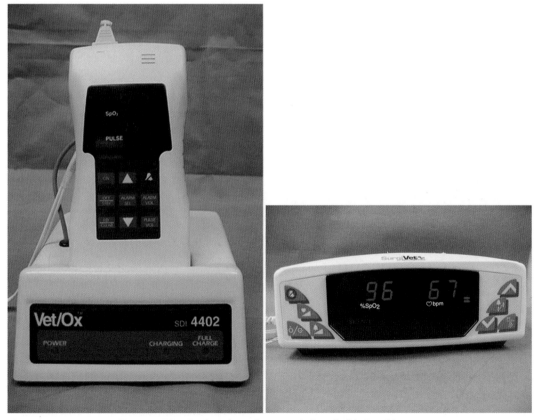

A   **B**

Figure 4-71   Basic pulse oximeters: **A,** handheld; **B,** tabletop.

tongue but can be used on the ear pinna, toe webbing, external genitalia (vulva or prepuce), or any body region with no hair. The *reflectance probe* can be used with a protective sleeve and placed in the rectum or used alone on the underside of the tail, at the base of the tail. The *universal C-clamp* sensor can be used on feet, hocks, and other areas. Regardless of what sensor is used, certain factors can affect the efficacy of the unit and the reliability of the information. Some factors are related to patient wellness, some are related to patient anatomy, and others are related to machine function. If at any time the information being displayed by the unit appears unreasonable, the factors listed here should be evaluated to ascertain the true status of the patient.

Unit Options

Some SaO₂ units provide only basic information, that is, a pulse rate and an SaO₂ readout. Even these basic units, however, also have a pulse bar graph to indicate the strength of the peripheral pulse being evaluated. Other models include additional information, such as noninvasive blood pressure (NIBP) monitoring, end-tidal CO_2 readings (capnography), and electrocardiograph readouts. The more parameters measured by the

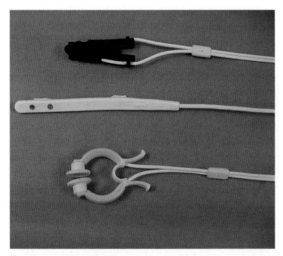

Figure 4-72   Pulse oximeter sensors. *Top to bottom,* Lingual sensor, reflectance probe, and universal C-clamp.

device, the more information acquired by the anesthetist, but there is also greater potential for machine malfunction.

Troubleshooting

Maintaining an appropriate level of oxygen in the patient's blood is paramount. With a patient attached to the anesthesia machine with 100% O_2 running, the SaO₂ reading should be greater than 95%. If the reported data fall below this level, the veterinary technician needs to evaluate the situation to determine if the machine is malfunctioning or if in fact the patient's SaO₂ levels are dropping. Assessing the patient and the equipment quickly is important to correct the problem appropriately. Sometimes the sensor has slipped from its original position, and simply repositioning it may correct the problem. If the machine appears to be functioning properly, the animal may have had a change in its physiologic status. If the animal is not exchanging gases well, even though a normal respiration rate is present, ventilation of the animal may need to be provided manually. Artificial ventilation will help to expand the lungs more completely, thereby allowing better gas exchange.

Capnometer or Capnograph

Capnometry is the measurement and evaluation of the level of CO_2 in the patient's exhaled breath, or the end-tidal CO_2 (ETCO_2). This component of anesthesia is important because it can aid the anesthetist in evaluating the patient's respiratory rate and the quality of the respirations, therefore allowing better interpretation of the patient's depth of anesthesia. An arterial blood gas sample evaluation is the best method to determine blood CO_2 levels, but this is not usually performed in most practices. The alternative, ETCO_2 monitoring, is an option that accurately reflects the arterial CO_2 levels.

Measurement

The capnometer can measure ETCO_2 levels by one of two methods (Figure 4-73). The sensors used are either a "main-stream" or a "side-stream" device. A main-stream device evaluates the patient's CO_2

levels as the breath passes through the airway. This sensor requires the patient to be intubated and correlates to the patient's breathing pattern. A side-stream device uses a vacuum to draw a portion of the exhaled breath down a tiny tube to the main unit for evaluation. The delay in the collection of the sample translates into a displayed pattern that is "out of sync" with the patient's breathing pattern.

Display Wave

The display on the *capnometer* is a digital readout of the ETCO2. The display of a *capnograph* is in the form of a wave. The incline of the wave indicates the exhaled portion of a breath. The plateau at the peak height of the wave indicates the ETCO2 level. As the patient begins to inhale, the wave begins the decline because inspired CO_2 levels should be close to zero (Figure 4-74). Some monitoring devices are capnometers, whereas others are capnographs. Either can combine the measurement of ETCO2 with other monitoring parameters to provide the anesthetist with the most complete picture of the patient and the anesthetic episode.

Normal Values

Normal levels of expired CO_2 are 35 to 45 mm Hg for both dogs and cats. Levels that alter from the accepted range require quick, efficient evaluation

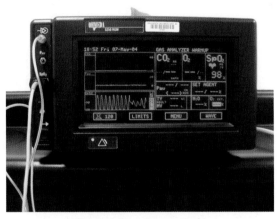

Figure 4-73   Capnograph.

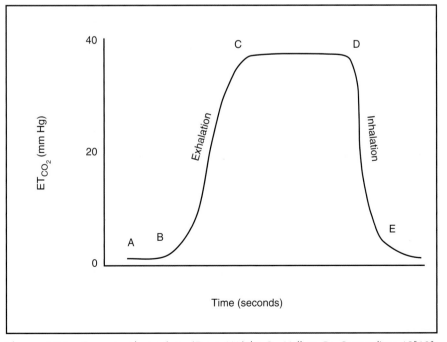

Figure 4-74   Capnograph tracing. (From Wright B, Hellyer P: *Compendium* 18[10]: 1083, 1996.)

by the anesthetist to determine the appropriate course of action. Values below 35 mm Hg, or *hypocarbia,* can be attributed to overzealous artificial ventilation, increased respiratory rate, too light of a plane of anesthesia, pain, or hypoxia. Administering analgesics, easing up on ventilation, increasing anesthetic depth, or treating an underlying hypoxia may help to resolve the hypocarbia. Values above 45 mm Hg are caused by hypoventilation, which leads to higher levels of CO_2. If more CO_2 is being produced than removed, a dangerous situation can quickly develop. *Hypercarbia* can be the result of a decreased respiratory rate, decreased respiratory minute volume, exhausted soda lime, malfunction of one of the unidirectional valves on the anesthesia machine, or a kinked endotracheal tube. Elevated CO_2 levels generally imply that some or all of the gas that was just exhaled has been rebreathed. Corrections to lower the CO_2 include checking the machine and increasing ventilation to remove the excess CO_2.

Blood Pressure Monitor

Blood pressure monitors are used to assess the blood pressure of a patient that is either awake or under anesthesia. It is important to monitor all aspects of physiology while an animal is anesthetized. Using only one monitoring device may only provide information on one parameter. Blood pressure monitors should be used in conjunction with other devices to enable the anesthetist to provide the best anesthetic care possible.

Indirect Monitoring

In private small animal hospitals, blood pressure is most often monitored by indirect methods (Figure 4-75). Doppler crystals are placed on the skin over arteries to produce an auditory assessment of pulse quality and blood pressure trends (Figure 4-76). A sphygmomanometer and a cuff can be added to the ensemble to allow estimated numeric assessment of diastolic and systolic pressure.

Noninvasive blood pressure machines are available (Figure 4-77), which eliminates the need for a manual sphygmomanometer. The units have

cuffs that are placed on the patient, and the cuff inflation line is attached to the machine. The machine inflates the cuff at either preset intervals or manually determined intervals, the cuff is deflated, and a blood pressure measurement is acquired. The reliability of the numeric value displayed depends on the use of an appropriately sized cuff. Cuffs that are either too large or too small will give inaccurate results. To ensure the

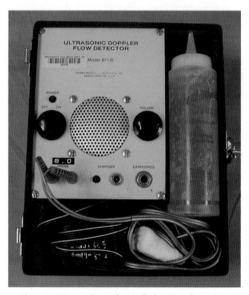

Figure 4-75   Doppler unit in carrying case.

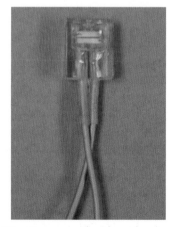

Figure 4-76   Concave side (the side placed next to animal) of Doppler crystal.

proper-sized cuff is being used, the following guidelines should be used: (1) the cuff width should be 40% of the circumference of the limb on which it is to be used, and (2) the length should be appropriate so as to fall into the securing range indicated on the cuff.

Direct Monitoring

Direct blood pressure monitoring is done by placing a catheter in an artery and then attaching a transducer to the catheter. The transducer is connected to an oscilloscope that can display the information being received through the transducer. Usually, numeric values for diastolic pressure, systolic pressure, and mean arterial pressure (MAP) and a waveform for the pulses are displayed. This procedure is more technically challenging than indirect monitoring and requires more expensive equipment. The advantage of direct monitoring is that a "true" evaluation of the pressure can be done. With indirect monitoring, only trends can be observed because accurate numbers are not available.

Electrocardiograph

Continuous electrocardiographic (ECG) monitoring of anesthetized patients provides valuable information. In addition to providing a heart rate and wave formation tracing, many ECG machines (electrocardiographs) are capable of monitoring other parameters, including pulse oximetry readings, temperature, and respiratory rate. "High-end" electrocardiographs can also provide direct blood pressure monitoring options and tracing printouts. Regardless of the additional functions provided with an ECG unit, the basic ECG tracing (electrocardiogram) is a valuable source of information for the anesthetist. Continuous, or even intermittent, monitoring of the heart rate and rhythm with an ECG can alert the anesthetist to current or impending problems that may be avoided. For example, the appearance of a premature ventricular contraction (PVC) alone may be an isolated incident, but repeated multiple PVCs can be a sign of impending, severe cardiac distress. Other situations, such as atrial dysfunction (evident by changes in the P wave), myocardial hypoxia, and electrolyte disturbances (evident by changes in the T wave), can be observed with continuous ECG monitoring.

SURGICAL "POWER TOOLS"

Many types of surgical cases require the use of "power tools." These tools can be powered by compressed nitrogen, batteries, or electricity. Fracture repair requires the use of a power drill to place implants. Neurosurgery requires the use of a burring drill to remove the vertebral body. Even soft tissue surgery sometimes requires power tools. For example, a sternotomy for a thoracic surgery requires a power saw to open the sternum.

Some power devices are sold as individually functioning pieces, whereas others are available in

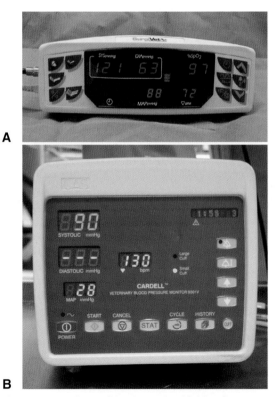

Figure 4-77   A, Combination unit with blood pressure monitor and pulse oximeter. **B,** Blood pressure monitoring unit.

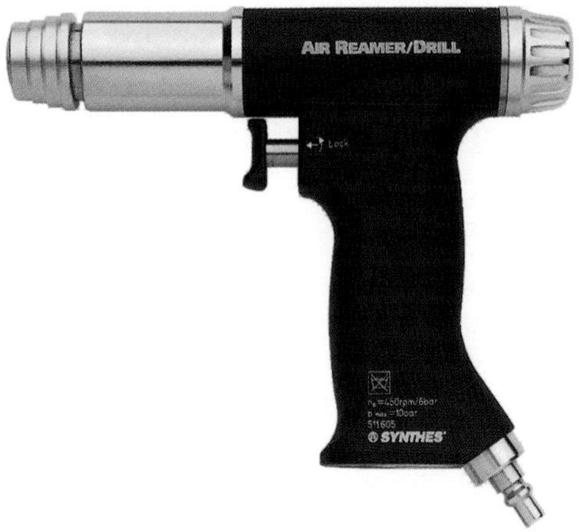

Figure 4-78   Orthopedic drill. (Courtesy Synthes, West Chester, Pa.)

sets that have interchangeable, multifunctional pieces. The Mini-Driver (3M) has a pin driver, sagittal saw, and power drill in one set. Check the manufacturer's recommendations for the best way to sterilize specific power tools, such as the Synthes orthopedic drill (Figure 4-78).

9. Appropriate scavenging of waste anesthetic gas is essential for the safety of the staff.
10. The use of a suture needle is determined by its shape.
11. All the characteristics of suture material should be considered before deciding which type of material to use in any particular case.
12. External warming devices should be employed to help maintain patient body temperature during anesthesia.
13. Cautery can be activated by hand or foot control devices and can be monopolar or bipolar in function.
14. Suction tip styles vary widely and have recommended intended uses.
15. A No. 40 or 50 clipper blade should be used to remove hair from the surgical site.
16. Pulse oximeters measure the level of oxygen saturation of the blood.
17. Capnometry is the measurement of the level of exhaled CO_2; a normal reading is 35 to 45 mm Hg.
18. Blood pressure can be monitored by direct or indirect methods.

KEY POINTS

1. Proper use of surgical instruments is vital to maintain the health and usefulness of the instrument.
2. Instruments need to be evaluated frequently to assess the ability of the instrument to function properly.
3. Each component of the anesthesia machine has a specific purpose and must be in good working order for the machine to function.
4. The flowmeter reduces the oxygen pressure to the atmospheric pressure of 15 psi, which is well tolerated by the patient.
5. The use of the fast flush valve should be avoided when using a non-rebreathing system.
6. Only the liquid anesthetic for which a vaporizer has been calibrated should be used in the vaporizer.
7. The pressure reading on the manometer should not exceed 20 cm H_2O when ventilating a patient.
8. The CO_2 absorber removes carbon dioxide from the exhaled breath of the patient.

REVIEW QUESTIONS

1. Why is it important to use surgical instruments only for their designed purpose?
   a. To avoid damaging them.
   b. To protect their useful life.
   c. The high-quality instruments are expensive and should be handled with care.
   d. All of the above.
   e. Both a and b.
2. Why is it important for ratchets to remain locked when the jaw is closed?
   a. The instrument needs to be a reliable mechanism of holding the target tissue (e.g., pedicle) or item (e.g., suture needle).
   b. If the ratchets do not remain locked, complications (e.g., hemorrhage) could result.
   c. Ratchets need to be protected by lock and key so that only the surgeon can unlock them when it is appropriate.
   d. Both a and b.
   e. All of the above.

3. Which scissors is finer and more lightweight and used on delicate tissues?
   a. Metzenbaum.
   b. Mayo.
4. Of the following hemostats, which is the smallest?
   a. Kelly.
   b. Crile.
   c. Rochester Carmalt.
   d. Halstead Mosquito.
5. Of the following needle holders, which ones have scissors included in the jaws?
   a. Olsen-Hegar.
   b. Mayo-Hegar.
6. Of the following thumb forceps, which has two rows of nine shallow teeth on both tips?
   a. Adson dressing.
   b. Adson-Brown.
   c. Russian.
   d. Debakey thoracic.
7. *True* or *False:* The Allis tissue forceps is considered a traumatic type of forceps.
8. *True* or *False:* The Gelpi retractor is a handheld retractor that is frequently used in orthopedic surgery.
9. *True* or *False:* The Balfour retractor is a self-retaining retractor that is frequently used during abdominal exploratory surgeries.
10. Which of the following is *true* regarding intramedullary (IM) pins?
    a. They must be used alone when used as a type of internal fixation for fractured bones.
    b. They can be combined with orthopedic wire, plates, and screws for orthopedic surgery.
    c. They can be placed in the fractured bone with Jacob's chuck or an electric drill.
    d. All of the above.
    e. Both b and c.
11. What part of the anesthesia machine converts the liquid anesthetic into a gas anesthetic?
    a. Pressure manometer.
    b. Oxygen flowmeter.
    c. Pressure-reducing valve.
    d. Vaporizer.
    e. Carbon dioxide canister.
12. *True* or *False:* The fast flush valve should never be used with a non-rebreathing system.

13. Which of the following have waferlike discs that flutter when the patient breathes?
    a. Unidirectional inspiratory valves.
    b. Unidirectional expiratory valves.
    c. Both a and b.
    d. None of the above.
14. Which valve allows for room air to enter the anesthesia system if negative pressure is detected in the system?
    a. Pop-off valve.
    b. Flowmeter.
    c. Negative-pressure relief valve.
    d. Pressure manometer.
15. When might a situation of negative pressure exist in the anesthesia system?
    a. When the oxygen source is depleted.
    b. During anesthesia induction.
    c. During recovery from anesthesia.
    d. Only during "high-flow" anesthesia.
16. *True* or *False:* The corrugated tubing used to connect the anesthesia machine to the patient's endotracheal tube determines the direction of gas flow through the rebreathing circuit.
17. Which part of the anesthesia machine indicates the amount of pressure in the system?
    a. Pressure-reducing valve.
    b. Flowmeter.
    c. Vaporizer.
    d. Carbon dioxide canister.
    e. Pressure manometer.
18. The pressure in the system should never exceed:
    a. 20 cm H_2O.
    b. 33 mm Hg.
    c. 100 pounds.
    d. All of the above.
    e. None of the above.
19. The rebreathing bag can:
    a. Be used to deliver an alveolar expanding "sigh" to the patient.
    b. Be used to manually ventilate the patient during CPR.
    c. Have a small leak in it causing the system to fail to maintain the patient at an acceptable plane of anesthesia for the given anesthetic setting on the vaporizer.
    d. Have a leak in it, but when it leaks it is always large and clearly visible.
    e. Answers a, b, and c.

20. When squeezing the rebreathing bag to ventilate the patient manually, the pop-off valve needs to be:
    a. Open and then closed after giving a breath.
    b. Closed and then opened after giving a breath.
    c. Open and to remain open after giving a breath.
    d. Closed and to remain closed after giving a breath.
    e. It makes no difference.
21. *True* or *False:* Carbon dioxide canisters contain granules that absorb the carbon dioxide the patient exhales.
22. *True* or *False:* Carbon dioxide canisters contain granules that never need replacing because they are made of inert crystals.
23. What part of the anesthetic system is responsible for conducting the exhaled and waste gases out of the operating room?
    a. Carbon dioxide canister.
    b. Scavenging system.
    c. Flowmeter.
    d. Pop-off valve.
    e. None of the above.
24. Which of the following is *true* regarding leak testing the anesthesia machine?
    a. It should be leak checked before every use.
    b. It only needs to be leak checked once each day it is in use.
    c. It needs to be checked with the patient's pre-selected rebreathing bag attached.
    d. Anesthesia machines need to be sent back to the manufacturer as soon as any leak is detected.
    e. Both a and c.
25. Which of the following generally uses higher oxygen flow rates?
    a. Rebreathing systems.
    b. Non-rebreathing systems.
26. Why is it important to confirm that the "pop-off" valve is completely open after checking the anesthesia machine and circuit for leaks?
    a. It can only reset if it is open.
    b. The next step is to connect the patient to the anesthesia machine, and if the pop-off valve is closed, the patient will not be able to exhale when connected.
    c. It is not important; the pop-off valve can be open or closed after checking the system for leaks.
    d. All of the above.
    e. None of the above.
27. A taper-point needle should be used:
    a. When a sealed suture line is needed.
    b. To close an incision in the urinary bladder.
    c. To suture the wall of the intestine closed.
    d. All of the above.
    e. None of the above.
28. *True* or *False:* Only multifilament suture material is absorbable.
29. Which of the following is *false* regarding patient warming devices?
    a. Electric heating pads are safe to use because they cannot burn the patient.
    b. Circulating warm water blankets are preferred over electric heating pads.
    c. Forced warm air is an acceptable means of warming patients.
    d. Combining methods of warming the patient should be used whenever available.
30. *True* or *False:* The surgeon can adjust the surgery lights when the handles have been autoclaved and are sterile.
31. *True* or *False:* Electrocautery is a method of providing intraoperative hemostasis.
32. Which of the following surgeries or circumstances can benefit from the use of suction?
    a. Joint lavage.
    b. Uroabdomen.
    c. Hemoabdomen.
    d. Abdominal lavage.
    e. All of the above.
33. Which of the following anesthesia monitoring devices is used primarily to measure the percentage of available hemoglobin that is saturated with oxygen?
    a. Capnometer.
    b. Electrocardiograph.
    c. Noninvasive blood pressure monitor.
    d. Direct blood pressure monitor.
    e. None of the above.
34. *True* or *False:* Capnometry is useful for measuring the patient's carbon dioxide levels in each breath.
35. *True* or *False:* Normal levels of expired carbon dioxide vary between cats and dogs.

36. Which of the following best describes the difference between direct and indirect (noninvasive) blood pressure monitoring?
    a. Noninvasive blood pressure monitoring is more accurate.
    b. Direct monitoring requires placing a catheter with a sensor in an artery, and indirect monitoring requires placing a catheter with a sensor in a vein.
    c. Noninvasive pressure monitors can be placed only by veterinarians.
    d. None of the above.
37. Which of the following is *true*?
    a. Changes in the P wave on an electrocardiogram (ECG) may indicate atrial dysfunction.
    b. Changes in the T wave on an ECG may suggest myocardial hypoxia.
    c. Changes in the T wave on an ECG may indicate electrolyte disturbances.
    d. Both a and b.
    e. All of the above.

ANSWERS

1. d
2. d
3. a
4. d
5. a
6. b
7. True
8. False
9. True
10. e
11. d
12. True
13. c
14. c
15. a
16. False
17. e
18. a
19. e
20. b
21. True
22. False
23. b
24. e
25. b
26. b
27. d
28. False
29. a
30. True
31. True
32. e
33. e
34. True
35. False
36. d
37. e

BIBLIOGRAPHY

Edwards NJ: *ECG manual for veterinary technicians,* Philadelphia, 1993, Saunders.

Fossum TW: *Small animal surgery,* ed 2, St Louis, 2002, Mosby.

Ko J: Anesthesia equipment: machine system, Spring 2004. *http://www.cvm.okstate.edu/Courses/vmed5412/default.htm.*

McCurnin DM, Bassert JM, editors: *Clinical textbook for veterinary technicians,* ed 5, Philadelphia, 2002, Saunders.

McKelvey D, Hollingshead KW: *Veterinary anesthesia and analgesia,* ed 3, St Louis, 2003, Mosby.

Monnet E: New suture materials offer more options for wound closures, *DVM* oct.1, 2002.

Simpson K: Let's talk about capnography, August 2003. *http://www.surgivet.com.*

Stromberg H: Mastersonics: frequently asked questions, 1999. *http://cleanosonic.com/ultrasonic_faq.htm.*

Thurman JD, Tranquilli WJ, Benson GJ: *Limb & Jones veterinary anesthesia,* ed 3, Baltimore, 1996, Williams & Wilkins.

PART II

Intraoperative Considerations

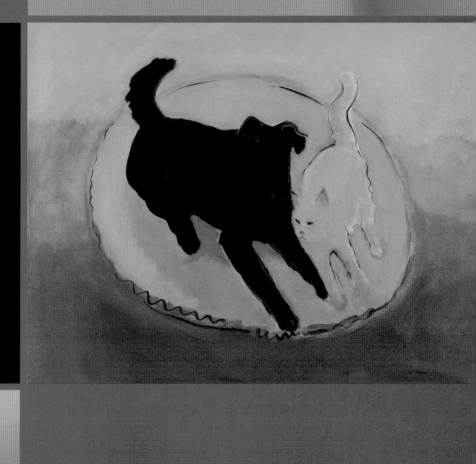

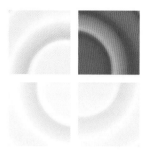

CHAPTER 5

The Intraoperative Patient

Gail Hartman, Nancy Shaffran

LEARNING OBJECTIVES

After studying this chapter, the reader should be able to do the following:

- Use appropriate techniques to conserve body heat.
- Secure the patient to the surgery table in a safe, accessible manner.
- Properly position the patient for various surgical procedures, providing access to the (1) surgical site, (2) intravenous (IV) catheter site, (3) endotracheal (ET) tube, (4) other venous access sites, and (5) monitoring sites.
- Perform a sterile preparation of the surgical site.
- Define a sterile field.

- Perform complete monitoring of the patient under anesthesia, assessing cardiovascular, respiratory, and neurologic parameters.
- Properly fill out and use an anesthesia form.
- Monitor the patient as part of the responsibilities of a scrubbed-in assistant.
- Know when additional intraoperative analgesics are indicated and what options are available for intraoperative analgesia.
- Understand the classifications of surgical wounds.
- Understand the concept of prophylactic antibiotic treatment.

The care and safety of an animal under anesthesia are the responsibility of all members on the veterinary health care team. The veterinary technician and veterinarian work together to ensure that the patient is safe and that the procedure is performed as efficiently as possible. Animals are anesthetized for diagnostic as well as therapeutic procedures. The success of the procedure depends on not only the skill of the surgeon or the competency of the technician performing the diagnostic test, but also the proper and vigilant monitoring of the patient under anesthesia.

Once the veterinary surgical patient has been positively identified and confirmed as an acceptable candidate for anesthesia and surgery (see Chapter 1), the veterinary technician's responsibilities as a surgical nurse begin. These responsibilities include surgical site preparation, patient monitoring, surgical assisting as performed by scrubbed-in personnel, monitoring during recovery, and delivery of postoperative treatments. Although having more than one veterinary technician perform these functions is desirable, it is sometimes necessary to have one technician cover all these responsibilities. This chapter discusses techniques to maintain body temperature, positioning on the surgical table, the sterile field, patient monitoring, intraoperative analgesia, and surgical wounds.

TECHNIQUES FOR MAINTAINING BODY TEMPERATURE

Once the surgical suite has been thoroughly cleaned before the first surgery of the day (see Chapter 3), the room is prepared for the scheduled surgery. This preparation includes setting up and warming up any devices available to help maintain the surgical patient's body temperature. Several of these devices require time to reach warm temperatures and therefore should be turned on before moving the patient into the operating room (OR). In addition, it is preferable to place a patient on a warming device rather than arrange a warming element underneath a patient already positioned on the surgery table.

Several factors contribute to hypothermia in the surgical patient, as listed later in this chapter. The following devices and techniques should be used as available and appropriate to prevent hypothermia:

1. A pad with circulating warm water is placed under the patient as soon as the animal is under anesthesia. Electric heating pads can become too hot and can burn the patient's skin and therefore should *not* be used. The circulating warm water pad avoids the risk inherent with electric heating pads because the water is constantly circulating between the pad under the patient and the warming unit (see Figures 4-55 and 4-56). Water bottles do not provide a constantly renewable source of heat and also carry the risk of leaking. A wet patient can quickly become a cold patient.

2. Warm air convection blankets consist of an electrical unit that warms air and pumps the warm air through a tube to a pad. The pad has a series of holes that allows the warm air to escape slowly. The pad is laid on top of the patient, or the patient rests on top of the pad; this creates a warm microenvironment. When used for the surgical patient, the unit is not activated until the surgeon has completed draping the patient (Figure 5-1).

3. Some stainless steel surgical tables are fitted with heating coils that warm the entire surface of the table to approximate body temperature. The need for warm water

blankets and bottles is eliminated while the patient is on the heated surgical table.

4. The Snuggle Safe disc is a flat plastic device that is placed in a microwave oven for a set number of minutes. This disc retains heat much longer than warm water bottles (Figure 5-2).

5. A plastic bottle (e.g., soda bottle) can be filled with dry, uncooked rice and heated in a microwave oven. The bottle with rice holds

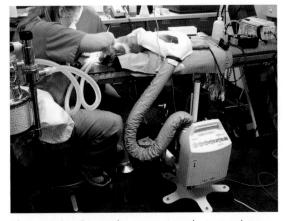

Figure 5-1   Convection-current patient-warming system (Gaymar). The disposable blanket is lying on top of the patient. Air is warmed and pumped into the blanket, through which the warmed air slowly diffuses around the patient.

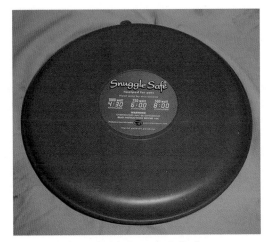

Figure 5-2   Snuggle Safe disc.

heat longer than a water bottle and eliminates the risk of leaking water on the patient.

6. The bag of intravenous (IV) fluids can be warmed in a microwave oven to approximately the same temperature as body temperature. The line for the IV administration set can run through a bowl of warm water to make the fluid warmer before going into the patient.

7. Plastic bubble wrap can be wrapped around the patient's extremities, including the head. The plastic wrap is light but provides warmth by retaining the body heat that would be lost through the extremities (Figures 5-3 and 5-4).

INITIAL PREPARATIONS AND POSITIONING

Finishing Preparation of Surgical Site

Surgical site preparation involves clipping the fur from the patient's intended surgical and incisional area and cleansing the skin with an antiseptic soap and solution. The initial surgical site preparation is generally performed outside the surgical suite in the surgery "prep" or treatment area (see Chapter 1).

After anesthesia is induced and initial preparation of the surgical site completed, the patient is moved from the prep area into the surgical suite.

The final sterile scrub is performed in the surgical suite after the patient has been positioned appropriately on the surgery table. It is difficult, if not impossible, to maintain asepsis of the intended site when moving the patient from the prep area into the surgical suite. Contaminated clothing or personnel will likely have some contact with the intended surgical site while transferring and positioning the patient, so the final sterile scrub is performed after the patient is positioned. Details for the final sterile scrub are covered later in this chapter. The patient needs to be positioned and secured appropriately to provide adequate exposure to the surgical site and adequate access to the patient for monitoring vital signs.

Securing Patient in Position on Surgery Table

Properly securing the animal to the table aids in the aseptic preparation of the surgical site and ensures that the surgeon has an immobile subject with adequate room for working. The techniques used are dictated by the surgical procedure. The animal's limbs may be tied to the table. The body may be braced in position by a V-trough or sandbags. The head, neck, or abdomen may need to be elevated through the use of a foam rubber tube or rolled towels. The patient's legs should not be forced to bend or extend beyond their natural

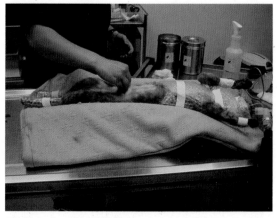

Figure 5-3   Plastic bubble wrap around the extremities, head, and thorax helps to maintain the body heat as this cat is being prepped for a spay procedure.

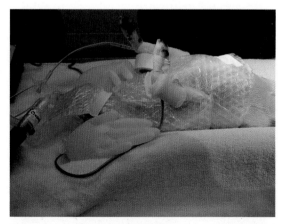

Figure 5-4   Plastic bubble wrap and latex gloves filled with warm water laid across the pinnas help to retain the body heat in the upper portion of this Chihuahua undergoing a spay procedure.

anatomic limitations. Bony prominences should be cushioned to protect against excessive compression.

The use of a sturdy, flexible cord is common practice for securing the animal's limbs in position to the table. Most surgery tables are fitted with four stays (supports) located near the corners of the table. Some tables have adjustable stays that are capable of sliding and thus accommodating patients of various sizes. The end of the cord can be wrapped in a figure-8 fashion around the stay with a half-hitch loop to secure the cord in place. It is important to tie the cord to the table with a quick-release method because the patient may need to be untied quickly. Wrap the cord around the stays only two or three times, and lock the cord with a half-hitch loop at the end (Figure 5-5). If the surgery table does not have stays to secure the cords, they can be tied to each other under the tabletop. The knot used should be a quick-release knot such as a bow tie (Figure 5-6).

It is best to spread out the distribution of pressure around the limb by placing two half-hitch loops, one proximal to and the other distal to the elbow, carpus, or hock (Figure 5-7). If the animal has a catheter in its leg, both loops should be placed distal to the catheter. The tie may prevent the administration of fluid to the animal during the procedure if the cord loop is placed proximal to the catheter. The paws should be checked throughout the surgical procedure. If the paw becomes swollen or the toes feel unusually cold compared with the

opposite paw, the ties are too tight and are cutting off circulation to the paw. In this situation the cord needs to be loosened and repositioned.

Positioning for Specific Procedures

Abdominal Surgery

For abdominal procedures the patient is placed in dorsal recumbency and secured by all four legs to the table. Keeping the patient in perfect dorsal

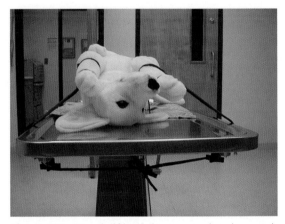

Figure 5-6   Two half-hitch loops are placed on each foreleg, then the end of each rope is extended underneath the tabletop and tied with a bow tie.

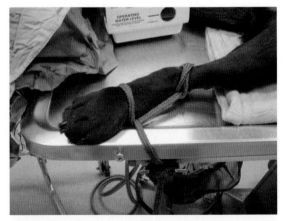

Figure 5-7   Two half-hitch loops are tied around the limb. This technique distributes the pressure on the limb evenly between the two hitches. Care is taken to keep all the joints of the leg in anatomic alignment; that is, the limb is not forced into an unnatural position that may strain or torque the joints.

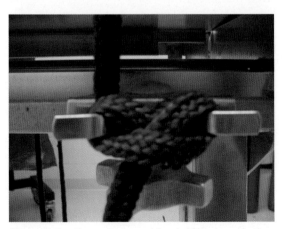

Figure 5-5   Figure-8 wrap with a half-hitch as the last loop.

recumbency is a challenge in the animal with a deep-chested conformation. Deep-chested dogs will need to be placed in a V-trough or braced up by sandbags (Figures 5-8 and 5-9). Some surgical tables are designed with built-in adjustability to form a V-trough (Figure 5-10). Another technique to keep the patient balanced on the table involves tying the forelegs crossed over the chest (Figure 5-11).

Castration

For canine castration the veterinary surgeon may prefer dorsal recumbency or a modified version of this position. For modified dorsal recumbency the hind legs are secured to the table. The forelegs are not tied, and the cranial half of the dog rolls toward the side on which the surgeon stands (Figure 5-12).

For feline castration the cat is placed in dorsal recumbency with the hind legs pulled toward the head. The legs may be taped into position, held by the assistant, or tied to the surgical table (Figure 5-13).

Orthopedic and Extremity Surgery

The patient is placed in lateral recumbency for procedures involving the extremities. If the left limb is the focus, the patient is positioned in right

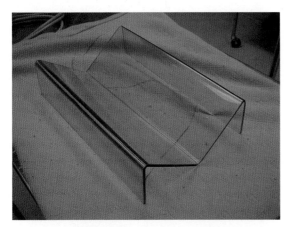

Figure 5-8   Plastic V-trough.

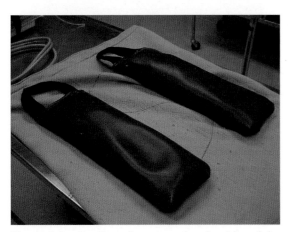

Figure 5-9   Sandbags for supporting the sides of the patient.

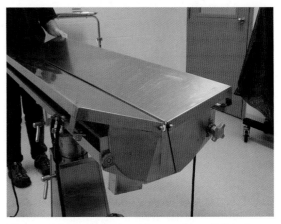

Figure 5-10   Surgical table capable of forming a V-surface to help stabilize the patient in position.

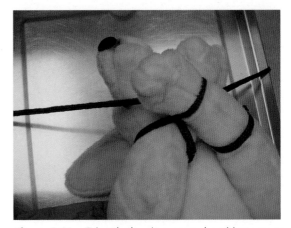

Figure 5-11   Tying the legs in a crossed position across the chest helps to stabilize the patient in dorsal recumbency. Care must be taken when this technique is used to avoid restricting chest excursions as the patient breathes.

lateral recumbency. If the right limb is the surgical site, the patient is placed in left lateral recumbency. The paw is wrapped in gauze and tape. The limb is suspended from above by tying the tape around the paw and tying the tape to an IV pole. The leg is clipped and scrubbed in this position. All sides of the leg are prepared (Figure 5-14).

Tail and Perianal Surgery

The patient is placed in ventral recumbency for procedures involving the tail or perianal area. The forelegs are secured to the table, with the hind legs hanging over the edge at the end of the table. A rolled towel is placed under the caudal abdomen for extra padding. A piece of adhesive tape is placed in a spiral on the tail, with a long extension of the tape attached above to an IV pole or other object (Figure 5-15).

Back Surgery

The patient having back surgery is placed in ventral recumbency. Positioning in a V-trough

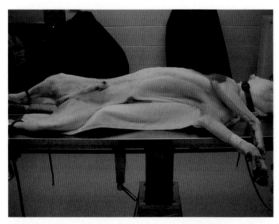

Figure 5-12   Canine patient in position for castration procedure.

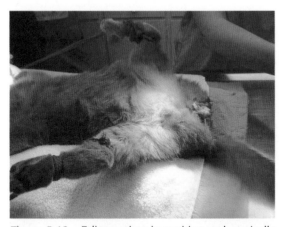

Figure 5-13   Feline patient in position and surgically prepared for castration. The legs are secured to the table with two half-hitches on each leg and then carefully pulled in a cranial direction.

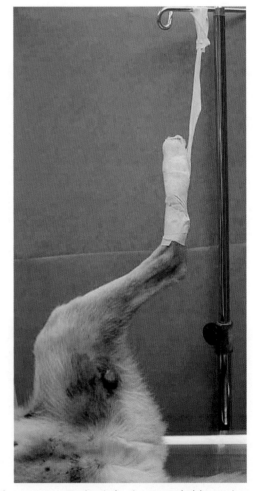

Figure 5-14   Patient's leg is suspended by a piece of tape secured to an IV stand. This patient has a skin mass on the medial aspect of the thigh, so suspending the leg from the IV pole facilitates the preparation process.

or placing sandbags on both sides helps to brace the patient and prevents listing to one side. The forelegs are extended cranially. The hind legs are bent in a natural sitting or squatting position. A strip of adhesive tape may provide additional stabilization across the shoulders (Figure 5-16).

Thoracic Surgery

The patient is placed in lateral or dorsal recumbency depending on the surgeon's intended approach. The forelegs are extended cranially as much as possible and secured to the table.

Preparation in the Operating Room

See Chapter 1 for initial surgical scrub preparation.

Final (Sterile) Surgical Site Preparation

Once the patient has been transported and appropriately positioned on and secured to the surgery table, the final surgical prep is performed in the OR.

Sterile bowls are prepared in advance. One bowl contains sterile gauze squares saturated with a mixture of sterile water and surgical scrub soap solution. The second bowl holds gauze sponges soaked in alcohol or sterile water. The bowls are aseptically prepared in the following manner:

1. Open the sterilized surgical bowl containing gauze sponges.
2. Pour off a small amount of surgical scrub solution into a trashcan to cleanse the lip of the container, then pour the soap on the gauze sponges.
3. Open container of sterile water and pour off a small amount into trashcan, then dilute the scrub soap in the bowl with sterile water.
4. Open second sterile bowl containing sterile gauze.
5. After pouring a small amount of "rinse" (70% rubbing alcohol or sterile water) into trashcan, carefully pour the rinse on the sterile sponges until they appear soaked.
6. Aseptically perform the open-gloving technique (see Chapter 2).
7. Once surgical gloves are donned, grasp a gauze sponge filled with scrub using your designated "clean hand," then squeeze out the excess liquid.
8. Transfer this sponge to your other hand, designated your "dirty hand," and start scrubbing. A new sponge is retrieved each time by the same (clean) hand, then transferred to the other (dirty) hand to do the scrubbing; thus the phrase "clean hand, dirty hand" technique. Only the clean hand goes into

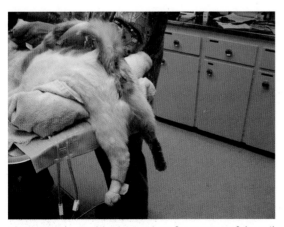

Figure 5-15   Positioning patient for surgery of the tail or perineal area. Note the rolled towel placed under the abdomen for extra cushioning.

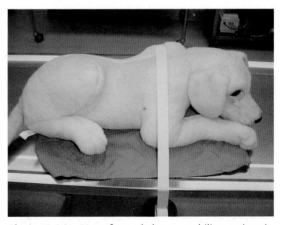

Figure 5-16   Use of tape helps to stabilize patient in ventral recumbency.

the sterile bowl, and only the dirty hand touches the patient. (Rather than clean and dirty, both hands are actually sterile because they are covered with sterile gloves.)

9. The surgical site is scrubbed for the appropriate length of time recommended by the manufacturer of the scrub product, usually about 5 minutes. Scrubbing is done in circles, starting from the intended incision site and working outward to the edge of the shaved area. The time can be adjusted according to the duration of the initial surgical scrub performed in the surgery prep area.

10. Begin at the center of the clipped area over the proposed surgical incision.

11. Without touching the hairline, scrub the length of the incision with long, straight strokes. Scrub outward toward the periphery while slightly overlapping the previously scrubbed line in a circular fashion.

12. Never go back to the center of the area with the same gauze sponge.

13. After scrubbing the skin at the margin of the clipped area, discard the used gauze sponges and start again.

14. The skin should be cleansed thoroughly but gently. Excessive friction can result in hyperemia and bleeding of the skin and subcutaneous tissues.

15. The surgical scrub must have an overall contact time as recommended by the manufacturer. After the appropriate duration has elapsed, wipe the scrub away by using the "rinse"-soaked gauze.

16. Apply a light mist of chlorhexidine gluconate or povidone-iodine solution from a spray bottle to the center of the proposed surgical site, and allow to dry.

Solutions ("Paint")

The final step (16 above) in the surgical site preparation is the application of the solution product, or "paint." Povidone-iodine solution is in the same chemical family as the scrub, but the paint does not contain a detergent. The solution also has a stronger concentration of iodine, therefore increasing its potential for staining. It is corrosive when it contacts metal. The full-strength solution is applied to the patient and remains on the surgical site. It has much better efficacy when allowed to dry on the patient's skin before the drapes are applied or the incision is made.

A second current option for a final solution is chlorhexidine gluconate. As with povidone-iodine, chlorhexidine as a solution contains no detergent. This product is diluted to a 0.2% solution (30 ml/gallon of distilled water) when used as a final paint. Chlorhexidine also has better efficacy when allowed to dry on the patient's skin before the incision is made.

It is important to remember that only povidone-iodine scrub should be followed by povidone-iodine solution. Likewise, only chlorhexidine scrub should be followed by chlorhexidine solution. Using a povidone-iodine scrub with a chlorhexidine solution, or vice versa, is counterproductive and strongly discouraged.

Maintaining Sterile Field

The *sterile field* is the area in which the scrubbed-in surgical team (e.g., surgeon and surgical assistant) can work. All sterile instruments and supplies must be kept within the boundaries of the sterile field. The top surface of the drapes on the patient and the drape on which the instrument tray rests define the boundaries of the sterile field. Supplies such as suture materials and the scalpel blade are aseptically dropped into the instrument tray.

The surgical instruments are wrapped in cloth or paper drapes. Usually the instruments are double wrapped. Non–scrubbed-in personnel aseptically unfold the outer wrapping, and sterile personnel unwrap the inner layer of the sterile packs (see Chapter 3).

The patient is covered with sterile field towels and a fenestrated drape. For most abdominal surgeries, four field towels (four-quarter draping method) are placed around the surgical site. One edge of the towel is folded over and grasped at each corner, with the fingers of the person placing the towel wrapped to protect them from touching the skin (Figure 5-17). Once the towels are placed and secured to the patient with towel clamps, a fenestrated drape is placed on top. Some surgeons may use two fenestrated drapes instead of towels, and others may use only one drape and no towels. Regardless of the number of drapes and layers used, all towels and drapes are attached and secured to the patient below by towel clamps to prevent them from shifting and possibly dragging contaminants into the surgical field during the surgery.

If an extremity is the surgical site, sterile field towels are placed around the base of the leg or tail where it attaches to the body. The surgeon grasps the distal end of the leg with sterile stockinette. The tie that supports the leg attached to the IV pole is cut by the nonsterile assistant near the paw. The surgeon then unrolls the sterile stockinette up the leg (Figure 5-18), stopping short of the surgical site. Some surgeons may prefer to cover the entire leg with sterile stockinette and simply make a hole by cutting a fenestration in the stockinette where it covers the intended skin incision. The stockinette is secured to the patient by a towel clamp.

PATIENT MONITORING

Role of Veterinary Technician Anesthetist

For surgical procedures it is desirable to have a veterinary technician anesthetist whose sole responsibility is to monitor the patient under anesthesia, as well as a circulating nurse to help transport the patient from the surgery prep area to the surgical suite. This team approach allows the surgeon and surgical assistant to be scrubbing while the anesthetist and circulating nurse arrange the patient, anesthesia machine, and monitoring devices in the OR. With the circulating nurse taking responsibility for positioning the patient on the surgery table, attaching the monitoring devices to the patient, and performing the final skin prep and paint in the OR, the anesthetist is able to focus on the most important task, monitoring the patient. Without the help of a circulating nurse, the veterinary technician would need to perform all these tasks alone in rapid succession. If the technician is working alone, the primary task is careful and constant monitoring of the surgical patient. This may mean delaying the final surgical scrub (or other less critical tasks) until the veterinary technician is confident that the patient is stable.

Constant monitoring of the animal under general anesthesia or sedation is an extremely important responsibility. The patient that is monitored closely is the patient that is safely anesthetized. Close and constant monitoring will allow the anesthetist to detect dangerous trends and to make appropriate adjustments. If the patient is showing signs of waking up, the anesthetist can increase the concentration of anesthetic. If the patient is showing signs of becoming too deeply anesthetized, the anesthetist can decrease the concentration of gas delivered. Table 5-1 summarizes the stages of anesthesia.

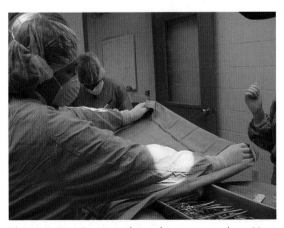

Figure 5-17   Surgeon places drape over patient. Note that the surgeon's hands are protected by the drape from possible contamination caused by accidental touching of the patient's fur.

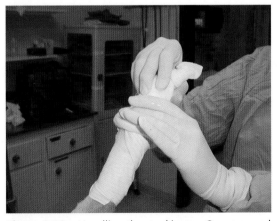

Figure 5-18   Unrolling the stockinette: Once covered with the sterile stockinette, the paw becomes part of the sterile field.

TABLE 5-1 Stages of Anesthesia

STAGE OF ANESTHESIA	BEHAVIOR	RESPIRATION	CARDIO-VASCULAR FUNCTION	RESPONSE TO SURGERY	DEPTH	EYE POSITION	PUPIL SIZE	PUPIL RESPONSE TO LIGHT	MUSCLE TONE	REFLEX RESPONSE
I	Disoriented	Normal, may be panting; respiration rate 20-30 breaths/min	Heart rate unchanged	Struggle	Not anes-thetized	Central	Normal	Yes	Good	All present
II "Excitement stage"	Excitement: struggling, vocalization, paddling, chewing, yawning	Irregular, may hold breath or hyperven-tilate	Heart rate may increase	Struggle	Not anes-thetized	Central, may be nystagmus	May be dilated	Yes	Good	All present, may be exaggerated
III— PLANE 1 Light anesthesia	Anesthetized	Regular; rate 12-20 breaths/min	Pulse strong: Heart rate >90 beats/min	May respond with move-ment	Light	Central or rotated, may be nystag-mus	Normal	Yes	Good	Swallowing poor or absent, others present but diminished

III—PLANE 2 Medium surgical anesthesia	Regular (may be shallow): rate 12-16 breaths/min	Heart rate >90 beats/min	Heart and respiration rates may increase	Moderate	Often rotated ventrally	Slightly dilated	Sluggish	Relaxed	Patellar, ear flick, palpebral, and corneal may be present; others absent
III—PLANE 3 Deep anesthesia	Shallow: rate <12 breaths/min	Heart rate 60-90 beats/min; CRT increased; pulse less strong	None	Deep	Usually central, may rotate ventrally	Moderately dilated	Very sluggish or absent	Greatly reduced	All reflexes diminished or absent
III—PLANE 4	Jerky	Heart rate <60 beats/min; prolonged CRT; pale mucous membranes	None	Overdose	Central	Widely dilated	Unresponsive	Flaccid	No reflex activity
IV Moribund	Apnea	Cardiovascular collapse	None	Dying	Central	Widely dilated	Unresponsive	Flaccid	No reflex activity

From McKelvey D, Hollingshead KW: *Small animal anesthesia and analgesia*, ed 2, St Louis, 1997, Mosby.

Beats/min, Beats per minute, *CRT*, capillary refill time.

Constant monitoring by a technician responsible solely for that patient is the preferred situation. Recommendations include checking the patient every 5 minutes and recording the findings on an anesthesia form. When using gas anesthetic agents that provide quick induction and recovery, such as sevoflurane, more frequent monitoring may be needed. The observant surgeon and surgical assistant can supplement intermittent and frequent monitoring by nonsterile personnel.

Several patient parameters should be monitored every 5 minutes, including heart rate and rhythm, respiratory rate and rhythm, capillary refill time, color of mucous membranes, eye position, muscle tone, and reflexes. The patient's temperature should be monitored at least every 15 minutes if possible. Several anesthetic and treatment parameters should be tabulated every 5 to 15 minutes, including volume of fluid administered, oxygen flow rate, oxygen tank pressure, and anesthetic gas concentration.

The most reliable way to monitor the patient is through personal, direct contact. The technician can *listen* for the heart rate and respiratory rate through the stethoscope. The pulse can be *palpated* to obtain a general impression of pulse strength and therefore of blood pressure (Figures 5-19 to 5-23). The reservoir bag can be *observed* for frequency and extent of movement. The color of the mucous membranes can be visually assessed, and the capillary refill time is directly measured.

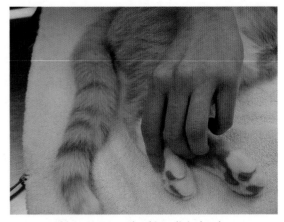

Figure 5-20   Checking digital pulse.

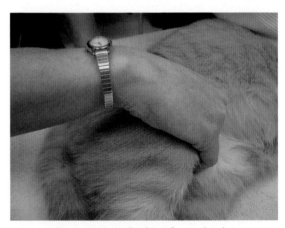

Figure 5-21   Checking femoral pulse.

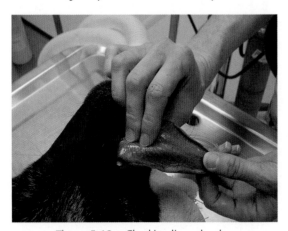

Figure 5-19   Checking lingual pulse.

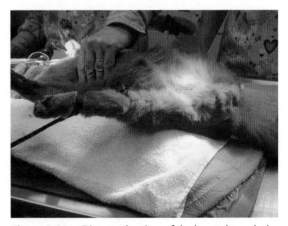

Figure 5-22   Direct palpation of the heart through the chest wall.

The technician's sense of *smell* can detect possible anesthetic leakage problems.

Heart Rate and Rhythm

The heart rate can be monitored through direct palpation of the thoracic wall or by listening through a stethoscope. The stethoscope can be the conventional type that is placed on the thoracic wall. However, the location of the surgical site may prevent the use of a conventional stethoscope. An *esophageal stethoscope* is a more convenient and less intrusive means of monitoring heart rate intraoperatively.

In positioning the esophageal stethoscope, special sensory plastic tubing is placed in the esophagus next to the heart. The tubing is passed through the mouth into the esophagus. The endotracheal (ET) tube prevents the esophageal stethoscope tubing from entering the trachea. The heart sounds can be heard through ear pieces, or an amplifier can be attached to broadcast the sound (Figures 5-24 and 5-25). If the end of the tubing is adjacent to the lung fields, breath sounds will be heard.

The heart rate of an anesthetized dog or cat is expected to be slower than the animal's rate when awake and excited about being examined by a stranger. Most anesthetic drugs have cardiac depressant effects. Hypothermia can also cause a decreased heart rate. When the heart rate falls below an acceptable limit, the surgeon should be notified. Suggested guidelines for acceptable lower limits are 50 beats per minute (beats/min) for a large dog, 70 beats/min for a small dog, and 100 beats/min for a cat. Rates lower than these warrant notifying the surgeon immediately.

Anticholinergic drugs such as atropine and glycopyrrolate are administered to help maintain the heart rate above the acceptable lower limits (see Chapter 1). Dissociative anesthetics such as ketamine and tiletamine can also elevate the heart rate.

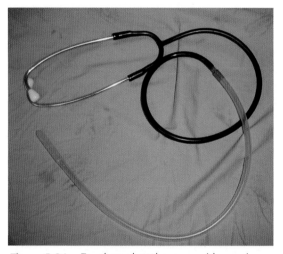

Figure 5-24 Esophageal stethoscope with ear pieces.

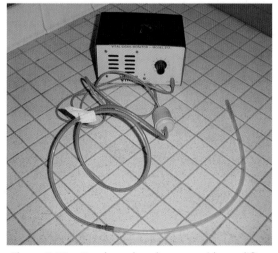

Figure 5-25 Esophageal stethoscope with amplifier.

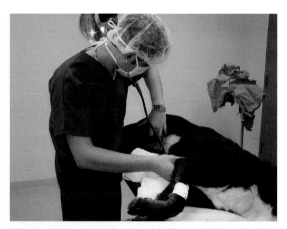

Figure 5-23 Auscultating the heart and monitoring the femoral pulse simultaneously.

When an animal is in shock or pain, the heart rate is usually rapid. Regardless of the reason, once the heart rate exceeds the acceptable limits, the surgeon should be notified. Suggested guidelines for acceptable upper limits are 180 beats/min for a large dog, 200 for a small dog and 220 for a cat.

An irregular heart rhythm may be detected through auscultation of the thorax or on an electrocardiogram (ECG). Some anesthetic agents sensitize the heart muscle to arrhythmias. When the heart beats arrhythmically, the heart is inefficient at pumping the blood through the body. This leads to poor tissue perfusion, acidosis, poor oxygen delivery to the tissues, and buildup of waste products in the body tissues. These irregular beats may spontaneously disappear. If the arrhythmic beats are frequent or continuous, the veterinarian should be alerted.

Detection of a pulse deficit is cause for concern. A *pulse deficit* occurs when the heart contracts (beats) but does not generate enough push to produce a palpable peripheral pulse. Pulse deficits are detected when the heartbeat is arrhythmic; tissue perfusion will be poor, and the patient may quickly go into shock. The veterinarian should be alerted immediately. "Skipped" beats are detected while listening to the heartbeat with a stethoscope, but being unable to palpate that individual beat simultaneously as a peripheral pulse. In this case the single skipped beat is a result of a single premature depolarization of the heart muscle.

Tissue Perfusion

To maintain healthy and functioning tissues and organs, adequate tissue perfusion must be maintained. If not, adverse long-term effects may be sustained. The kidneys are particularly sensitive to states of low perfusion. During inadequate perfusion states, waste products from cellular metabolism are not removed, and nutrients such as oxygen and glucose are not delivered to the cells.

Mucous Membranes

The color of the mucous membranes is a general indicator of tissue perfusion. The pink color of the mucous membranes results from the color of the blood in the capillaries seen through the nonpigmented areas. Mucous membrane color may be evaluated by looking at the gums, conjunctiva, and mucosal surface of the vulva or prepuce.

Pale mucous membranes may indicate a state of poor tissue perfusion or anemia (Figure 5-26). Preanesthetic diagnostic blood tests such as complete blood count (CBC), hematocrit, and hemoglobin will identify the anemic patient. Preferably, the severely anemic patient will not go to surgery before receiving appropriate blood component therapy.

Dark-red mucous membranes may be seen if an animal is *septic,* which means the patient has a severe blood infection. Bacteria may be cultured from the blood. The immune system is reacting to the infection by releasing vasoactive chemicals that cause postcapillary venous dilation and increased permeability in the vessel walls. This can lead to congestion in the capillary beds and thus the brick-red color to the mucous membranes.

A bluish color to the mucous membranes (called *cyanosis*) suggests that the red blood cells are not carrying adequate oxygen. The red cells may not have exchanged oxygen in the lungs, suggesting respiratory problems such as obstruction of oxygen flow to the lungs or lack of breathing. The ET tube should be evaluated immediately for a kink or obstruction. A bluish color in the buccal mucosa may also result from a tie on the ET tube being too tight around the cheeks, causing

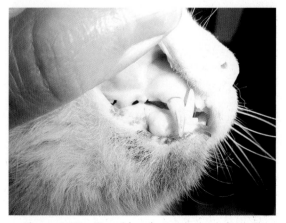

Figure 5-26   Cat with pale mucous membranes.

stagnant blood flow. The buccal mucosa should be compared with the conjunctival mucosa to determine if a tight tie could be the cause of the bluish color and needs to be loosened.

Capillary Refill Time

The capillary refill time (CRT) normally should be less than 2 seconds. The same areas used to assess the color of mucous membranes may be used to assess CRT. When CRT is longer than 2 seconds, perfusion in these tissues is poor. This may be caused by low arterial blood pressure or peripheral vasoconstriction. Release of epinephrine can cause peripheral vasoconstriction, and slow CRT is often seen in nervous and frightened animals. Alpha$_2$-adrenergic agonist drugs such as medetomidine will cause significant peripheral vasoconstriction, thus slowing the CRT. A normal CRT can be detected shortly after some animals are deceased, which reinforces the importance of constant monitoring of several vital signs, not just one.

Pulse and Blood Pressure

Pulse strength can be defined as the ease or difficulty in palpating the blood flowing through the artery. Pulse strength is a general indicator of the blood pressure. If the patient's pulse becomes more difficult to palpate, the blood pressure has fallen. If the patient's pulse becomes more easily palpable or bounding, the blood pressure has increased. Pulses can be monitored at the following sites: lingual (under the tongue), femoral (medial thigh), carotid (neck), dorsal metatarsal (hind foot), and digital (ventral paw) (see Figures 5-19 to 5-21). The heart may be palpated directly through the chest wall. In cats the thumb and fingers are placed on either side of the chest, and light pressure is applied. The beating heart may be felt through the chest wall (see Figure 5-22). Obese patients and larger patients, such as medium-sized to large dogs, are more difficult to palpate.

An ultrasonic Doppler or oscillometric device is needed to assess arterial blood pressure accurately (see Chapter 4). Normal mean arterial pressure (MAP) ranges from 85 to 120 mm Hg. MAP should be maintained above 70 mm Hg while the patient is under anesthesia.

Hypotension

Hypotension (low blood pressure) in an anesthetized patient may be caused by the following:

1. *Hypovolemia.* Excessive blood loss or dehydration reduces the volume of the vascular space. With little blood to pump through the vessels, the blood pressure will be low.
2. *Cardiac insufficiency.* Patients with preexisting heart disease may have a weak myocardium or leaking heart valves, which can lead to inefficient pumping action.
3. *Excessive vasodilation.* Many preanesthetic and anesthetic drugs cause vasodilation to varying degrees. The effects can be additive and significant. When the blood vessels dilate, the blood pools, venous return to the heart is decreased, and blood pressure drops.
4. *Anesthetic depth.* In general, as the patient goes deeper under anesthesia, the blood pressure drops. The correlation between blood pressure and anesthetic depth is quite accurate.

Respiratory Rate and Rhythm

One inhalation and one exhalation are considered one breath. Counting only the inhalations or only the exhalations is necessary to determine the correct respiratory rate (RR). The number of breaths counted in 15 seconds is multiplied by 4 to calculate the breaths per minute, or the respiratory rate. A dog or cat in the surgical plane of anesthesia will have a rate of 8 to 20 breaths/min. A respiratory rate of less than 8 breaths/min is cause for concern and most likely indicates an excessive anesthetic depth. As anesthetic depth becomes dangerously deep, respiration will cease before the heart stops beating.

The respiratory rate can be determined by watching the patient's chest movement. The reservoir bag on the anesthesia machine can also be observed. The reservoir bag will collapse and fill synchronously with the patient's breathing. The anesthetist can listen for breath sounds through the stethoscope and should note their character and intensity. An increase in intensity, crackles, or wheezing indicates pulmonary airway narrowing through constriction or the presence of fluid. Devices such as the capnograph display the respiratory rate on a digital display (see Chapter 4).

The depth and rhythm of the respirations should also be assessed. The inspiratory phase is about half as long as the expiratory phase. A short pause occurs before the next inspiration. If the animal feels pain during the surgery, the respiratory rate will increase. Dissociative anesthetic agents will cause the animal to inhale, hold its breath, then exhale. This irregular breathing pattern is characteristic of dissociative anesthetics. As anesthetic depth increases, respiratory rate usually decreases. Gasping or labored breathing is of particular concern. An obstruction of the trachea or ET tube or a lack of fresh gas flow can cause exaggerated respiratory effort. Check the patency of the ET tube, check for the appropriate oxygen flow rate on the anesthesia machine, and confirm that the pressure in the reservoir bag is not too high. If the ET tube is not patent, it may need to be suctioned, or the patient may need to be reintubated. If the setting on the oxygen flowmeter is not maintaining the desired setting, the oxygen tank supplying the anesthesia machine may need to be changed. If the reservoir bag is overinflated and has a high pressure, open the "pop-off" valve (pressure relief valve), and consider decreasing the oxygen flow rate on the anesthesia machine.

The animal that spasmodically contracts its diaphragm may be exhibiting *agonal* ("death agony") breathing. Agonal breathing, or agonal gasping, is not "real" breathing; that is, no physiologic exchange of gases is occurring in the lungs. Agonal gasps can be mistaken for deep breaths if the respiratory rate has not been sufficiently monitored. Agonal gasps typically occur after a long period of apnea and are often detected as rapid movement in the patient's diaphragm, jaw, or larynx. Agonal gasps occur after cardiac arrest, and the veterinarian must be alerted immediately.

The practice of manually ventilating the patient every 5 to 10 minutes during the anesthetic period is recommended. Assisted ventilation ("bagging") opens up collapsed alveoli, preventing atelectasis. Anesthetized patients tend to breathe more shallowly; combined with the weight of other internal organs on the lungs, this contributes to atelectasis. The technique for administration of a ventilating breath is as follows:

1. The pressure relief valve is closed.
2. The reservoir bag is squeezed while ensuring that the manometer does not exceed 20 cm H_2O or that the chest does not exceed a normal excursion.
3. The pressure relief valve is opened.

While administering a ventilating breath, the anesthetist should listen at the animal's mouth for any sound of air rushing past the ET tube. Some anesthetic agents, such as isoflurane, have a pungent odor, which indicates leakage if detected. If a sound is heard or the odor of gas detected, the cuff seal is incomplete. The cuff on the ET tube should be further inflated or the patient reintubated with a larger ET tube.

Body Temperature

Body temperature is monitored before and during the anesthetic period. Monitoring every 15 minutes is common practice.

In rare instances, *hyperthermia* may develop when inhalation anesthetics are used. Dangerously high body temperatures spontaneously manifest in patients that develop *malignant* hyperthermia. If the high temperature goes unnoticed, life-threatening cerebral edema can develop. Genetic predisposition may play a role in the phenomenon of malignant hyperthermia, which has been documented in humans, pigs, and dogs. If an abnormally high body temperature is detected, or if a temperature significantly higher than the preanesthetic body temperature is recorded, the anesthetic procedure should be terminated as soon as possible.

The development of *hypothermia* is common and a constant concern in patients undergoing general anesthesia. The following factors contribute to the decrease in body temperature:

1. Anesthetic drugs relax muscles, significantly diminish the shivering response, and decrease the overall metabolic rate. Production of body heat decreases.

2. The surgical site is shaved, washed with soap and water, then rinsed with alcohol. Evaporation from the skin surface has a cooling effect on the body.
3. Room-temperature fluids are administered.
4. Cold gases are inspired.
5. A body cavity may be opened, and internal organs are exposed to ambient temperatures.

Measures to prevent body heat loss should be taken, as discussed earlier.

Neurologic Parameters

Reflexes

As anesthetic depth increases, reflex activity diminishes and eventually disappears. A *reflex* is an automatic reaction to a stimulus made by the animal without conscious awareness of the reaction. These reflex actions protect the animal from harm. For example, the swallowing reflex is triggered by the presence of saliva or other matter in the pharynx. The animal swallows the material into the gastrointestinal system rather than aspirating it into the respiratory system. Most reflexes monitored during anesthesia are located around the face, eyes, and throat. The return of the reflex or increasing strength of the reflex response indicates that the level of anesthesia is becoming lighter. The technician anesthetist may monitor the following reflexes:

- *Auricular (ear flick) reflex.* The fully conscious animal will flick its ear when the pinna is lightly touched or tickled. The intensity of the reaction varies among individuals. If the reflex is tested in rapid succession, the reaction to the stimulus may diminish quickly. Although this reflex can persist well into a moderate level of anesthesia, its variable nature renders it somewhat unreliable. It is best to monitor all available reflexes.
- *Pedal (withdrawal) reflex.* When pressure is applied to a toe, the limb is withdrawn. The pressure applied should be significant. The withdrawal reflex is useful when the animal is being masked. The mask interferes with the ability to monitor other reflexes around the face. Once the pedal reflex disappears, the animal may be sufficiently anesthetized to attempt intubation.
- *Palpebral (blink) reflex.* The blink reflex protects the globe from injury by the eyelids quickly closing. The reflex can be elicited by lightly touching the medial canthus of the eye. The reflex disappears or is significantly diminished as the animal enters the surgical plane of anesthesia. The palpebral reflex usually returns just before the laryngeal reflex as the animal is recovering.
- *Corneal reflex.* The animal will blink or retract the globe when the cornea is touched. This reflex persists well into the deep levels of anesthesia. The corneal reflex is seldom used when monitoring anesthesia; it is used more often to help assess the point of death during euthanasia.
- *Laryngeal (swallow) reflex.* When saliva, food, or water is in the pharynx, the epiglottis and arytenoid cartilage will close the entrance to the trachea, and the animal will swallow. The laryngeal reflex can also be initiated by rubbing the ventral throat. The swallow reflex must be lost in order for intubation to proceed easily.

Cats tend to retain the laryngeal reflex longer than dogs, so they need to be more deeply under anesthesia before intubation can be accomplished. If intubation is attempted too soon, the larynx may go into a spasm and remain closed. Cats also are more likely to develop laryngeal spasm than dogs during the intubation process. To prevent this, many anesthetists drip 0.1 ml of 2% lidocaine on the vocal cords, then wait a moment before attempting intubation.

Muscle Tone

Muscles usually relax as the animal goes deeper under anesthesia. Dissociative anesthetics cause muscle rigidity, however, so muscle relaxants such as benzodiazepines (e.g., diazepam, zolazepam) are usually added when these anesthetics are used. The most import muscles to relax are those that control the opening of the mouth. Once the mouth can be easily opened, intubation can be performed more easily.

It is important to monitor the intensity of the *jaw tone* during anesthesia. When jaw tone increases, the animal's depth of anesthesia is becoming lighter. Test the resistance to opening the mouth by carefully prying apart the upper and lower teeth with just two fingers (Figure 5-27).

Depending on the procedure being performed, jaw tone may not be available for monitoring by the anesthetist. If the animal is undergoing a dental procedure or oral surgery, a mouth speculum may be placed in the mouth to keep it open. In such cases the anal opening may be inspected because it can indicate the degree of muscle relaxation the patient is experiencing. In the conscious animal the anal opening is closed. In general, as the animal goes deeper under anesthesia, the anal tone becomes more relaxed and the anus opens more.

Eyes

The position of the eye in the socket, the pupil size, and the eye's responsiveness to light can be used to assess anesthetic depth. Although the responses may vary depending on the individual animal and the drugs given, the following general observations can be useful in assessing anesthetic depth:

- The eye will rotate ventrally when the animal is in a moderate or surgical level of anesthesia (Figure 5-28).
- At light and deep levels of anesthesia, the eye will be in a central position.

- When dissociative anesthetics are given, the eye position may never change (Figure 5-29).
- As the anesthetic depth increases, the pupil constricts more slowly in response to a light shined at it (pupillary light response [PLR]).
- Deeper stages of anesthesia and anticholinergic drugs will cause pupillary dilation (mydriasis). The use of these drugs in the preanesthetic protocol will interfere with the reliability of this reflex.

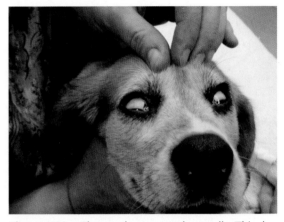

Figure 5-28   The eyes have rotated ventrally. This dog is in stage III (plane 2) of anesthesia.

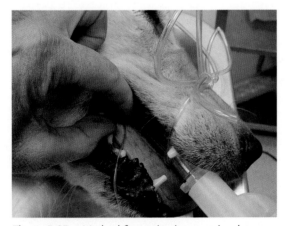

Figure 5-27   Method for testing jaw tone involves prying the mouth open with just two fingers barely inserted into the mouth.

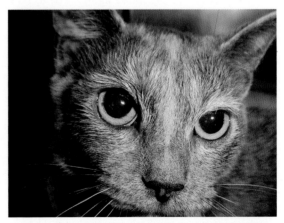

Figure 5-29   Glycopyrrolate and Telazole were administered intramuscularly to this cat 15 minutes ago. Eye ointment should be applied as soon as possible to protect the eyes from drying out. Tear production and the blink reflex are diminished. Note the widely dilated pupils.

It should be noted here as well that when a patient arrests and expires, the pupils are fully dilated.

Anesthesia Form

The anesthesia form "tells the story" of the anesthesia event from beginning to end. It is an important piece of the patient's medical record and can serve as a legal document. It can help guide the choice of anesthetic protocols to follow in the future. The anesthesia form documents vital signs and their trends intraoperatively. For example, a graph of the patient's blood pressure may be a line that goes down over time, with an occasional spike as the surgery proceeds, indicating that the trend for the overall blood pressure is dropping, a cause for concern.

The anesthesia form should be filled out completely and accurately. The following discussion provides the information typically found in each section of the form.

Demographics

```
Client Name:_____

Pet's Name:_____

Species:_____Breed:_____

Sex:_____DOB:_____
```

This section records the owner's name and the patient's signalment, with date of birth (DOB). Fill in the blanks using the information from the medical record.

Preanesthetic Values and Disposition

This section records the date and patient's weight, identifies the clinician, and lists the surgical procedure(s) to be performed.

DATE	Weight lb.	Clinician				
	Kg	Anesthetist				
Procedure			Pre-anes. disposition			
1.			Alert Recumbent			
2.			Excited Caution			
3.			Depressed Painful			
			Nervous Other			
Pre-anes. values	Temp	HR	RR	MM/CRT	PCV	TP
				Renal Function	Hydration	ASA Status I II III IV V

TABLE 5-2   American Society of Anesthesiologists (ASA) Rating System for Anesthetic Risk (ASA Status)*

CATEGORY	PHYSICAL CONDITION	EXAMPLES OF POSSIBLE SITUATIONS
Class I **Minimal risk**	Normal healthy patient with no underlying disease.	Ovariohysterectomy; castration; declawing operation; hip dysplasia radiographs
Class II **Slight risk**	Patient with slight to mild systemic disturbances. Patient able to compensate; no clinical signs of disease.	Neonatal or geriatric patients; obese patients; fracture without shock; mild diabetes; compensating heart or kidney disease; full-blown estrus
Class III **Moderate risk**	Patient with moderate systemic disease or mild clinical signs.	Anemia; anorexia; moderate dehydration; low-grade kidney disease; low-grade heart disturbances, heart murmur, or cardiac disease; moderate fever
Class IV **High risk**	Patient with preexisting systemic disease or severe disturbances.	Severe dehydration; shock; anemia; uremia or toxemia; high fever; uncompensating heart disease; diabetes; pulmonary disease
Class V **Grave risk**	Surgery often performed in desperation on patients with life-threatening systemic disease or disturbances, not often correctable by surgery; includes all moribund patients not expected to survive 24 hours.	Advanced cases of heart, kidney, liver, lung, or endocrine disease; profound shock; major head injury; severe trauma; pulmonary embolus

*ASA recommends that all patients with ASA status of III, IV, or V have a responsible person solely dedicated to managing this patient during the anesthetic period. However, more veterinarians are finding it advantageous to have an anesthetist assigned to *all* patients under anesthesia.

1. **Weight.** Be sure to enter both pounds (lb) and kilograms (kg).
2. **Procedures.** More than one procedure may be done. List the procedures in the order they will be performed.
3. **Preanesthetic values** *(Pre-anes. values).* Temperature *(Temp),* heart rate *(HR),* respiratory rate *(RR),* mucous membrane color and capillary refill time *(MM/CRT),* packed cell volume *(PCV),* total protein *(TP),* renal function, and hydration are the values obtained *just before* premedication is given.
4. **ASA status.** The American Society of Anesthesiologists (ASA) rating system is used to assess a particular patient's risk for an anesthetic procedure, helping to define the patient's anesthetic risk category (Table 5-2).
5. **Preanesthetic disposition** *(Pre-Anes. disposition).* Circle the descriptive term that

best describes how the patient appears *before* any premedication is given.

Preanesthetics

Preanesthetic drugs are usually given intramuscularly (IM) or subcutaneously (SQ, SC) to relax and sedate the patient. This relaxed state generally allows for a more willing patient when it is time to place the IV catheter and induce anesthesia.

Preanesthetic Drugs			
Drug	Dose	Route	Time

1. **Drug.** Write out full name of drug.
2. **Dose.** Write in a weight unit, such as milligrams (mg). It is important here to avoid units of volume, such as milliliters (ml), because one drug may be available in different concentrations. Depending on which concentration of the drug is used, the amount of milligrams in 1 ml of the same drug will vary. The important amount to know is how many milligrams of the drug the patient received, *not* how many milliliters, which depends on the concentration.
3. **Route.** IM, IV, or SC (SQ).
4. **Time.** Note the time when the drugs are administered.

Anesthetic Induction

Anesthetic induction drugs are generally given intravenously (IV) and have a rapid onset and short duration. Anesthesia induction should be a

	Anesthetic Induction		
Drug	Dose	Route	Time

rapid and smooth event that brings the patient to a level of anesthesia that will allow the patient to be quickly and safely intubated with an ET tube.

1. **Drug.** Full name of drug.
2. **Dose.** Use a weight unit (e.g., mg) only. Remember that this cannot be filled in before the drug is given. IV induction agents are given to effect. The desired *effect* is sufficient muscle relaxation of the jaw and diminished gag reflex such that the patient can be intubated. For example, the calculated IV dose may be 2 ml, but the patient may require only 1 ml for sufficient relaxation to be intubated. The amount of milligrams of induction drug in the 1 ml administered is what needs to be recorded here. This underscores the

importance of filling out the dose box *after* the induction drug was administered. Induction agents given by the IM or oral (PO) route are based on the calculated dosage rate.
3. **Route.** This is the route of administration of the induction drug.
4. **Time.** Note the time the drug was administered. In the case of gas induction, note the time the anesthetic gas was first turned on.

Premedication Results

Pre-med Results

Sedation		Resistance
☐	None	☐
☐	Slight	☐
☐	Moderate	☐
☐	Marked	☐

1. **Sedation.** Record results after administration of premedication. How well did the patient seem to be sedated?
2. **Resistance.** How much did the patient resist manipulation, such as catheter placement?

Breathing System

Circle ☐	Non-reb ☐
Closed ☐	Semi-closed ☐
Mask ☐	Intubated ☐

Size tube

Recumbency:

1. **Breathing system.** Check that appropriate breathing system is used (*Non-reb,* non-rebreathing system).
2. **Size tube.** Record size of ET tube used. The size is stamped on the side of the ET tube. If a patient's medical history includes recent general anesthesia, the anesthesia form for that procedure may help in tube selection for this procedure.
3. **Recumbency.** Enter the position in which the patient is placed for the procedure. For example, "LL" may be entered here for "left lateral" recumbency (patient's left side is in contact with surgery table). Recumbency is important to note, especially if a complication occurs (e.g., nerve paralysis in a limb, burn from heating pads). If more than one procedure is performed, the patient may be in more than one position during this anesthetic period.

Postoperative Values

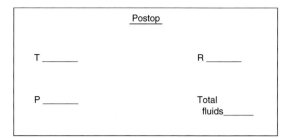

1. **T:** Temperature
2. **P:** Pulse
3. **R:** Respiration
4. **Total Fluids:** Total volume administered and type of fluids given.

Measure these values after extubation.

Time	
Start anesthesia	When the vaporizer is turned on.
Start proc. 1	Time of first incision by surgeon.
Start proc. 2	When second procedure starts.
Start proc. 3	
End surgery	When surgeon has finished closing.
End anesthesia	When vaporizer is turned off. May be a minute or two before the surgeon finishes depending on the depth of patient.
Extubated	Important to note. Especially if charging for anesthetic gas use.
Sternal	The time when the animal is able to support itself in sternal recumbency.
Standing	The time when the animal is able to stand without assistance.

Intraoperative Updates

It is important to keep the anesthesia form as current as possible throughout the surgical procedure. Record all information every 5 minutes (heart and respiratory rates, level of anesthetic, oxygen flow rate, patient's depth of anesthesia); fluids need to be updated every 15 minutes.

Figure 5-30 describes the graph component of the anesthesia form.

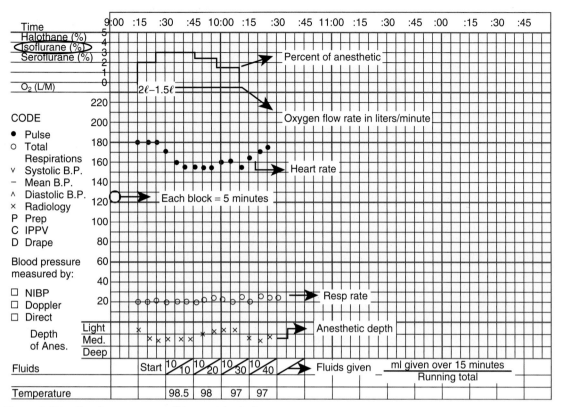

Figure 5-30   Graph component of the anesthesia form.

Time: Each block (or small square) represents 5 minutes. If "start anesthesia" time is 9:15, start recording all the parameters at the 15-minute mark (see graph).

Percent of anesthetic: This is a record of the percentage of anesthetic gas being delivered to the patient. It corresponds to the settings on the vaporizer (%).

Oxygen flow rate: This is a record of the flow of oxygen throughout the procedure. This corresponds to the rate of flow at which the flowmeter is set on the anesthesia machine.

Heart and respiratory rate: Record every 5 minutes. See codes at far left.

Anesthetic depth: Subjective assessment of the patient's depth of anesthesia graphed over time reveals whether the patient may be "getting light" or "too deep" for the specific procedure. Assessment is affected by trends in heart and respiratory rate, pupil position, and presence or absence of reflexes.

Fluids given: This is a record of how many milliliters (ml) of fluid the patient received throughout the procedure. *Top number* is the amount of ml given over 15 minutes (ml/hour divided by 4). *Bottom number* is a running total of how much the patient has received at that particular point in the procedure, again in 15-minute blocks. First box is usually written as "start," but "0/0" is also acceptable.

Temperature: This is measured every 15 minutes; however, you may not be able to obtain a body temperature measurement once the surgery has started and the patient has been draped.

Role of Scrubbed-in Surgical Assistant

Manual Monitoring

The observant surgeon and surgical assistant can help monitor the surgical patient. Pulsing arteries may be noted within the surgical field. The color of the patient's skin and the dryness of the cut edges provide important information about the adequacy of tissue perfusion.

Scrubbed-in personnel can note movements of the patient's chest. An audible heart and respiratory monitor is recommended to aid the sterile personnel in monitoring the patient.

Surgical Site Bleeding

A decrease in the amount of bleeding at the surgical site should alert the surgeon of a possible problem with the patient. If the surgical site is dry of blood and the color of skin and mucous membranes is pale to white, tissue perfusion is poor. Collecting blood for intraoperative monitoring of PCV and total solids (TS), turning up the IV fluid drip rate, and decreasing the anesthetic gas concentration may be required to assess and help this patient. If the intraoperative PCV and TS values are dropping (compared with preanesthetic blood results), the patient may need blood component therapy.

INTRAOPERATIVE ANALGESIA

Good preemptive pain management protocols are designed to transition the patient through the surgical period and into the recovery phase. However, patients undergoing surgical procedures of greater than several hours' duration often require additional analgesia intraoperatively. In addition, patients undergoing procedures necessitating major tissue or nerve damage (e.g., back, knee, hip, amputation, multiple anastomoses, ear or rectal surgeries) will benefit from intraoperative analgesia and analgesic techniques. Finally, patients with poor tolerance for gaseous anesthesia can be effectively managed with constant-rate infusions of opioids, which can greatly decrease the inhalant requirements.

In any of these cases, increased duration or intensity of surgical pain, often evidenced by sudden elevation in heart or respiratory rate, should not be addressed by merely increasing the concentration of inhaled anesthesia. Although "turning up the gas" will keep the patient immobile on the table, it will not manage acute pain, which will become evident as soon as the patient returns to consciousness.

Options for Delivery

Bolus

Administration of additional bolus doses of opioids is determined by the patient's response to surgical stimulation. Such responses include movement, audible sounds such as growling or crying (if patient is not intubated), and increased heart rate, blood pressure, or respiratory rate. Intraoperative boluses should be delivered intravenously for fastest onset of action. The full opioid agonists morphine, hydromorphone, and oxymorphone are optimum choices. Fentanyl is not recommended for one-time bolus use because of its short half-life, and it is best administered as a constant-rate infusion.

Constant-Rate Infusion

Intraoperative analgesia is best administered by constant-rate infusion (CRI). Many agents can be delivered by this method, but the drug groups most often given by CRI are local anesthetics (lidocaine), opioids (morphine or fentanyl), and *N*-methyl-D-aspartate (NMDA) antagonists (ketamine). Regardless of the drug, a loading dose is typically given immediately before beginning CRI. These drugs can be used as single agents or in combination with one another.

Specific Analgesics

Morphine

The main advantage of giving morphine as a CRI is the avoidance of the peaks and valleys typically seen with opioid bolus dosing. The use of morphine as an intraoperative CRI also allows a reduction in inhalant anesthesia, which can be advantageous in patients with adverse reaction to gaseous agents. Finally, a lower dose of morphine can be used in CRI than in bolus dosing, which can reduce the unwanted side effects of morphine (e.g., dysphoria, panting). Morphine CRI is useful to manage any severe surgical pain and can be safely combined with ketamine or lidocaine.

The CRI dose for morphine follows:

- *Dogs:* 0.2-0.5 mg/kg *slow* IV loading bolus, followed by 0.1-0.3 mg/kg/hr CRI.
- *Cats:* 0.05-0.1 mg/kg IV loading bolus, followed by 0.025-0.2 mg/kg/hr CRI.

Fentanyl

Fentanyl is a full opioid agonist with similar properties to morphine. The main advantages of fentanyl over morphine are rapid onset of action and short half-life, which allow for rapid cessation of unwanted side effects. The major disadvantage is that fentanyl is considerably more expensive than morphine.

The CRI dose for fentanyl follows:

- *Dogs:* 2-5 μg/kg IV loading dose, followed by 5-20 μg/kg/hr CRI intraoperatively.
- *Cats:* 1-2 μg/kg IV loading dose, followed by 5-20 μg/kg/hr CRI.

Lidocaine

Lidocaine is a local anesthetic that provides excellent systemic analgesia when delivered intravenously. Because it is safe for use in patients with gastrointestinal disturbances lidocaine is a good choice for intraoperative analgesia in patients with gastric dilatation and volvulus (GDV) or similar disorders. Lidocaine seems to also provide benefit for patients undergoing procedures with excessive nerve trauma, such as complicated back surgeries or limb amputations. IV lidocaine is extremely short acting and can be discontinued without residual effect almost immediately. Lidocaine CRI should be discontinued if the patient shows signs of toxicity (e.g., muscle tremors, seizures, nausea or vomiting).

The CRI dose for lidocaine follows:

- *Dogs:* 2 mg/kg IV followed by 20-50 μg/kg/min.
- *Cats:* Not recommended.

There are reported lidocaine CRI dosages for cats, but lidocaine usually is not recommended for use in cats because of the potential for severe cardiotoxic effects.

Ketamine

Ketamine is a dissociative anesthetic and NMDA antagonist. Stimulation of NMDA receptors in the spinal cord results in firing of neurons that transmit pain signals. Prolonged bombardment of these receptors, as occurs with intense surgical pain or chronic pain, results in amplification of the signals; the spinal neurons become more easily excited by less stimulation, a condition called *hyperalgesia*. A second phase called *allodynia* follows, in which even nonpainful stimuli are perceived as painful by the spinal cord neurons. This phenomenon, collectively called "wind-up," will be most evident in the postoperative period once the patient has regained consciousness. As an NMDA receptor antagonist, however, ketamine given as an intraoperative CRI binds at these central nervous system (CNS) receptors and prevents wind-up.

Because of its mechanism of action, ketamine is best used to manage neuropathic pain, particularly when the pain has been longstanding and the patient has not responded well to other analgesics. Ketamine should always be given in combination with an opioid, and both can be delivered in the same infusion.

The CRI dosage for ketamine follows:

- *Dogs and cats:* 0.5 mg/kg IV loading bolus, followed by 10 μg/kg/min CRI during surgery and 2 μg/kg/min for 24 hours after surgery.

SURGICAL WOUND CLASSIFICATION

An important intraoperative consideration is whether or not the surgery patient needs intraoperative antibiotics, and if antibiotics are indicated, which type is appropriate. If the surgery is an elective procedure and a possible break in sterility during the surgery is not a concern, antibiotics are generally unnecessary. However, if the surgical procedure is done specifically to treat contaminated or infected wounds, or if possible contamination during an elective procedure is a concern, intraoperative antibiotics may be indicated. Specific guidelines for prophylactic antibiotic use follow this section on wounds.

When determining if antibiotics are indicated, it is helpful to know what type of wound is present. Wounds are classified by several means. One method of classification is by etiology, or cause. In this scheme a surgical wound is called an *incisional wound*; that is, the soft tissue damage (or wound) is caused by the surgeon's scalpel. Another method of classification is based on the duration and degree of wound contamination. *Class 1* wounds are 0 to 6 hours old with minimal contamination; most surgical wounds fall into this class. *Class 2* wounds are 6 to 12 hours old with significant contamination. *Class 3* wounds are over 12 hours old with profound (gross) contamination. However, this system fails to address the contaminated wounds that are new or a few hours old, such as traumatic wounds sustained in animal fights or automobile accidents.

A more useful classification scheme is based only on the *degree of contamination*. Age of the wound is not part of this system. Using degree of contamination to classify wounds helps to guide the veterinarian in making decisions regarding wound management. There are four classes: clean, clean contaminated, contaminated, and infected.

Clean Wound

Surgical wounds made under aseptic conditions are considered "clean." Surgical sites of castration or ovariohysterectomy are considered examples of "clean" wounds (Figure 5-31).

Clean Contaminated Wound

Surgical wounds that are contaminated with contents from the gastrointestinal (GI), respiratory, or urinary tract are considered clean contaminated wounds. The contamination is minimal and easy to remove. Traumatic wounds can be

considered clean contaminated wounds after lavage and debridement (Figure 5-32).

Contaminated Wound

These types of wounds have heavy contamination. Foreign material (e.g., grass, asphalt) and compromised tissue are incorporated in the wound. The wound can become contaminated when there is major spillage from the GI tract. Wounds sustained in fights are another example of contaminated wounds. Wounds located within the mouth cavity are immediately contaminated by oral cavity flora (Figure 5-33).

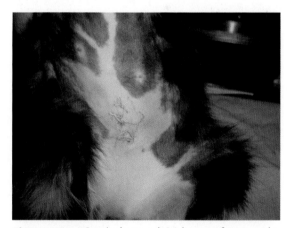

Figure 5-31   Surgical wound 24 hours after completion of procedure; clean wound.

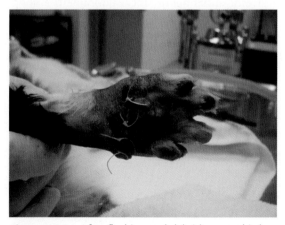

Figure 5-32   After flushing and debridement, this lacerated paw was sutured closed; clean contaminated wound.

Infected Wound

Infected wounds are inflamed, contaminated with many bacterial organisms (by definition greater than 100,000/gram of tissue), purulent discharge (pus), and varying amounts of necrotic (dead) tissue. Traumatic or surgical wounds can progress to become infected if treatment is inadequate or nonexistent (Figure 5-34).

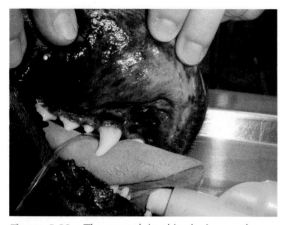

Figure 5-33 The wound in this dog's mouth was caused by a spider bite. Dark red tissue is necrotic. Wound was flushed with sterile saline, and dog received regimen of broad-spectrum antibiotics. Because the wound was located in a contaminated area, in this case the mouth, the wound was initially classified as a "contaminated" wound.

Wounds heal quickest when sutured closed. Depending on the level of contamination, however, the wound may not be sutured closed immediately. If a wound is sutured closed immediately, this is known as *primary closure*. If a wound is left open for a few days, protected with dressings, and sutured closed later, this is known as *delayed primary closure*. If the wound is left open for a longer period (5-7 days) and then sutured closed, this is known as *secondary closure*. It is important to appose healthy skin edges that have an adequate blood supply with sutures or staples. Apposing necrotic skin edges or compromised skin edges together (as opposed to healthy skin edges) will result in dehiscence (sutures pull apart) and delayed healing.

Some wounds may be left to heal close without suturing. This is known as *second-intention healing* (Figure 5-35). Scarring is most likely to occur in second-intention healing. The management of various surgical wounds is addressed in more detail in Chapter 8.

PERIOPERATIVE ANTIBIOTICS

Prophylaxis refers to the measures taken in the prevention of disease. The administration of antibiotics just before and during surgery is known as *perioperative prophylaxis*. The purpose of this practice is to decrease the chances of postoperative infection of the surgical site. Few surgical cases or

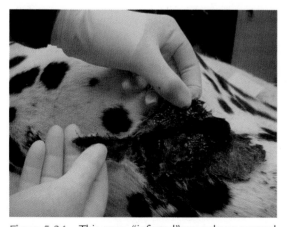

Figure 5-34 This open, "infected" wound was covered with a thick layer of dried, purulent fluid, blood, and fur.

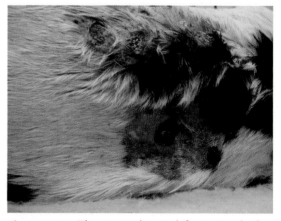

Figure 5-35 These wounds were left unsutured. They healed as open wounds.

circumstances warrant prophylactic antibiotic treatment; one example is an orthopedic procedure involving the placement of implants.

The choice of antibiotic depends on the type of bacterial contamination expected. For example, staphylococci from the skin are of concern in orthopedic procedures. Gram-negative bacteria (e.g., *Escherichia coli*) are of concern in large-bowel procedures. The antibiotic's spectrum of activity should be narrow and limited to the predicted bacterial contaminant.

The antibiotic must be administered by IV injection just before induction. The dose may be repeated during the surgical procedure to ensure adequate serum levels throughout the surgery. The antibiotic administration is usually *not* continued after the procedure is completed. Antibiotics that cannot be administered intravenously are not used as prophylactic antibiotics.

When contamination occurs during surgery, such as leakage from a bowel loop, copious lavage with sterile saline solution is important. Thorough lavage in such cases is often more effective than antibiotic treatment. Diluting the number of bacterial contaminants is the most effective measure to ensure that the animal's immune system can handle the insult. Remember the saying, "The solution to pollution is dilution."

If an animal is taken to surgery with an infection that is already established, the clinician may have prescribed antibiotics for a period before the surgery. This situation is not considered "prophylactic" in nature. The antibiotics have been prescribed in response to an already-established infection. In this case, it is important to continue the administration perioperatively and postoperatively, during the recuperative period. The antibiotic may need to be administered by injection (SQ, IM, or IV) immediately before the surgery. Oral antibiotic administration can be reinstituted as soon as the animal can tolerate ("keep down") food and water after the surgery.

When reconstituting injectable antibiotics, it is important to follow the manufacturer's directions carefully. If sterile water is specified, use it. Do not substitute sterile saline. If the bottle is not packaged under a vacuum, the pressure in the bottle may reach high levels as the diluent (liquid) is

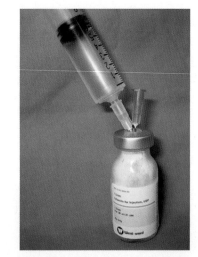

Figure 5-36   When injecting fluid into a stopper bottle, if the bottle is not vacuum-sealed, a vent for the displaced air in the bottle must be created. Here a vent is created by simply inserting a small-gauge (e.g., 22-gauge) hypodermic needle through the stopper.

added. If the content of the bottle is under pressure, some contents may spew from the hole in the rubber stopper as the needle is pulled out of the vial. This is unacceptable and can be prevented by placing a second hypodermic needle through the cap as a vent (Figure 5-36).

KEY POINTS

1. It is important to position the animal on the surgery table in the most natural position possible that does not put excess stress on joints, severely compress blood vessels and nerves, or compromise the well-being of the patient in any way.
2. Quick-release knots are tied so that the patient can be easily and efficiently untied.
3. The cords securing the animal to the table can cause problems if wrapped around the legs too tightly. Check the paws repeatedly throughout the procedure.
4. "Light and lively" is better than "deep and dead." It is safer to keep the patient in a light to moderate plane of anesthesia.
5. Hands-on monitoring can be more reliable than mechanical device monitoring. Mechanical

devices can register incorrect readings. Do not rely exclusively on mechanical monitoring devices.

6. For a full evaluation of the patient's condition and stage of anesthesia, the anesthetist should assess multiple parameters, including reflexes.

7. There is a direct correlation between progression of hypotension and progression of anesthetic depth.

8. To determine a decreasing or increasing trend in body temperature, pulse, and respiratory rate (TPR), the technician must be sure to measure these preanesthetic values of the patient. Preanesthetic TPR is invaluable information.

9. Patients undergoing long surgical procedures may need intraoperative doses of analgesia. "Turning up the gas" is often not sufficient.

10. Intravenous (IV) boluses or constant-rate infusions (CRIs) of analgesics can provide intraoperative analgesia.

11. CRI of the local anesthetic lidocaine provides systemic analgesia to dogs but is generally not used in cats.

12. CRI of the NMDA antagonist ketamine can be an effective way of preventing "wind-up."

13. The best way to prevent infection is to help the patient's immune system by decreasing the exposure to high numbers of microorganisms that could overwhelm the immune system. The use of proper aseptic technique decreases exposure to these microorganisms.

14. Lavage techniques are effective in reducing the number of microorganisms in contaminated or infected wounds; "the solution to pollution is dilution."

15. Antibiotic prophylaxis is a supplement to proper aseptic technique, not an alternative.

REVIEW QUESTIONS

1. What are some safe techniques for preventing hypothermia in small animal surgical patients?
   a. Circulating warm-water pads.
   b. Electric heating pads.
   c. Snuggle Safe discs.
   d. All of the above.
   e. Both a and c.

2. Which of the following is next in the order of events after the patient has been induced with anesthesia, clipped, and had the initial prep applied to the intended surgical site?
   a. The patient is moved to the surgery room, positioned on and secured to the table, then draped, and the surgeon begins surgery by making an incision.
   b. The final prep is applied, and the patient is moved to the surgery room and positioned on and secured to the table.
   c. The patient is moved to the surgery room, the final prep performed, and the patient is positioned on and secured to the table.
   d. The patient is moved to the surgery room, positioned on and secured to the surgery table, and the final prep is performed.
   e. None of the above.

3. Which of the following is *true* regarding positioning patients on the surgery table?
   a. The particular position of the limbs is insignificant because the patient is anesthetized and cannot feel any pain that might be associated with awkward positioning.
   b. Bony prominences should be cushioned to protect against excessive compression.
   c. The patient's legs should not be forced into unnatural anatomic alignment.
   d. All of the above.
   e. Both b and c.

4. What position is the patient placed in for abdominal exploratory surgery?
   a. Sternal recumbency.
   b. Dorsal recumbency.
   c. Right or left lateral recumbency depending on which side of the abdomen needs to be accessed.

5. What can be done to help prevent deep-chested dogs from tilting to the side while in dorsal recumbency?
   a. Using a V-trough.
   b. Bracing the chest with sandbags.
   c. Tying the forelegs crossed over the chest.
   d. All of the above.
   e. Both a and c.

6. *True* or *False:* For orthopedic surgeries of the extremity, only the side of the limb to be incised needs to be clipped and prepped.

7. What position is the patient placed in on the surgery table for thoracic surgery?
   a. Dorsal recumbency.
   b. Right lateral recumbency.
   c. Left lateral recumbency.
   d. Any of the above may be appropriate.
   e. None of the above.

8. *True* or *False:* When scrubbing the skin of the intended surgical site, sufficient friction should be generated to cause hyperemia.

9. *True* or *False:* Chlorhexidine scrub or solution can be used as the final, sterile surgical paint.

10. Which of the following is *true* regarding the sterile field?
    a. Only the surgeon and scrubbed-in surgical assistant are allowed to work in the sterile field.
    b. All sterile instruments must be kept within the boundaries of the sterile field.
    c. The sterile field includes the top surface of the drapes on the patient.
    d. The sterile field includes the top (inner) surface of the surgical pack wrap, which is maintained on or above the instrument table.
    e. All of the above.

11. How frequently should physiologic parameters be recorded in the anesthesia log during a surgery?
    a. Every minute.
    b. Every 5 minutes.
    c. Every 10 minutes.
    d. Whenever the technician has the time.
    e. None of the above.

12. In addition to monitoring the patient's physiologic parameters, what other anesthetic parameters should be tabulated?
    a. Fluid volume administered.
    b. Oxygen flow rate.
    c. Oxygen tank pressure.
    d. Anesthetic gas concentration.
    e. All of the above.

13. If the patient is covered with sterile drapes, making it impossible to auscultate the patient's chest without contaminating the sterile field, what option is available to the anesthetist to monitor heart and lung sounds?
    a. None; other parameters will have to suffice.
    b. Pulse oximeter.
    c. Esophageal stethoscope.
    d. Palpation of peripheral pulses.
    e. None of the above.

14. Which of the following contributes to hypotension?
    a. Hypovolemia.
    b. Fluid overload.
    c. Cardiac insufficiency.
    d. Anesthetic depth.
    e. Answers a, c, and d.

15. *True* or *False:* A cat in the surgical plane of anesthesia will breathe between 8 and 20 breaths per minute.

16. *True* or *False:* "Bagging" the patient by providing assisted ventilation prevents atelectasis.

17. Which of the following contributes to hypothermia in the anesthetized patient?
    a. Anesthetic-induced muscle relaxation.
    b. The surgical prep using water and alcohol.
    c. Administering room-temperature IV fluids.
    d. Breathing cold gases from compressed cylinders.
    e. All of the above.

18. What neurologic parameters can be monitored in the anesthetized patient?
    a. None, because with the patient anesthetized, the neurologic parameters are not valid.
    b. Reflexes.
    c. Muscle tone.
    d. Eye position.
    e. Answers b, c, and d.

19. *True* or *False:* A constant-rate infusion of an intraoperative opioid can greatly reduce the gas anesthetic requirements of the anesthetized patient.

20. When might a patient need an IV bolus of an analgesic drug?
    a. If the patient moves during surgical stimulation.
    b. If the heart rate rapidly increases.
    c. If the blood pressure markedly rises.
    d. All of the above.
    e. None of the above.

21. Which of the following is done if contamination occurs intraoperatively?
    a. Copious lavage of the contaminated area is indicated.
    b. The veterinarian will likely prescribe systemic antibiotics postoperatively.

c. Irrelevant, because under sterile surgical conditions where aseptic technique is practiced, intraoperative contamination cannot occur.
d. Both a and b.

ANSWERS

1. e
2. d
3. e
4. b
5. d
6. False
7. d
8. False
9. False
10. e
11. b
12. e
13. c
14. e
15. True
16. True
17. e
18. e
19. True
20. d
21. d

BIBLIOGRAPHY

Birchard SJ, Sherding RG: *Saunders manual of small animal practice,* ed 2, Philadelphia, 2000, Saunders.

Fossum TW et al: *Small animal surgery,* ed 2, St Louis, 2002, Mosby.

McKelvey D, Hollingshead KW: *Small animal anesthesia and analgesia,* ed 3, St Louis, 2003, Mosby.

Muir WW et al: *Handbook of veterinary anesthesia,* ed 3, St Louis, 2000, Mosby.

Slatter D: *Textbook of small animal surgery,* ed 3, Philadelphia, 2003, Saunders.

CHAPTER 6

Surgical Assisting

Teri Raffel

LEARNING OBJECTIVES

After studying this chapter, the reader should be able to do the following:

- Discuss personal preparation for duties as a surgical assistant.
- Describe the procedure for performing an instrument count.
- Describe the procedure for performing a sponge count.

- Discuss the correct method of loading and passing a scalpel blade and handle.
- Discuss the techniques used to pass various types of surgical instruments safely to the surgeon.
- Discuss the role of the sterile surgical assistant as related to care of the surgical field.

For the veterinary technician with a passion for surgery, performing duties as the surgical assistant (or "scrubbing-in") is a coveted job. The technician performs a critical service for the surgeon in providing retraction of tissue, lavaging the surgical field with sterile fluid, and managing ("running") the instrument table. For the surgeon, having a skilled, qualified assistant can significantly affect the duration and outcome of the surgical procedure.

NUTRITION, HYGIENE, AND APPEARANCE

Before scrubbing-in, the technician must review some personal considerations. If personnel know in advance that they will be assisting on a surgical case, they should consume a meal of substance. Complex carbohydrates (e.g., bagel, bread) and

protein (e.g., peanut butter, meats) will sustain a person longer than a candy bar or other sugar food. The technician should also consume plenty of fluids to combat dehydration, as well as be sure to visit the restroom before the case begins. Who knows how long the surgery will last?

The closeness of the surgical team and the risk of patient infection require consideration of personal hygiene and appearance. All members of the surgical team mutually appreciate daily showers and hair washing. Fingernails need to be kept shorter than the fingertips and free of nail polish. The use of perfume or cologne should be avoided. When working in close quarters, it is respectful to remember that people are becoming increasingly sensitive to smells. More importantly, the smell from perfume or cologne may mask odors from the inhalation gas. It is critical that the anesthetist be able to detect any leaks in the system through odors.

SURGICAL ATTIRE

Proper attire in the operating suite is paramount. Wearing clean scrubs with the shirt tucked in is the first step in dressing appropriately for a surgical case. Tucking in the shirt helps to reduce the amount of normally shed skin deposited at the level of the surgical site. A surgical cap that completely covers the hair should be worn. If facial hair is present (beard, mustache), a beard cover must be worn. Personnel should wear a surgical mask whenever in the surgery room; the mask must be applied properly to work as intended.

Having a dedicated pair of shoes for the surgical area is recommended. If dedicated footwear is not an option, disposable shoe covers should be used. Personnel should remove shoe covers as soon as they exit the operating area.

If eyeglasses are worn, an elastic band or head strap will prevent the glasses from slipping down the nose during surgery. Fogging of the eyeglasses may be a problem for personnel in sterile attire. Simple remedies include applying a no-fog solution to the glasses, taping the glasses to the face, and pinching the mask tightly across the bridge of the nose.

Cell phones and pagers should be removed from pockets and given to the circulating technician. These devices should be available to nonsterile members of the team in the event that a response to a page or call is needed.

For more information on the proper attire of surgical personnel, see Chapter 2.

RESPONSIBILITIES

Once scrubbed-in, maintaining sterility and monitoring the patient must be the primary concerns of the surgical assistant. In addition, the surgical assistant needs to manage the instrument table (i.e., arrange the instruments on the table, count instruments and gauze squares [sponges] before opening and closing a body cavity), pass instruments to the surgeon, retract and moisten tissues, and maintain hemostasis. With all these duties, assistants can easily forget to be considerate of their own body. To avoid becoming weak in the

knees or nauseated during surgery, it is important to avoid locking the knee joints while assisting and to eat before scrubbing-in. Slowly shifting the weight from leg to leg and slightly bending the knees help to prevent blood from pooling in the assistant's feet and to keep the assistant alert.

Instrument Count

The first duty that the surgical assistant should perform is an instrument count. An instrument count documents how many instruments are present at the onset of the case. Before the surgical site is closed, a repeat count of the instruments should be done. Most anesthesia logs have a space to record the initial surgical instrument count and the instrument and "sharps" count at closure. The circulating nurse helps the surgical assistant keep track of how many instruments (if any) were removed from the sterile field and how many sharps were used.

Sponge Count

Next, the assistant should perform a sponge count. Only radiopaque sponges should be used in surgical situations (Figure 6-1). These gauze sponges have a radiopaque string woven into the fiber.

The initial quantity of sponges in the pack is counted before any sponges are used. As the

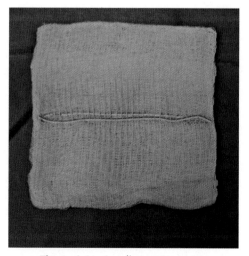

Figure 6-1   A radiopaque sponge.

sponges are used, they should be discarded in a dedicated sponge bowl or kick bucket. The sponge bowl should be a basin located off the sterile field on a back table. As the sponges are discarded, the circulating nurse can unfold and count each sponge. It is important to unfold the sponges to avoid the possibility of two or more sponges sticking together. All sponges, whether gauze squares or laparotomy ("lap") pads, subsequently added to the sterile field must be accounted for as well.

Before the surgical site is closed, the sponges on the sterile field must be counted (by the surgical assistant) and the number of discarded sponges counted (by the circulating nurse), then totaled. The sum of these two groups of sponges must equal the number of sponges documented as entering the sterile field. If the numbers do not agree, the hunt for the missing sponge(s) begins. First, other trash receptacles in the room should be checked to see if a sponge was discarded in an inappropriate place. If the missing sponge is not found there, the sterile team should evaluate the surgical field. Sponges may accidentally become tucked between the folds of the drapes. If the missing sponge is still not recovered, an intraoperative radiograph should be taken. If radiology is not an option, the wound should be closed and a radiograph taken in the immediate postoperative period. Using only radiopaque sponges intraoperatively aids in identifying sponges left in the patient.

The incident must be thoroughly documented in the medical record in the event the sponge(s) is not recovered.

Instrument Handling and Passing

The surgical assistant is responsible for properly passing the instruments to the surgeon, maintaining the instrument (or back) table, and ensuring the working order of the instrumentation throughout the procedure. Setting up and managing the instrument table allows the technician to assist the surgeon more efficiently. An organized table makes it easier for the technician to find the requested instrument quickly. Instruments should be laid out so that the ring handles

(or shafts) of the instruments are closest to the assistant. Where the technician stands in relation to the table and patient dictates which direction the instruments will face.

Some technicians scrub into a procedure with the sole responsibility of managing the instrument table (e.g., for cardiovascular cases, total hip replacements). Cases with extensive instrumentation and equipment will greatly benefit from having a technician "run the table." At other times the technician may be required to scrub-in to assist the surgeon with the procedure.

Properly passing the instruments to the surgeon is a skill that must be mastered not only for efficiency in movement, but for safety as well. The shape and purpose of the instrument will determine the method used to pass the instrument safely and properly to the surgeon.

Scalpel Blades and Handles

Scalpel blades should be handled with the greatest respect. Needle holders are the only instrument that should be used to place the blade onto and to remove the blade from the scalpel handle. The use of any other instrument or device (e.g., hemostat, finger) is inappropriate and can be dangerous. Needle holders are designed to hold metal and therefore can withstand the stress of clamping a metal blade and then placing it on the handle. Hemostats are designed to grasp tissue or vessels and will be damaged by the metal if used to place a blade on a scalpel handle.

When loading a handle with a scalpel blade, the needle holder should firmly grasp the blade on the noncutting edge and slip it onto the handle (Figure 6-2). Once loaded, the handle and blade should be passed to the surgeon in a specific manner. Holding the scalpel handle in hand, the technician should have the blade facing away from the technician's hand, with the point toward the technician (Figure 6-3). The thumb and index finger should be holding the handle with the hand in a supinated position. Pronation of the hand follows as the handle is passed into the waiting hand of the surgeon (Figure 6-4). As the surgeon grasps the handle, the technician should maintain the forward momentum of the hand so as not to contact the cutting edge of the blade.

This method of passing the instrument allows the cutting edge of the blade to face away from the assistant as well as the surgeon for optimal safety and handling.

Threading Eyed Needles

The needle holder should be placed at about two-thirds the needle's curve for secure and controlled handling. The suture to be passed through the eye of the needle should pass from the inside of the needle's curve to the outside. This orientation in the eye will allow the short end of the suture to

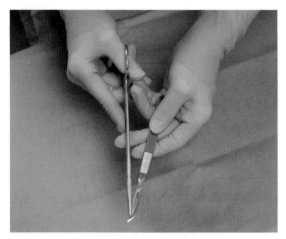

Figure 6-2   Loading the scalpel blade onto the scalpel handle.

fall away from the outside curve of the needle, reducing the chance that the suture will pull out of the needle. When loading a needle holder with a needle and suture, whether threaded or swaged, it is important for the assistant to remember which hand is the surgeon's dominant hand. The needle and suture should be placed in the needle holder so that the surgeon can use it immediately without having to adjust the needle's position. A right-handed surgeon will need the point of the needle facing to the left, whereas a left-handed surgeon will need the needle point facing to the right (Figure 6-5).

Passing Ring-Handled and Other Instruments

When passing an instrument to the surgeon, it is important to remember to place the instrument *firmly* in the palm of the waiting hand to decrease the chance that the instrument will be dropped. The surgeon needs to know that the instrument is in hand without having to look up from the field.

Ring-handled instruments should have the first ratchet closed before the instrument is passed. The ring handles should be facing the floor and the tip of the instrument facing the ceiling. The box lock should be held between the thumb and index finger, with the shaft of the instrument stabilized by the remaining fingers of the delivering hand (Figure 6-6).

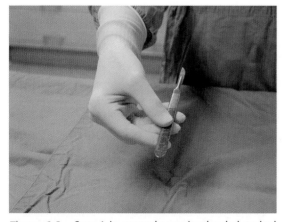

Figure 6-3   Step 1 in properly passing loaded scalpel handle. Scalpel blade is pointed toward assistant, with cutting edge of blade away from hand.

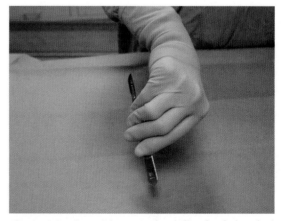

Figure 6-4   Step 2 in properly passing loaded scalpel handle. Assistant pronates hand and places handle firmly in waiting hand of surgeon.

The technician should hold instruments with a curved tip with the curve facing the thumb holding the instrument (Figure 6-7). When held in this fashion, after being passed to the surgeon, the instrument will be positioned for immediate placement on the tissue.

When passing an instrument without ring handles, such as a thumb tissue forceps, the instrument should be held with the tips facing the floor. The other end of the instrument should be held firmly with the thumb and index finger, while the remaining fingers stabilize the instrument (Figure 6-8). When held in this manner, once placed in the hand of the surgeon, the instrument is ready to be used.

Tissue Handling

The careful handling of tissue in the surgical field is an extremely important responsibility of the surgical assistant. Healthy tissue needs to be handled appropriately so as not to cause trauma.

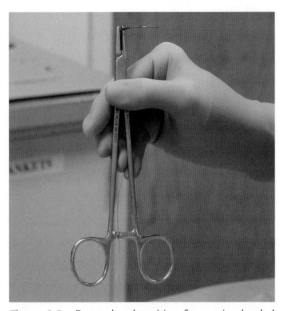

Figure 6-5   Proper hand position for passing loaded needle holder. Needle is loaded for a right-handed surgeon.

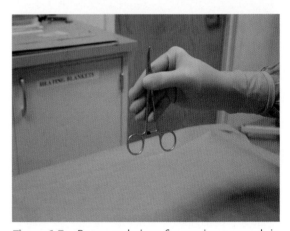

Figure 6-7   Proper technique for passing a curved-tip instrument.

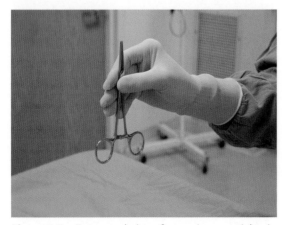

Figure 6-6   Proper technique for passing a straight-tip instrument.

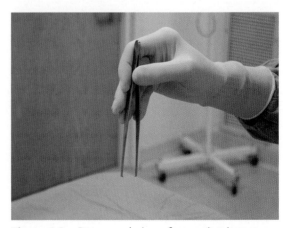

Figure 6-8   Proper technique for passing instrument without a ring handle.

Unhealthy tissue requires extreme care when being handled so as not to compromise its viability further. The surgical assistant must be aware of the status of the tissue in the field and must be familiar with appropriate methods of tissue retraction. Healthy tissue may withstand the pressure of a handheld retractor, but too much pressure may cause vascular tissue damage. If too little retraction is provided, however, the surgeon will not be able to see clearly, and the procedure may be compromised. "Finding a happy medium" is the job of the surgical assistant.

Self-retaining retractors (e.g., Balfour retractor for abdomen, Finochetto retractor for chest) have moist lap pads placed between the blades of the retractor and the tissue. The lap pad acts as a cushion to alleviate excessive pressure on the tissue and helps keep the tissues moist. For some situations the surgeon may choose to place stay sutures in an organ to facilitate retraction or manipulation of the organ. Assistants holding stay sutures must be careful not to hold them too firmly because of the risk of ripping the suture from the tissue.

Keeping Tissues Moist

Another important duty of the surgical assistant is to keep the exposed tissues moist. Systemic hydration should be achieved and maintained through the infusion of intravenous (IV) fluids, but the tissue must be kept moist topically as well. Generally, an isotonic solution such as lactated Ringer's solution or 0.9% normal saline is used as a lavage fluid. Depending on the surgical case, an antibiotic may be added to the solution for topical application.

One of the most important guidelines in surgical assisting states that "moist tissue is happy tissue." If the tissues are kept moist, rather than allowed to dry out, the circulation will be less compromised and tissue function will remain intact. The heat from lights and exposure to room air make tissue vulnerable to adverse conditions.

A bowl on the sterile field can be filled with warm isotonic solution. A single gauze square can be soaked in this lavage solution, then squeezed while suspended above the exposed tissues to drip the lavage solution onto the tissues. It is important to avoid wiping or rubbing the gauze sponge on the tissue directly. The friction created even with gentle wiping or rubbing irritates the tissue and promotes the formation of adhesions between the irritated surface of the affected tissue and other abdominal organs or body tissues. Adhesions may become problematic for the patient, requiring more surgery later to correct. The bowl containing the warm lavage solution should be kept at the back of the instrument table, preferably on a separate tray, so that if spillage does occur, there will be no contamination of the sterile field. Any spilled solution will remain on the tray and will not soak the covering on the table.

Maintaining Hemostasis

Maintaining hemostasis on the surgical field is also an important duty of the scrubbed-in surgical assistant. If vessels are cut, the assistant should be ready to pass the necessary hemostat. Blotting the hemorrhaging site before the surgeon places the hemostat will help the surgeon place the clamp on the vessel and not include excessive tissue in the hemostat. It is important to remember that bleeding tissue should be *blotted*, not wiped, when trying to achieve hemostasis. Wiping with a sponge may cause coagulation already initiated to be wiped away. Firm, but not excessive, pressure blotting is more effective. The blood-soaked sponge count can serve as an estimate of blood loss. A 3 × 3–inch sponge holds approximately 6 ml of blood. A 4 × 4–inch sponge holds approximately 10 ml of blood. Ideally, only radiopaque sponges should be included in surgical packs. Less expensive, nonradiopaque sponges can be used for routine external use.

Hemostasis can also be achieved by the use of electrocautery. The assistant, at the direction of the surgeon, may cauterize tissue or a vessel or may elevate the hemostat that is on the vessel so that the surgeon can activate the cautery.

KEY POINTS

1. Eating before scrubbing-in to assist on a surgical procedure will help prevent the technician from experiencing nausea and hypoglycemia while assisting in surgery.

2. Personal hygiene and proper attire are important factors to address before entering the surgical suite as an assistant.
3. It is the usually the surgical assistant's responsibility to perform both an instrument count and a sponge count before the procedure begins and again before the incision is closed.
4. Proper technique, for safety and efficiency reasons, must be used when passing various types of surgical instruments to the surgeon.
5. Tissue handling is a delicate process and must be properly performed by the surgical assistant.
6. Keeping exposed tissues moist intraoperatively is an essential task of the surgical assistant.
7. Effectively assisting the surgeon includes providing hemostasis on the surgical field.

REVIEW QUESTIONS

1. *True* or *False:* Going into surgery with an empty stomach is the best way for the surgical assistant to avoid experiencing nausea and hypoglycemia should the surgery be unexpectedly long.
2. For which of the following is the surgical assistant responsible?
   a. Monitoring the patient.
   b. Maintaining sterility.
   c. Maintaining hemostasis.
   d. All of the above.
   e. Both b and c.
3. What does managing the instrument table involve?
   a. Keeping the instruments organized for quick retrieval.
   b. Counting instruments and gauze squares at the beginning and end of surgery.
   c. Loading the needle holders with suture needle.
   d. All of the above.
   e. Only a and c.
4. Why is it important to perform an instrument count and a sponge count at the beginning and end of the surgery?
5. Why should radiopaque sponges rather than plain gauze sponges be used in abdominal or thoracic surgery?
   a. They are more absorptive.
   b. They are less abrasive.

c. They can be more easily seen on survey radiographs should they be left in the body cavity.
   d. All of the above.
   e. None of the above.
6. Which of the following should be used to place a scalpel blade on a scalpel handle?
   a. Thumb and index finger of the assistant's nondominant hand.
   b. Any hemostat with secure ratchets.
   c. Needle holder.
   d. All of the above.
   e. None of the above.
7. *True* or *False:* When passing ring-handled instruments to the surgeon, the rings should be firmly placed into the surgeon's palm.
8. *True* or *False:* When passing ratcheted instruments to the surgeon, it is important to remember to keep the ratchets open.
9. Proper tissue handling involves which of the following?
   a. Knowing how much tension the tissue can safely tolerate (without damaging the tissue) while retracting the tissue.
   b. Keeping the tissue moist.
   c. Maintaining hemostasis.
   d. All of the above.
   e. None of the above.
10. *True* or *False:* Rubbing or wiping a "bleeder" with a gauze square is the best means of maintaining hemostasis.
11. *True* or *False:* A 3×3-inch sponge can absorb about 6 ml of blood, and a 4×4-inch sponge can absorb about 10 ml of blood.
12. Why is it important to know the approximate volume of blood a sponge can absorb?

ANSWERS

1. False
2. d
3. d
4. Because if the numbers at the end of the surgery do not match the number of instruments and sponges at the beginning of the surgery, it is possible that an instrument or sponge was accidentally left in the patient's body cavity and will need to be removed before closure is completed

5. c
6. c
7. True
8. False
9. d
10. False
11. True
12. To estimate the amount of blood volume the patient lost intraoperatively

BIBLIOGRAPHY

Fossum TW et al: *Small animal surgery,* ed 2, St Louis, 2002, Mosby.

McCurnin DM, Bassert JM: *Clinical textbook for veterinary technicians,* ed 5, Philadelphia, 2001, Saunders.

CHAPTER 7

Specific Procedures

Michael McCallum, Marta Bates, Zoe Ramagnano,
Marissa Richio, Paula Emma

LEARNING OBJECTIVES

After studying this chapter, the reader should be able to do the following:

- Understand and give a description of each surgical procedure discussed.
- Properly position patients for specific surgical procedures.
- Identify surgical instruments and supplies that may be used for specialized surgical procedures.
- Properly identify the bones and joints of the dog and cat.
- Identify different types of fractures.
- Identify the different types of fixation devices related to fracture repair.
- Discuss the different repair options for cruciate ligament rupture.
- Identify specific biopsy instruments and understand tissue preservation techniques for biopsy samples.
- Discuss minimally invasive options to general surgery, such as endoscopy, laser surgery, and laparoscopy.
- Discuss surgical options for various ophthalmic conditions.
- Discuss surgical options for aural hematomas.
- Drape the patient for specific surgical procedures.
- Discuss the advantages and disadvantages of specific surgical procedures.

RESPONSIBILITIES OF SURGICAL TECHNICIAN

Over the years the role and responsibilities of the surgical technician have increased in numerous ways. In most surgical cases the technician is responsible for preoperative, intraoperative, and postoperative duties. Preoperative duties may include the setting up and breaking down of the operating room (OR), preparation of the OR for specific surgical procedures, maintenance and sterilization of surgical instruments, and preparation of the surgical patient for surgery. Other preoperative duties may include examination of the patient, diagnostic workup, and anesthetic induction.

The intraoperative duties usually involve assisting the surgeon during surgery as a "scrub nurse" (scrubbed-in, gowned, and gloved) or a circulating nurse. As a scrub nurse, assistance may be required for retraction of tissues, bone reduction, wound sponging, suction, and hemostasis. As a circulating nurse, nonsterile circulating assistance may be required. In many practices the technician may also be responsible for monitoring the anesthetized patient while acting as a scrub nurse or surgical assistant.

Postoperatively, the technician's duties may include monitoring of the patient's recovery, as well as care and treatment of the patient while in the hospital. Other postoperative duties may include the cleaning and maintenance of the OR and cleaning, maintenance, and sterilization of the instruments.

In all these roles, the technician is responsible for adhering to strict aseptic and sterile technique. This chapter mainly focuses on the role of the surgical technician intraoperatively.

Being a competent surgical technician, or scrub nurse, requires (1) proficient knowledge of (a) the surgical procedure, (b) the surgical instruments, and (c) aseptic and sterile technique, as well as (2) anticipation of the surgeon's needs. The intraoperative responsibilities of the scrub nurse entail the following:

1. Assist in the sterile draping of the patient.
2. Maintain an orderly surgical field while preventing its contamination by adhering to the strict practice of sterile technique.
3. Organize the instrument table and instruments; the table should be arranged in an orderly and consistent manner.
4. Count sponges and instruments at the beginning of surgery and just before closure of the cavity.
5. Pass instruments and other supplies in an appropriate manner so that the surgeon is not required to turn away from the site to receive them.
6. Assist the surgeon with proper tissue handling, retraction, bone reduction, hemostasis, suture cutting, fluid evacuation, and wound sponging (see Chapter 6).
7. Keep tissues moist throughout the surgery.
8. Practice "running the suture," or holding the suture of a continuous pattern out of the surgeon's way.
9. Save and label all specimens collected during surgery.
10. Collect all "sharps" and related materials throughout the procedure.

ABDOMINAL PROCEDURES

Ovariohysterectomy

Definition: Ovariohysterectomy (OHE, OVH), also called *spay* or *neuter,* refers to the surgical excision of the ovaries and uterus.

Indications: The primary indication for OHE is to sterilize the animal so that it can no longer reproduce. Other indications include the following:

- Neoplasia of reproductive tract
- Treatment of neoplasia elsewhere in the body influenced by reproductive hormones (e.g., mammary tumors)
- Trauma or injury to reproductive tract
- Dystocia (difficult birth)
- Uterine torsion
- Abolition of heat cycle
- Stabilization of other systemic diseases (e.g., diabetes)
- Congenital abnormalities

The OHE is one of the most common surgical procedures performed in small animal practice. Clients may inquire about ovariohysterectomies more than any other surgical procedure. The veterinary technician should be able to communicate to clients the advantages and disadvantages of having their pet spayed or neutered. Clients may have preconceived notions about spaying their pet, and the technician may be responsible for explaining to the client the importance of OHE and correcting any misconceptions.

Common questions that owners may ask the technician about OHE are listed next with appropriate responses.

• "Is it beneficial for my pet to have at least one litter before an ovariohysterectomy is performed?"

There is no benefit for a pet to have at least one litter before an OHE is performed. Many structures of the reproductive tract can become enlarged after the first heat cycle, especially the reproductive vessels. The vascular and organ swelling may require a lengthier surgery. In actuality, it is better to spay your pet before the pet's first heat cycle. Spaying the pet before the first ovarian cycle decreases the incidence of mammary gland tumors to less than 0.5%. If an OHE is performed after the first ovarian cycle, the risk of mammary gland tumors increases to 8%, and after two ovarian cycles, the risk increases to 26%. Intact female cats have a sevenfold higher risk of mammary cancer than that of spayed females. Another obvious argument for spaying a pet is that thousands of unwanted puppies and kittens are euthanized each day at shelters because of overpopulation.

• **"Will my dog or cat become obese after an ovariohysterectomy?"**
Some dogs and cats may gain weight after being spayed, but this is generally caused by inactivity or overfeeding by the owner, not from the spay itself. The technician must tell the owner to adjust the food offered to the pet according to its physical activity level.

• **"Is my dog or cat too old to be spayed?"**
Age can sometimes be a factor with any surgical procedure, but the more important factor is the overall health of the animal. Preoperative blood tests should be considered before performing any surgical procedure (see Chapter 1). Results of preoperative testing may change the anesthesia protocol or cancel an elective surgery.

• **"Does my pet have to be 6 months old to be spayed?"**
There are many factors to consider when deciding what the appropriate age is for an animal to be spayed or neutered. The surgeon's preference is one factor; some surgeons have a personal preference to work with larger, more mature organs, whereas others prefer working with smaller reproductive organs. The individual health of the patient, as determined by the physical examination and pre-anesthetic blood work, is another factor. Another factor to consider is having the appropriate means to prevent or address hypoglycemia or hypothermia, which may be more problematic when spaying or neutering a puppy or kitten less than 5 months old.

• **"Is an ovariohysterectomy free of risk?"**
Any anesthetic or surgical procedure is a risk and this fact should be conveyed to the client.

Every precaution should be taken to avoid a potential disaster (e.g., appropriate preoperative blood tests performed and analyzed, thorough preoperative exams, careful and continuous intraoperative monitoring). Ovariohysterectomies have the same potential complications as any abdominal procedure: complications from anesthesia, delayed wound healing, suture abscesses or tissue reaction to the sutures, and self-inflicted trauma to the surgical wound. Hemorrhage is reported to be the most common cause of death after OHE.

Any long-term disadvantages relating to OHE should also be discussed with the owner. The lack of estrogen circulation can result in urinary incontinence in older spayed females. Some spayed females are more prone to skin disorders as well.

Special Instruments
Surgeons may or may not use a spay hook ("Snook Hook") for OHE. The hook is used to exteriorize the uterine horn. This may allow the surgeon to make a smaller abdominal incision if desired. Spay hooks come in an assortment of sizes; the technician should pick the size appropriate for the animal (Figure 7-1).

Patient Positioning
Most patients are positioned in dorsal recumbency for OHE. This positioning is best suited for a ventral midline incision. Some surgeons may prefer a lateral (flank) approach to the abdomen for an OHE, which requires positioning the patient in lateral recumbency.

Patient Draping
The type of drape used for OHE is the surgeon's preference. Because this is an abdominal procedure,

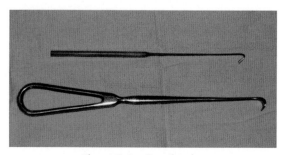

Figure 7-1   Spay hooks.

a four-quarter draping method should be considered (Figure 7-2).

Canine and Feline Ovariohysterectomy Procedures

The ventral abdomen should be clipped and aseptically prepared from the xiphoid process to the pubis. In dogs the start of the incision can be made just caudal to the umbilicus. In cats the incision should be made a bit more caudally. An incision should be made through the skin (Figure 7-3) and the subcutaneous tissue and linea alba (Figure 7-4). The length of the incision is the surgeon's preference.

The left abdominal wall is raised and the spay hook is slid down against the abdominal wall to grasp the horn of the uterus. The hook should be turned to trap the uterine horn, which can then be elevated from the abdomen. In dogs the suspensory ligament should be torn without tearing the ovarian vessels; this allows exteriorization of the ovary. Tearing the suspensory ligament is generally not necessary to exteriorize a cat's ovary. The method of ligation and transection of the pedicle is the surgeon's preference. Surgeons may decide to use clips, the two-clamp method, or the three-clamp method (Figure 7-5). Carmalt, Kelly, or Crile forceps (see Chapter 4) may be used for clamping the pedicles. The forceps used will depend on the size of the pedicle. Two clamps should be placed across the ovarian pedicle, proximal (deep) to the ovary, and one clamp should be placed across the ovarian ligament.

The technician should be knowledgeable about what type of suture the surgeon will be using and have it loaded and ready for use on the instrument table, before it is needed. An absorbable suture material is usually used for pedicle ligation. The size of the suture is the surgeon's preference and will depend on the size of the pedicle. If clips are being used, the technician should have the clip applicator loaded and accessible for the surgeon.

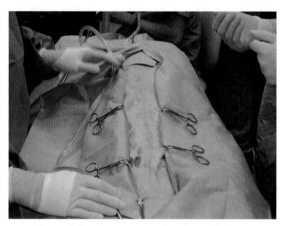

Figure 7-2   Four-quarter draping technique.

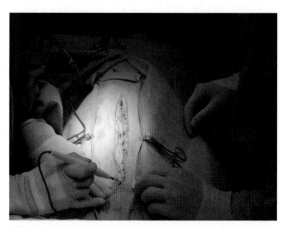

Figure 7-3   Abdominal skin incision. Electrocautery is used for hemostasis of small vessels.

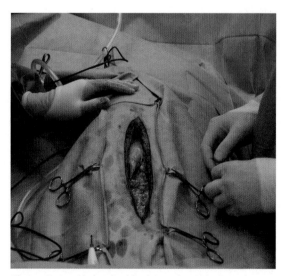

Figure 7-4   Abdominal incision through the subcutaneous tissue and linea alba.

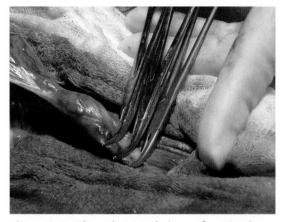

Figure 7-5 Three-clamp technique of uterine horn. Note ovary caudal to hemostats.

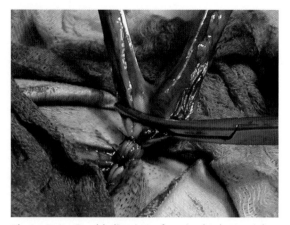

Figure 7-6   Double ligation of uterine body, cranial to cervix.

The surgeon then places a ligature proximal to the ovarian pedicle clamp and securely ties the ligature. One clamp may be removed or "flashed" (unclamping and then reclamping) while the surgeon tightens the ligature. Flashing is done to compress the pedicle and secure the ligature so that it is less likely to slide off once the pedicle is transected. If the ligature is not secure and slides off the pedicle, the pedicle will bleed, and the patient could lose a significant amount of blood and die. If the ligature slides off, the pedicle needs to be isolated (this may require extending the incision more cranially) and the ligature replaced. A second ligature is placed proximal to the first (therefore flashing is not necessary to secure the second ligature) to provide additional security in preventing hemorrhage. The pedicle can then be transected at the level of the third clamp, between the clamp and the ovary. The same procedure can be done for the opposite uterine horn.

The body of the uterus should then be exteriorized, and a two-clamp or three-clamp method can be used. The clamps are placed onto the uterine body, cranial to the cervix. A ligature is placed closer to the cervix (Figure 7-6). A clamp should be placed distal to the ligatures. The surgeon then transects the uterine body between the clamp and the ligatures. The uterine stump should be checked for hemorrhage.

The number of layers closed and the suture pattern used for closure are the preference of the surgeon. In dog spays, most surgeons close the abdominal wall in a three-layer or four-layer closure: (1) linea alba (fascia), (2) subcutaneous tissue, (3) subcuticular tissue, and (4) skin. The linea alba is frequently closed using a simple interrupted suture pattern. The subcutaneous and subcuticular layers are frequently closed using a simple continuous suture pattern.

Surgery Report

A surgery report should be completed for each surgical procedure performed at the hospital. This will be valuable information for any future procedures that may be performed on the animal, as well as any legal issues that could arise. The surgery report provides patient information as well as protection for the hospital. The surgery report should consist of the hospital's name; the owner's name, address, and phone number; the patient's name, date of birth (DOB), species, breed, and hospital identification number, if applicable. A complete record of the surgery performed should be recorded on this form and placed in the animal's record. Box 7-1 shows an example of a surgery report for an ovariohysterectomy.

Cesarean Section

Definition: Cesarean section, also referred to as "cesarotomy" or "hysterotomy," is delivery of a fetus or fetuses by incision through the abdominal wall

BOX 7-1   Surgery Report: Ovariohysterectomy

Animal Hospital Name

Owner: John Doe   **Animal Name:** Sasha

Address: 555 Sterling Lane   **Animal #:** 65656501

        Jupiter, NY 55555   **Species:** Canine

Phone number: 555-5555   **Breed:** Labrador

                                            DOB: 05/05/04

Date of Surgery: 01/03/2005

Primary Surgeon: Dr. Vet

Assistant: Nurse Scrub

Diagnosis or Preoperative Signs: None

Surgical Procedure: OHE

Description of Surgical Procedure

Surgical Approach: A ventral midline skin incision was made from the umbilicus 7 cm caudally toward the pubis. The subcutaneous tissue and fascia were gently incised until the linea alba was visualized.

Surgical Pathology: Intact female. No abnormalities noted on gross examination.

Surgical Procedure: A stab incision was made into the linea alba 1 cm caudal to the umbilicus. The linea was incised over the length of the incision using forceps as a guard. The uterine body was isolated and traced up to the right ovary. The suspensory ligament was strummed loose and the right ovary exteriorized. Using the three-clamp technique, the ovarian pedicle, including the artery and vein, was ligated with two encircling ligatures using 2-0 chromic gut. The ovary was then excised from the pedicle. The pedicle was observed receding into the abdomen with no significant hemorrhage. This procedure was repeated on the left side. The broad ligament was manually broken down on both sides, and the cervix was visualized. Using the three-clamp method, a ligature was placed around the uterine body. An incision was made between the clamps, and the uterine stump was observed for hemorrhage. The ovarian pedicles were located and rechecked for hemorrhage before closing.

Closure:
Linea alba: 2-0 polydioxanone (PDS) in simple interrupted suture pattern.
Subcutaneous tissue: 3-0 PDS in simple continuous suture pattern.
Subcuticular tissue: 3-0 Monocryl in simple continuous suture pattern.
Skin: 3-0 nylon in simple interrupted cruciate suture pattern.

and uterus. The word "cesarean" has no relation to the birth of Julius Caesar, as some believe.

Indications: The primary indication for a cesarean section is *dystocia* (difficult birth). Dystocia can develop from the following situations:

- Maldeveloped fetuses
- Oversized fetuses
- Malpositioned fetuses
- Small pelvic canal size of dam
- Previous pelvic trauma of dam
- Insufficient dilation
- Uterine inertia (lack of contractility of uterus; can result from overstretching of uterus, toxemia, obesity, or exhaustion)

The objective of a cesarean section is to remove all the fetuses from the uterus as swiftly as possible. Although it may be performed as an intervention in an emergency, cesarean section is frequently planned for brachycephalic breeds (e.g., boxers, bulldogs, Pekingese, pugs) or animals with a history of dystocia. Published reviews indicate that 60% to 80% of dystocia cases require surgery.

Stages of Labor

Stage 1 of labor, commonly referred to as the "nesting stage," begins with the onset of uterine contractions and can last 6 to 12 hours. This stage ends when the cervix is dilated.

Stage 2 of labor begins with full dilation of the cervix, entry of the first fetus into the birth canal, and rupture of the fetal membranes. Abdominal contractions begin at this stage. It may take up to 4 hours for the first fetus to be delivered and up to 2 to 3 hours for subsequent fetuses. If delivery of subsequent fetuses takes longer than 4 hours, or if there are strong abdominal contractions for more than an hour without delivery of a fetus, the owner should contact the veterinarian.

Stage 3 of labor is passage of the placenta.

Special Instruments

A general-use soft tissue surgery pack should provide the surgeon with the necessary instruments needed for cesarean section. Extra hemostats should be available. Extra hands will also be needed to help warm and resuscitate the puppies or kittens.

Patient Positioning

For cesarean section the patient should be positioned in dorsal recumbency.

Patient Draping

A four-quarter draping technique should be used for cesarean section.

Cesarean Section Procedure

Cesarean sections can be performed in three different ways, as follows:

1. Cesarean without an ovariohysterectomy. The owner may elect not to spay the animal. The veterinarian should inform the owner of the possibility of future dystocia in this pet. In addition, the surgeon may open the abdomen, inspect the uterus, and discover that the uterus has deteriorated to such an extent that leaving it in the abdomen is no longer an option.
2. Cesarean followed by an ovariohysterectomy. An indication to perform this procedure may be to prevent the animal from having dystocia in the future.
3. En bloc resection (radical resection of the uterus; neonates removed after resection of uterus). En bloc removal of the uterus may be optional or essential because of possible fetal compromise or uterine viability.

For all three procedures, the ventral abdomen should be clipped, preliminary abdominal preparation performed, and urinary bladder emptied before entering the OR. The animal should be rapidly anesthetized in the OR, and a final surgical "prep" should be performed while the surgeon and scrub assistant are preparing for surgery. After the animal is draped, a ventral midline incision should be made into the skin and subcutaneous tissue, from just cranial to the umbilicus and continuing caudally to the pubis. The external rectus sheath should be elevated with forceps before making the stab incision into the abdomen, to avoid lacerating the uterus.

Cesarean Without Ovariohysterectomy

The uterine horns should be gently exteriorized from the abdomen (Figure 7-7). It is extremely important that this process be done carefully to avoid tearing the uterine vessels. The uterus should be isolated with moistened laparotomy ("lap") sponges to help prevent contamination of the abdomen. The scrub nurse should have the sponges moistened in warm saline and ready to place under and around the uterus.

The surgeon then incises the uterine body. The uterine body should be tented on incision to avoid damage to the fetuses. The incision is made on the ventral aspect of the uterus and can be extended using Metzenbaum scissors (not a blade). Each horn should be emptied by squeezing each fetus cranially toward the incision (Figure 7-8). The fetus can then be gently lifted out of the uterus (Figure 7-9) and the amniotic sac manually ruptured. The scrub nurse should have hemostats available for clamping off the umbilical cord of each neonate. Once clamped, the surgeon then severs the cord.

Care should be taken at this point to make every attempt to avoid contamination of the abdomen and surgical field with amniotic fluid. An abundance of lap sponges will aid in this endeavor. If the placenta easily separates from the uterus, it will be removed with the neonate. Each neonate should be passed to a nonsterile assistant. When the fetuses are being passed to the nonsterile assistant, breaks in sterility can occur

and should be monitored closely by a nonsterile technician.

The scrub nurse should always be focused on the surgical procedure and the patient in front of him or her. After removal of all obvious fetuses, a meticulous examination of the uterus should be performed from the ovaries to the cervix to make certain that no fetuses remain. A local lavage of the external uterus should be performed after closure of the uterine incision. The specific technique used for closure of the abdomen ("closure") and the suture used to close the incision are the choice of the surgeon. An absorbable suture

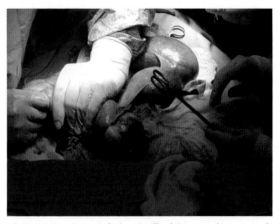

Figure 7-8   Fetus is being "milked," or gently squeezed, toward the hysterotomy incision.

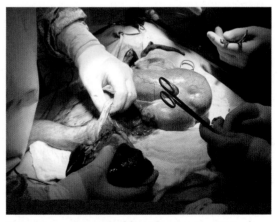

Figure 7-9   Removal of fetus from uterus. Note abundance of laparotomy sponges isolating uterus from abdomen.

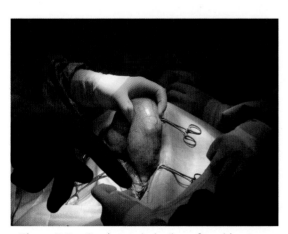

Figure 7-7   Gentle exteriorization of gravid uterus.

172   Part II   *Intraoperative Considerations*

should be used for closure of the uterus. After closure of the uterine body, the abdominal cavity should be lavaged with warm saline in case the abdomen was contaminated with uterine contents (amniotic fluid). "The solution to pollution is dilution" holds true for any surgical case in which bacteria may have entered the sterile abdomen (e.g., gastrointestinal tract).

Cesarean Followed by Ovariohysterectomy

An OHE may be performed after the cesarean section, as previously described.

En Bloc Resection

The first step in an en bloc resection is to isolate the ovarian pedicles. Separation of the broad ligament from the uterus is done at the point of the cervix. Any fetuses within the vagina will have to be directed back into the uterine body. The uterine body should be clamped at the cranial aspect of the cervix. Once the ovarian pedicles and the uterine body are clamped, the surgeon transects between the clamps, and the ovaries and uterus are removed. The uterus is handed off to nonsterile personnel. Again, breaks in sterility can easily occur at this time and should be monitored. The nonsterile personnel need to remove the fetuses from the uterus (see following discussion). Once the uterus is removed en bloc ("as a whole"), the surgeon ligates the ovarian and uterine pedicles with two ligatures. The pedicles should be examined for bleeding before closing. A warm lavage of the abdomen will help with any contamination of the abdomen from uterine spillage and will also help warm the dam.

Closure of the abdomen is done according to the surgeon's preference. Some surgeons may close the abdomen in three layers, and others may choose to close in four layers (linea alba, subcutaneous, subcuticular, skin). Some surgeons may finish with a subcuticular layer or intradermal layer rather than placing skin sutures (closing in three layers). This is done to avoid irritation of the neonates from the skin suture ends during the nursing process.

Neonatal Care

The care of the neonates generally is the responsibility of the nurse or technician. This job can be extremely rewarding, especially if the neonates are able to be resuscitated successfully and can leave the hospital with their mother. If the neonates are transferred still in the uterus, the technician will need to incise the uterus, as by tenting the uterus and using Metzenbaum scissors. Extreme caution must be used when incising the uterus so as not to injure the neonates. The amniotic sac on each neonate will need to be broken as well.

The technician should have a warm, dry area prepared for the neonates before surgery. The area should include some or all of the following: plenty of clean, warm towels; a radiant lamp; hair dryer; and circulating warm water heating pads. Drugs to have available include naloxone (opioid antagonist), doxapram (respiratory stimulant), and epinephrine (cardiovascular stimulant). Suture and scissors should also be available to ligate the umbilical cords. The neonates should be dried off immediately with warm towels (Figure 7-10). A heating unit should be used to aid in the warming process. The neonates should be briskly rubbed to initiate spontaneous respiration. Some hospitals recommend firmly grasping the neonate and swinging downward (making sure the head and neck are held securely). The centrifugal force helps remove fluid from the nasopharyngeal region.

The nurse or technician also must ensure that the clamp on the umbilicus is secure and there is no unnecessary pulling on the umbilicus. Strain on the umbilical cord can cause abdominal herniation

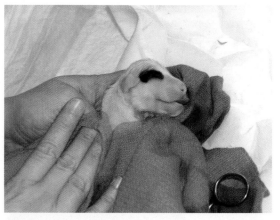

Figure 7-10   Initiation of tactile stimulation for neonate.

from the umbilical site. An infant suction bulb can be used to help aspirate fluid from the oropharynx and nares (Figure 7-11). If opioids were used as a premedication for the dam, a drop of naloxone can be placed under the tongue of each neonate to reverse the effects of the opioids on the neonates. If respiratory efforts of the neonate are slow to commence, a drop of doxapram placed under the tongue can be used to aid in respiratory stimulation. If the newborn has an appropriate heart rate (120-150 beats/min) but is still having respiratory-related issues, tactile stimulation and administration of oxygen by mask may be successful in instituting respiration. If respiratory efforts do not commence within about 30 seconds, or if bradycardia occurs, the nurse may need to administer positive-pressure ventilation by mask. The newborn may need to be intubated and ventilated until it starts to take breaths on its own (Figure 7-12).

Once respiration has been achieved, cardiovascular stability must be addressed, especially if the patient is bradycardic or has a weak heartbeat. If no heartbeat can be identified, chest compressions should be administered using fingers across the lateral chest wall. If chest compressions appear unsuccessful, epinephrine can be administered under the tongue.

Some neonates never achieve respiration or a heartbeat once retrieved from the uterus, but every attempt should be made to revive the newborn.

A newborn's survival can depend on each individual situation. How long the fetus was wedged in the canal or how long the dam was in labor can determine the outcome. Whimpering and crying sounds from the newborns are always a good sign.

Once the newborn has been stabilized with an adequate respiratory rate and an adequate heart rate, the umbilical cord can be ligated and transected approximately 1 to 2 cm from the body (Figure 7-13). The newborns should be kept in a warm environment (about 90° F) until the mother's surgery is complete, and oxygen supplementation may be a necessary part of a successful resuscitation (Figure 7-14).

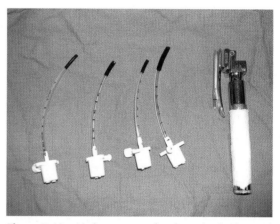

Figure 7-12 Various neonatal endotracheal tubes and pediatric laryngoscope.

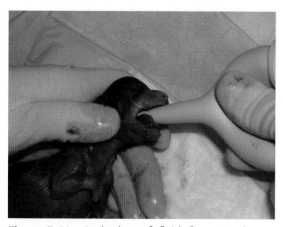

Figure 7-11 Aspiration of fluid from oropharynx using an infant suction bulb.

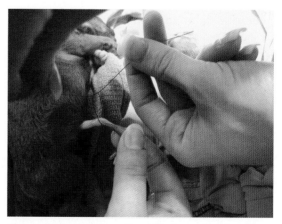

Figure 7-13 Ligation of umbilical cord 1 to 2 cm from body wall.

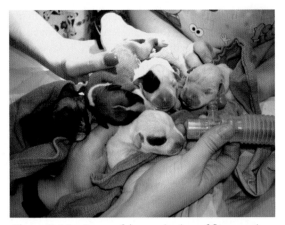

Figure 7-14   Successful resuscitation of five puppies.

The mammary glands of the dam should be cleaned after surgery to remove any surgical prep solutions as well as any blood. The newborns should be reunited with their mother, and nursing should commence as soon as possible. The mother's behavior toward the newborns should be observed during the first few hours. Care should be taken not to return the newborns with their mother too soon. She could inadvertently injure them if she is not fully recovered. Some mothers may reject or kill their young, so careful observation is important.

To reduce stress and exposure to pathogens and nosocomial infections, the bitch and the newborns should be released from the hospital as soon as possible.

Box 7-2 shows an example of a surgery report for a cesarean section.

Abdominal Exploratory Surgery

Definition: Abdominal exploratory surgery refers to surgical exploration of the abdominal cavity. Related terms include the following:

- **Celiotomy:** Surgical incision into the abdominal cavity.
- **Laparotomy:** Flank incision into the abdominal cavity. Laparotomy is typically used interchangeably with other terms to describe any approach into the abdomen.

Indications: Exploratory surgery may be indicated for a variety of reasons. Most often an exploratory surgery is indicated for diagnostic or curative purposes. Diagnostic purposes include obtaining surgical biopsies of abdominal organs for analysis because of a chronic disease process. Curative surgery may be required because of an *acute abdomen,* which refers to a sudden onset of clinical signs associated with the abdomen. Some causes of acute abdomen can be life threatening and may require an emergency exploratory laparotomy. Common indications for abdominal exploratory surgery include abdominal masses and traumatic injury to the abdomen.

The veterinarian must distinguish whether a patient requires abdominal exploratory surgery or can be medically managed. To make this determination, the veterinary team begins by first collecting a history on the patient from the owner. After a history, a thorough physical examination is performed. The results of the physical examination may lead the veterinary team to proceed to the diagnostic testing stage. Diagnostic tests may include radiographs, ultrasound, and laboratory analysis. All these findings will help the veterinary team in determining the patient's status and whether the patient is a candidate for surgery.

Special Instruments
The Balfour retractor is a self-retaining abdominal retractor (Figure 7-15). The Balfour retractor holds the abdomen open and allows for full exposure of abdominal contents. Balfour retractors are available in different sizes, and selection of the appropriate size is based on the size of the patient. Other special instruments may be needed depending on the results of the abdominal exploratory surgery. A routine surgical instrument pack should be sufficient for this procedure.

Patient Positioning
For abdominal exploratory surgery the patient should be positioned in dorsal recumbency for a ventral midline approach.

Patient Draping
Because this is an abdominal procedure, a four-corner draping method should be considered.

BOX 7-2   Surgery Report: Cesarean Section

Animal Hospital Name

Owner: John Doe

Address: 555 Sterling Lane

Juniper, NY 55555

Phone number: 555-5555

Animal Name: Sasha

Animal #: 656565

Species: Canine

Breed: Labrador

DOB: 05/05/03

Date of Surgery: 1/05/2005

Primary Surgeon: Dr. Vet

Assistant: Nurse Scrub

Diagnosis or Preoperative Signs: Dystocia

Surgical Procedure: Cesarean section

Description of Surgical Procedure

Surgical Approach: A ventral midline skin incision was made cranial to the umbilicus and extended caudally 10 cm.

Surgical Pathology: Three neonates were removed from the uterus.

Surgical Procedure: An incision was made through the subcutaneous tissue and linea alba into the peritoneal cavity. The fetus-distended uterus was identified, exteriorized, and packed off with moistened lap sponges. A 5-cm longitudinal incision was made into the ventral aspect of the uterine body, and three puppies were milked out one by one. A hemostat was placed on the umbilical cords, and the umbilical cords were transected. The puppies were handed to the assistants. The remaining placenta was grasped with forceps and removed from the uterine body. The uterus was closed, and the abdomen was lavaged with sterile saline before closure of the peritoneal cavity. Hemostasis was maintained throughout the surgery with the aid of monopolar cautery.

Closure:
Uterine body: 3-0 PDS in two continuous layers.
Linea alba: 2-0 PDS using simple interrupted suture pattern.
Subcutaneous tissue and subcuticular layer: each closed with 2-0 PDS using simple continuous suture pattern.
Tissue adhesive was applied to the skin.

Abdominal Exploratory Procedure

The ventral abdomen should be clipped from just above the xiphoid process to the pubis. Adequate hair clipping is important because the incision may need to be extended either cranially or caudally for better exposure. A blade is used to incise the subcutaneous tissues, and the abdominal wall should be tented to make a sharp incision into the linea alba. The falciform fat attachments can be digitally broken down on one side of the body wall, or electrocautery can be used to remove them together. The removal of the falciform fat may allow for better exposure of the abdominal organs. The technician can moisten laparotomy sponges and place them on either side of the incision. The Balfour retractor should be placed to allow full exposure of the abdominal cavity. When placing a Balfour retractor, the assistant should visualize the insertion on the side of the surgeon, and the surgeon should visualize insertion on the side of the assistant. This is done to avoid entrapping any organs within the Balfour retractor.

The surgeon then performs a systematic exploration of the entire abdomen and its contents. Most surgeons have a system for exploring the abdomen and conduct the exploration the same way each time they perform the procedure. This is done to ensure that all organs and structures are observed and a possible disease process is not overlooked. The scrub nurse should note any abnormalities seen within the abdominal cavity and record the findings in the pathology section of the surgery report (Box 7-3).

Gastric Foreign Bodies and Gastrotomy

Definition: A gastric foreign body is any ingested foreign object that becomes lodged in the stomach and is unable to be digested; it may also be referred to as a "gastric obstruction." A distinction

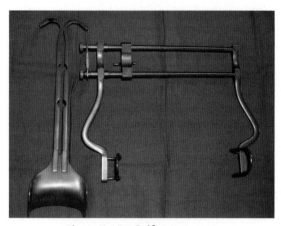

Figure 7-15   Balfour retractor.

BOX 7-3   Systematic Exploration of the Abdominal Cavity

1. Explore the cranial quadrant.
   - Examine the diaphragm (including the esophageal hiatus) and the entire liver (palpate the liver).
   - Inspect the gallbladder and biliary tree; express the gallbladder to determine its patency.
   - Examine the stomach, pylorus, proximal duodenum, and spleen.
   - Examine both pancreatic limbs (palpate *gently*), the portal vein, hepatic arteries, and caudal vena cava.
2. Explore the caudal quadrant.
   - Inspect the descending colon, urinary bladder, urethra, and prostate or uterine horns.
   - Inspect the inguinal rings.
3. Explore the intestinal tract.
   - Palpate the intestinal tract from the duodenum to the descending colon, and observe the mesenteric vasculature and nodes.
4. Explore the "gutters."
   - Use the mesoduodenum to retract the intestine to the left, and examine the right "gutter." Palpate the kidney, and examine the adrenal glands, ureter, and ovary.
   - Use the descending colon to retract the abdominal contents to the right. Examine the left kidney, adrenal gland, ureter, and ovary.

From Fossum TW et al: *Small animal surgery,* ed 2, St Louis, 2002, Mosby.

is made between *gastric* foreign bodies, which are found in the stomach, and *intestinal* foreign bodies, which are found anywhere in the intestines (duodenum, jejunum, ileum, or large intestine). *Linear* foreign bodies are objects that usually consist of string or thread and are seen most often in felines. With linear foreign bodies, a part of the foreign object may become lodged under the tongue or in the stomach, while the rest of the object continues through the intestines. Linear foreign bodies may cause *plication* (pleating or folding) of the intestines.

Indications: A primary reason to perform a gastrotomy (incision into the stomach) is to remove a foreign body. In dogs, foreign bodies include rocks, plastic, toys, bones, coins, corncobs, and cassette tapes. Dogs tend to be indiscriminate eaters and will eat or swallow an assortment of objects. Another indication to perform a gastrotomy is for the retrieval of full-thickness gastric biopsies or neoplasia removal. Common gastric neoplasias in dogs and cats include adenocarcinoma, lymphosarcoma, leiomyosarcoma, and leiomyoma.

Common foreign bodies in cats include *trichobezoars* (hairballs), string, yarn, and thread. In cats, linear foreign bodies are frequently affixed under the tongue or at the pyloric sphincter and may cause intestinal plication. If a linear foreign body is suspected, the base and underside of the tongue should be inspected for the presence of a foreign object. Younger animals present most often with foreign bodies because of their behavior, but an animal of any age can present with a gastric or intestinal foreign body. Animals at higher risk for foreign bodies are those that have a history of foreign body ingestion or have conditions that predispose them to *pica* (craving for unnatural articles of food).

The most common clinical sign associated with a foreign body is vomiting. Vomiting may be intermittent, and some animals may otherwise act normal. Vomiting may be absent if the object is in the fundus of the stomach rather than obstructing the pyloric sphincter. Other clinical signs include lethargy, abdominal pain, anorexia, and depression. Clinical signs can be much worse

if the foreign body has perforated the stomach and caused peritonitis.

Diagnostic testing for gastric foreign bodies should include radiographs of the abdomen. Radiopaque foreign bodies may be apparent on survey films. Many foreign bodies are radiolucent and therefore may require contrast medium to identify. One common contrast study is the *barium study*. The patient is administered barium orally, then a series of films is taken at predetermined intervals. The foreign body either becomes highlighted by the surrounding barium, or the barium discontinues movement through the gastrointestinal (GI) tract. By comparing the time required for the barium to move through the stomach and into the intestine to normal gastric emptying time, a delay in gastric emptying can be identified and a foreign body suspected. Barium should not be used if a perforation of the stomach is suspected.

Endoscopy should be considered, if available in the practice and if a gastric foreign body is suspected, because it can be highly diagnostic and minimally invasive. Endoscopy allows the veterinarian to look at the inside lining of the stomach as well as the contents. A flexible scope is passed through the mouth of an anesthetized patient down the esophagus and into the stomach to view the contents. If the foreign object is small and blunt, the veterinarian may be able to retrieve the object through endoscopy. If the object is too large to bring back through the esophagus or has sharp edges that could perforate the esophagus, gastric surgery is indicated. A large object may become lodged in the esophagus on retrieval. Because esophageal surgery includes more risks than gastric surgery, performing a gastrotomy is preferred.

Special Instruments

A general soft tissue surgical pack should be sufficient for this surgery if only a gastrotomy is required. A Balfour abdominal retractor should be available. The technician should ensure that all instruments used within the stomach are kept away from the rest of the surgical instruments. The technician and surgeon must avoid contaminating the sterile abdomen with bacteria from the stomach. A good way to approach this situation is to have a sterile towel on which all gastric instruments can be placed during the gastrotomy. Once the gastrotomy is complete, gloves should be changed, and the gastrotomy instruments should be removed from the instrument table and replaced with new, sterile instruments.

Patient Positioning
The patient should be positioned in dorsal recumbency to perform a ventral midline incision.

Patient Draping
A four-quarter draping method should be considered for gastrotomy.

Gastrotomy Procedure
The entire ventral abdomen should be clipped from a few inches cranial to the xiphoid process and extend caudally to the pubis. This is done so that the veterinarian can make an incision long enough to inspect the entire GI tract during the surgery for linear foreign bodies or other possible intestinal foreign bodies.

Once the patient has been positioned and prepared for surgery, a ventral midline incision through the skin, subcutaneous tissue, and linea alba is made from the xiphoid process caudal to the umbilicus. This incision may need to be extended caudally for more exposure. Removal of falciform fat and placement of a Balfour retractor may also allow better exposure to the abdominal organs. The surgeon should inspect the abdominal contents before proceeding with the foreign body removal. The stomach should be identified and isolated. The scrub nurse can isolate the stomach by packing it off from the rest of the abdominal contents. The surgeon will locate the area of the stomach to incise (Figure 7-16). Stay sutures are placed on either side of the proposed incision site (Figure 7-17). Stay sutures allow for manipulation of the stomach as well as prevent leakage of gastric fluid into the abdomen. A stab incision is made with a new scalpel blade (not the same one used to make the initial skin incision) between the stay sutures, in a hypovascular region of the ventral stomach. The incision is generally made between the greater and lesser

curvatures of the stomach. The scrub nurse should have the suction ready to place into the stab incision and drain the gastric fluid. The surgeon then extends the incision with Metzenbaum scissors. An Allis tissue forceps can generally be used to grasp the foreign body and remove it from the stomach (Figure 7-18).

The stomach can be closed in two layers. The first layer is a simple continuous pattern of a 2-0 or 3-0 absorbable suture. This suture pattern provides apposition. The second layer is a continuous inverting pattern of 3-0 absorbable suture.

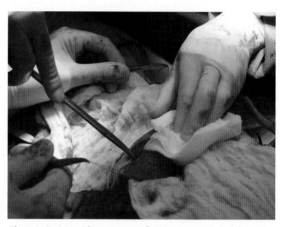

Figure 7-16   Placement of stay sutures in the gas-distended stomach of a dog with a gastric foreign body.

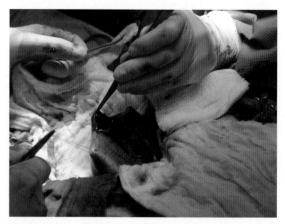

Figure 7-17   Gastrotomy incision is made between the stay sutures. Note that stay sutures are gently lifted upward to avoid leakage of gastric fluid.

It may be beneficial to perform a local lavage of the gastric incision site to help dilute any pollutants. The gloves of the scrub team should be changed, and all instruments that were used within the stomach should be removed from the table. Any instruments used to close the abdomen should be instruments that were kept out of the stomach during surgery. A warm lavage of the entire abdomen should be performed, and the abdomen can be closed routinely.

Postoperative Considerations and Instructions

One goal postoperatively for gastrotomy patients is to correct any prior fluid loss or electrolyte imbalance. If the patient continues to vomit after surgery, food and water should be withheld and intravenous fluids should be continued. Centrally acting antiemetics can be administered to help control the vomiting. In the absence of vomitus, a bland diet can be introduced 12 to 24 hours postoperatively. Prognosis for the gastrotomy patient should be considered good if there were no perforations in the stomach from the foreign body. If perforations were evident, and peritonitis (inflammation of the peritoneum) was present, the prognosis may be considered guarded. On discharge of the patient, postoperative instructions for the client should include the same general discharge instructions listed in Chapter 11.

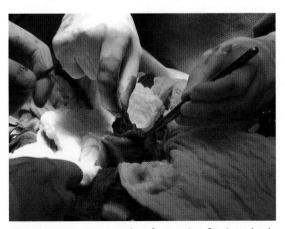

Figure 7-18 Removal of gastric foreign body (peach pit).

Box 7-4 shows an example of a surgery report for a gastrotomy.

Intestinal Foreign Bodies and Enterotomy

Definition: Foreign bodies of the intestines are any intraluminal obstruction of intestinal contents caused by an ingested object or objects; these bodies may also be referred to as "intestinal obstructions."

Indications: A primary indication to perform an enterotomy (incision into the intestines) is to remove a foreign body. Some foreign bodies have the ability to pass through the esophagus and stomach but are too large to pass through the intestines. The objects found in dogs and cats as gastric foreign bodies can also be found in the intestines (e.g., corncobs, balls, bones, peach pits, linear objects such as string). Intestinal foreign bodies may cause a partial or complete obstruction of the intestinal bowel. Some foreign bodies may slowly make their way through the intestinal tract, causing damage or perforations along the way. Others may become lodged in a segment of intestine where they cause a complete obstruction. A *complete* obstruction will prevent intestinal chyme (intestinal contents) to proceed beyond the obstruction. A *partial* obstruction may allow some intestinal contents to move beyond the point of the foreign object.

The most common clinical signs associated with an intestinal foreign body include abdominal pain, vomiting, diarrhea, depression, anorexia, and weight loss. The location (proximal vs. distal), type (partial vs. complete), and duration of the obstruction can be related to the clinical signs. Complete obstructions cause more acute and serious signs. More proximal obstructions may cause persistent vomiting and dehydration. Clinical signs of distal (e.g., ileum) and partial obstructions may include lethargy, intermittent anorexia, and intermittent vomiting.

Linear foreign bodies can present with any or all of these clinical signs. A portion of the linear foreign body may become embedded at the base of the tongue or pylorus, while the rest of the object moves down the intestinal tract due to

BOX 7-4   Surgery Report: Gastrotomy

Animal Hospital Name

Owner: John Doe

Address: 555 Sterling Lane

        Jupiter, NY 55555

Phone number: 555-5555

Animal Name: Sasha

Animal #: 656565

Species: Canine

Breed: Labrador

DOB: 05/05/04

Date of Surgery: 01/03/2005

Primary Surgeon: Dr. Vet

Assistant: Nurse Scrub

Diagnosis or Preoperative Signs: Gastric foreign body

Surgical Procedure: Gastrotomy

Description of Surgical Procedure

Surgical Approach: A ventral midline skin incision was made extending from approximately 2 cm below the xiphoid process to approximately 6 cm cranial to the pubis. Subcutaneous tissue was bluntly dissected to expose the linea alba. The linea alba was incised to expose the abdominal cavity and viscera.

Surgical Pathology: Foreign bodies (tennis ball remnants) were present in the stomach. No perforations or necrosis of the stomach were noted. All other organs were grossly unremarkable.

Surgical Procedure: The abdominal cavity was thoroughly explored for any gross abnormalities or perforations in the gastrointestinal tract. Stay sutures were placed in the stomach using 3-0 PDS. The stomach was gently retracted from the abdominal cavity, where an incision approximately 5 cm long was made over a relatively avascular area of the gastric body between the greater and lesser curvatures of the stomach. All foreign material was removed from the stomach. The abdominal cavity was lavaged with 3 liters of warm saline and closed routinely.

Closure:
Gastric mucosa and submucosa: 3-0 PDS in simple continuous suture pattern.
Gastric seromuscular layer: 3-0 PDS in Cushing pattern.
Linea alba: 2-0 PDS in simple continuous suture pattern.
Subcutaneous tissue: 3-0 PDS in simple continuous suture pattern.
Subcuticular layer: 3-0 Monocryl in simple continuous suture pattern.
Skin: skin staples.

peristaltic movement. Continuous peristalsis and resultant plication of the intestines (folding or bunching up of the intestines on themselves along the length of the linear foreign body) can cause the linear foreign body to be pulled tightly. This tightly pulled string now acts as a knife along the compromised intestinal tissue and cuts into the mucosa of the intestines, causing perforations along the way. The damage to the mucosa and the perforations can result in peritonitis.

The intestinal plication and peritonitis cause great abdominal pain. When the abdomen is palpated on a patient with plicated intestines and peritonitis, the abdominal muscles will frequently tighten, indicating abdominal pain.

Another indication to perform an enterotomy is biopsy retrieval from an intestinal segment. Malignant intestinal tumors are common and can cause partial or complete obstruction. The different types of intestinal neoplasias are mentioned in the following section on intestinal resection and anastomosis.

Diagnostic tests should include radiographs and blood work. Blood analysis will help determine hydration status as well as electrolyte imbalances that may be present. Radiographs may frequently reveal a complete obstruction. Radiographs may also indicate air-distended loops of bowel, which are common in foreign bodies lodged in the intestines. Contrast studies may be necessary to outline an intestinal foreign body. Ultrasound may also be useful in identifying foreign objects. Endoscopy is usually not recommended for a diagnosis of intestinal foreign body because the scope can rarely be advanced beyond the descending duodenum.

Special Instruments

A general-use soft tissue surgery pack in conjunction with Doyen intestinal clamps will be needed for an enterotomy. The Doyen clamps allow the surgeon to clamp the intestines on either side of the incision site (Figure 7-19). Doyen clamps are considered nontraumatic and prevent intestinal contents from leaking into the abdomen while performing the procedure. If Doyen clamps are unavailable, the fingers of the assistant can serve the same purpose. The scrub nurse must ensure that all instruments used within the intestines are kept away from the rest of the surgical instruments. This will aid in avoiding contamination of the abdomen with intestinal bacteria. All instruments used in the intestines should be placed on a sterile towel during the enterotomy and then removed from the instrument table, once the intestines are closed. The other option is to have an instrument set solely used for the GI tract, then replaced with a clean set after the intestinal closure.

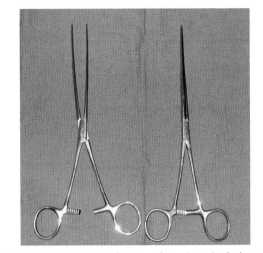

Figure 7-19 Doyen clamps. These intestinal clamps are considered nontraumatic to the intestines.

Once the enterotomy is complete, all scrubbed personnel should change gloves, and a new set of instruments can be introduced for closure of the abdomen. A Balfour retractor should also be available for better exposure of the abdomen.

Patient Positioning

The patient should be positioned in dorsal recumbency to perform a ventral midline incision.

Patient Draping

A four-quarter draping method should be considered for an enterotomy.

Enterotomy Procedure

The patient should be clipped and prepared for an abdominal procedure. The skin, subcutaneous tissue, and linea alba can be incised from the xiphoid process to just cranial to the pubis. Once the abdominal cavity is opened, moistened lap sponges can be placed on either side of the body wall, and a Balfour should be inserted for maximum exposure. A full exploratory procedure should be performed before beginning an enterotomy. The GI tract should be examined completely. Once the intestinal foreign body is located (Figure 7-20), the affected intestine can be isolated from the abdomen by packing off with lap sponges.

The surgeon will need to decide if an enterotomy or a resection and anastomosis should be performed based on analysis of the intestine. If necrosis or perforations of the intestinal segment are absent, an enterotomy may be sufficient. The intestinal contents should be milked away from the foreign body site. Doyen clamps or fingers of an assistant can be placed a few centimeters away on either side of the proposed enterotomy. The enterotomy incision should be made just distal to the foreign body on the antimesenteric border (the side of the intestine without the attached mesentery) of the intestine (Figure 7-21). This region is selected because the viability of the intestines proximal to the foreign body may be in question, and it is preferable to suture healthy intestine. The incision may need to be extended with Metzenbaum scissors to allow the removal of the foreign body (Figure 7-22). Allis tissue forceps may be useful in grasping and slowly removing the object.

Once the foreign body is removed, the enterotomy incision can be closed (Figures 7-23 and 7-24). An absorbable monofilament suture in a simple interrupted suture pattern may be used to close the incision. Multifilament suture should never be used in the GI tract; the braid of the suture can act as a wick for bacteria. A local lavage of the enterotomy site is warranted, as well as a warm abdominal lavage of the entire abdomen. All scrubbed personnel should change gloves, and the instruments used to perform the enterotomy should be placed aside. Clean instruments (those not used in the intestines) should be used to close the layers of the abdominal cavity. The abdominal cavity can be closed in three or four layers.

Postoperative Considerations and Instructions

One postoperative goal for enterotomy patients is to correct any previous fluid loss or electrolyte

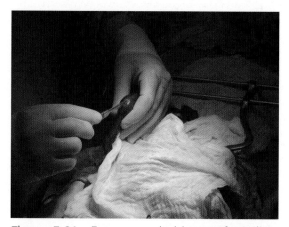

Figure 7-21 Enterotomy incision performed at antimesenteric border of jejunum. Incision is made over distal aspect of the foreign body.

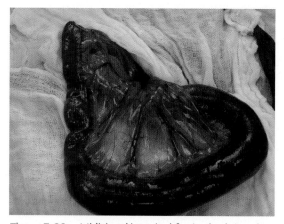

Figure 7-20 Midjejunal intestinal foreign body in a dog.

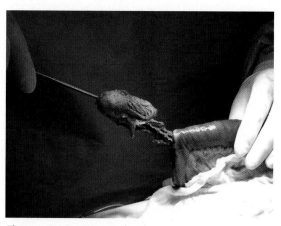

Figure 7-22 Removal of intestinal foreign body (cloth) in jejunum of a dog.

imbalances. The owner should be informed of possible complications that could arise postoperatively. Complications include necrosis and perforations of the bowel, as well as leakage and dehiscence of the intestines. All these complications can lead to peritonitis. The prognosis for a patient with peritonitis may be considered "guarded." If a simple enterotomy was performed and the bowel appeared healthy intraoperatively, a good prognosis can be given. Early identification of an intestinal foreign body is important for a positive outcome. On discharge of the patient, postoperative instructions for the client should include the same general discharge instructions listed in Chapter 11. Box 7-5 shows an example of a surgery report for an enterotomy.

Intestinal Resection and Anastomosis

Definition: Intestinal resection and anastomosis (R and A) is the excision of a segment of bowel followed by the reestablishment of the two remaining segments.

Indications: A primary indication for performing an intestinal resection and anastomosis is to remove a section of dead or diseased bowel. Causes of diseased bowel include foreign bodies, neoplasia, intussusception, necrosis, and ischemia. As stated previously, foreign bodies in dogs generally include rocks, plastic, toys, bones, corncobs, and cloth. In cats, foreign bodies generally include trichobezoars, string, yarn, and thread. All these conditions, if left untreated, may cause ischemia of the intestines, which can lead to necrosis. Ischemia or necrosis of the intestines can lead to peritonitis and a poor prognosis. Peritonitis is an inflammatory process that involves the serous membrane of the abdominal cavity. Leakage of GI contents is a main source of peritonitis.

Neoplasias of the GI tract of the dog and cat can include leiomyoma, leiomyosarcoma, fibrosarcoma, hemangiosarcoma, adenomas, mast cell tumors, lymphosarcoma, and GI adenocarcinoma. Adenocarcinoma and lymphosarcoma are considered the most common intestinal tumors in the dog and cat. An intestinal resection and anastomosis is required for neoplasia involving an intestinal segment.

As previously mentioned, common clinical signs associated with foreign bodies of the intestinal tract include vomiting, lethargy, abdominal pain, anorexia, and depression. Common clinical signs of neoplasia of the intestinal tract include vomiting, weight loss, flatulence, and melena. If an intestinal leakage has occurred and peritonitis is present, some common signs are abdominal pain, vomiting, shock, fever, and tachycardia.

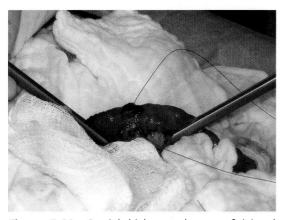

Figure 7-23 Partial-thickness closure of jejunal enterotomy site in a dog.

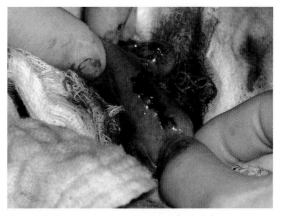

Figure 7-24 Complete closure of jejunal enterotomy site using absorbable suture material in simple interrupted suture pattern.

BOX 7-5   Surgery Report: Enterotomy

Animal Hospital Name

Owner: John Doe

Address: 555 Sterling Lane

Jupiter, NY 55555

Phone number: 555-5555

Animal Name: Sasha

Animal #: 65656501

Species: Canine

Breed: Labrador

DOB: 05/05/04

Date of Surgery: 01/03/2005

Primary Surgeon: Dr. Vet

Assistant: Nurse Scrub

Diagnosis or Preoperative Signs: Intestinal foreign body

Surgical Procedure: Enterotomy

Description of Surgical Procedure

Surgical Approach: A 15-cm ventral midline incision was made from the umbilicus to the pubis through the skin, subcutaneous tissues, and linea alba.

Surgical Pathology: All abdominal organs were examined. A foreign body was palpable at the proximal jejunum region. All other organs were unremarkable.

Surgical Procedure: A 4-cm incision was made through the antimesenteric border of the proximal jejunum at the distal end of the foreign body. The area was packed off with lap sponges to protect the abdomen from any intestinal spillage. A stocking material (approx. 12 cm long) was removed through the enterotomy incision. The incision was closed with 3-0 PDS in a simple interrupted appositional suture pattern. The abdomen was lavaged with warm sterile saline. The enterotomy site was surrounded with omentum and replaced into the abdomen.

Closure:
Linea alba: 2-0 PDS in simple interrupted suture pattern.
Subcutaneous: 3-0 Monocryl in simple continuous suture pattern.
Skin: 3-0 nylon in simple interrupted suture pattern.

Diagnostic tests should include radiographs and ultrasound (if available) of the abdomen, as well as a complete blood analysis. If peritonitis is suspected and an abdominal effusion is identified in the abdomen, an *abdominocentesis* (puncture of abdominal cavity to obtain fluid) should be performed. This will determine the type of fluid present. Bacteria seen in the abdominal fluid indicate a possible GI leak.

Special Instruments
A general-use soft tissue surgical pack will be needed for the R and A procedure. A Balfour retractor will aid in abdominal exposure. Doyen

clamps should be available for holding off intestinal contents. If Doyen clamps are unavailable, the fingers of an assistant can be used. As with enterotomy, the scrub team wants to avoid contaminating the abdominal cavity with intestinal contents, so sufficient laparotomy sponges should be available to pack off the intestinal segment. The scrub team will need to change their gloves as well as their instrument pack before closure of the abdomen.

Patient Positioning

The patient should be positioned in dorsal recumbency to perform a ventral midline incision.

Patient Draping

A four-quarter draping method should be considered for the R and A procedure.

Intestinal Resection and Anastomosis Procedure

A ventral midline abdominal incision from the xiphoid process to the pubis should be made so that a full exploratory laparotomy can be performed. Moistened lap sponges can be applied to either side of the incision and a Balfour retractor placed for better abdominal exposure. A full examination of the GI tract should be performed. The segment of diseased bowel should be identified, exteriorized, and packed off with lap sponges (Figure 7-25).

The surgeon will need to assess the viability of the intestinal segment in question. The presence of peristalsis, vascular pulses, and intestinal color may aid in determining intestinal viability. If the intestinal segment is questionable, it may be the surgeon's preference to resect that region. Neoplasia and necrosis of the intestines are conditions that would require resection. The blood vessels from the mesentery to the intestinal segment need to be ligated and transected. The intestinal contents (chyme) should be milked away from the area to be resected. The diseased region can be clamped with a crushing forceps (e.g., Carmalt). The area of the intestines to remain can be clamped with Doyen clamps, which are considered nontraumatic and should be gentle on the

intestinal tissues. If Doyen clamps are unavailable, the fingers of an assistant will provide the same effect.

The surgeon then transects the intestines with a scalpel blade along the outside of the Carmalt forceps, and the intestinal segment along with the forceps is removed. A few millimeters of healthy tissue should be removed with the diseased segment to ensure the anastomosis site will be closed with healthy intestine (Figure 7-26). The technician holds the two segments of intestine close to each other so that they are aligned correctly. A single-layer, simple interrupted suture pattern is frequently used for an end-to-end anastomosis because it produces minimal stenosis or leakage and heals rapidly. A 3-0 or 4-0 monofilament absorbable suture should be used for the anastomosis site. The first sutures are placed at the mesenteric border, followed by the placement of sutures at the antimesenteric border. Subsequent sutures can be filled in a few millimeters apart. The surgeon will be certain to identify the submucosa when suturing because it is the holding layer of the intestines.

After the anastomosis has been completed, sterile saline can be injected into the surgical site to check for any leakage from the suture site (Figure 7-27). The intestines should be moderately distended with fluid while maintaining intestinal occlusion. Additional sutures can be placed in the event that leakage occurs. The mesenteric defect should then be closed in a simple continuous or interrupted suture pattern. If peritonitis was present, a closed suction drain may need to be placed to allow drainage of the abdominal cavity. A local lavage of the anastomosis site as well as a full abdominal lavage with warm saline should be performed in the event that leakage of the intestinal contents has occurred. If peritonitis was present, bacterial cultures of the abdomen should be obtained before closure. The anastomosis site should be wrapped with omentum before closure. The scrub team will need to change gloves and receive a new instrument set to close the abdomen. The abdomen should be closed routinely in a three- or four-layer closure.

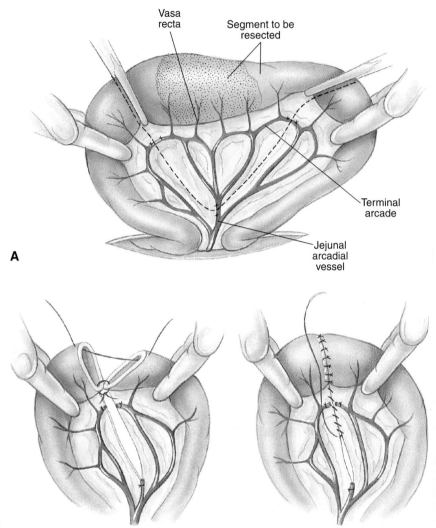

Figure 7-25   Jejunal resection and anastomosis. **A,** Carmalt forceps are placed on the region to be resected to avoid leakage of intestinal chyme. Fingers are used as Doyen clamps to help prevent leakage as well. Mesenteric vessels (jejunal arcadial and terminal arcade vessels) are ligated. **B,** After ligation, mesenteric vessels are transected. Diseased portion of bowel is removed and interrupted sutures are placed, starting at mesenteric border first. **C,** Additional interrupted sutures are placed at antimesenteric border and continued around the bowel segment until the anastomosis is complete. (From Fossum TW: *Small animal surgery,* ed 2, St Louis, 2002, Mosby.)

Postoperative Considerations and Instructions

Animals with peritonitis during the surgery are usually more critical cases and will need more supportive care. If the patient is debilitated, intravenous (IV) nutrition may be warranted. IV antibiotics and fluids should be continued. Peritonitis has a high rate of morbidity, and this should be explained to the owner. The patient's clinical signs should be closely monitored postoperatively. Any signs of depression, vomiting, fever, abdominal pain or tenderness, or discharge

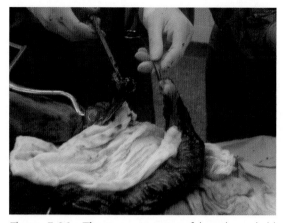

Figure 7-26   The two segments of bowel are held appositional from each other to begin the anastomosis.

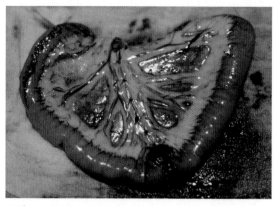

Figure 7-27   Completed anastomosis of jejunum.

from the incision site could be the result of a dehiscence of the intestinal suture and the presence of peritonitis. Other complications associated with intestinal surgery are leakage of the surgical site, stenosis of the intestinal lumen, perforation, and death. A large intestinal resection (approximately 80% or more) can lead to short-bowel syndrome. The clinical signs of short-bowel syndrome include malnutrition, weight loss, and diarrhea. Treatment of short-bowel syndrome is based on the clinical signs but includes correction of fluid loss and electrolyte imbalances.

Nutritional support must be provided until the intestines adapt. Prognosis for the patient receiving an intestinal resection and anastomosis can be considered good if peritonitis was absent and removal of large amounts of intestine was averted. The healing process of the intestines is generally rapid but can be interrupted by associated factors, such as debilitation of the patient. Prognosis of the patient with peritonitis should be considered "guarded." On discharge of the patient, postoperative instructions for the client should include the same general discharge instructions listed in Chapter 11. Box 7-6 shows an example of a surgery report for an intestinal resection and anastomosis.

Gastric Dilatation and Volvulus

Definition: A gastric dilatation and volvulus (GDV) refers to the swelling (specifically gaseous distension) and rotation of the stomach on its mesenteric axis. *Dilatation,* or *dilation,* refers to an organ being stretched beyond its normal dimensions. *Volvulus* refers to the rotation of an organ. A small animal patient can have a gastric dilatation without the volvulus, commonly referred to as a "simple gastric dilatation." The generic term "bloat" does not distinguish between a simple gastric dilatation and gastric dilatation with a volvulus.

Indications: A GDV is considered a true surgical emergency. The treatment for a GDV includes the following:

1. Decompression of the stomach.
2. Correction of fluid and electrolyte imbalances, correction of arrhythmias, and treatment for shock in most cases.
3. Correction of the malpositioned stomach and partial gastrectomy of devitalized tissue, if warranted.
4. Gastropexy procedure, which involves surgically attaching the stomach to the body wall to prevent future GDVs.

GDVs usually occur in deep-chested, large-breed animals but are sometimes seen in smaller breeds and rarely in cats. A GDV may occur at any age but is generally noted in middle-aged to older dogs. The precise etiology of GDV is unknown, but many occur after ingesting a large meal followed by strenuous exercise. Diet, amount of

BOX 7-6   Surgery Report: Intestinal Resection and Anastomosis

Animal Hospital Name

Owner: John Doe

Address: 555 Sterling Lane

        Jupiter, NY 55555

Phone number: 555-5555

Animal Name: Sasha

Animal #: 65656501

Species: Canine

Breed: Labrador

DOB: 05/05/04

Date of Surgery: 01/03/2005

Primary Surgeon: Dr. Vet

Assistant: Nurse Scrub

Diagnosis or Preoperative Signs: Intestinal foreign body

Surgical Procedure: Intestinal resection and anastomosis, exploratory laparotomy

Description of Surgical Procedure

Surgical Approach: A 20-cm ventral midline incision was made through the skin from the xiphoid process to the pubis. The incision was carried through the underlying subcutaneous tissues and linea alba.

Surgical Pathology: A purulent and serosanguineous discharge oozed out of the tissues when the incision was made. Approximately 200 ml of serosanguineous fluid was removed from the abdominal cavity. The mesentery and omentum were grossly inflamed. A foreign body was located mid-jejunum. The region of intestines where the foreign body was located was inflamed and thickened. Perforations were evident at the mesenteric border of the jejunum. The rest of the bowel and the abdomen were unremarkable.

Surgical Procedure: The abdomen was explored and the entire length of bowel examined. The affected portion of the jejunum was exteriorized and the abdominal cavity packed off with lap sponges. Approximately 5 cm of grossly normal jejunum was resected proximal and distal to the abnormal segment. First, the appropriate jejunal mesenteric vessels were double-ligated with 3-0 PDS and divided between the ligations. Intestinal contents were milked away from the surgical site. Crushing forceps were placed across the small intestines about 2 cm from the proposed site of transection of the intestine. The intestine was transected between each set of crushing and Doyen forceps with a scalpel. The mesentery attached to the resected portion of the bowel was incised, and the abnormal jejunum was completely removed from the surgical site. The bowel edges were apposed with 4-0 PDS in a simple interrupted suture pattern, beginning first at the mesenteric border and taking bites through the submucosal layer. The mesentery was apposed with 4-0 PDS in a simple continuous suture pattern. The abdomen was thoroughly lavaged with sterile saline. Aerobic and anaerobic cultures were collected of the abdomen. A closed suction drain was placed through the skin and into the cranial abdomen. The external portion was attached to the skin with 3-0 nylon. The abdomen was closed routinely.

Closure:
Linea alba: 0-PDS in simple interrupted suture pattern.
Subcutaneous tissues: 2-0 PDS in simple continuous suture pattern.
Subcuticular layer: 3-0 Monocryl in simple continuous pattern.
Skin: 3-0 nylon in simple interrupted suture pattern.

food ingested, frequency of feeding, feeding behavior, and exercise after a meal may all be contributing factors for the development of gastric dilatation and volvulus. Other contributing factors may include anatomic predisposition, ileus, trauma, primary gastric motility disorders, vomiting, and stress. The classic clinical sign of a GDV is severe abdominal distention past the rib cage (Figure 7-28). Other signs include restlessness, hypersalivation, abdominal pain, nonproductive attempts to vomit (retching, "dry heaving"), and signs of shock.

The first step in the correction of a GDV is to stabilize the patient and reverse shock. Compression of vessels by the distended abdomen decreases venous return to the heart (effectively decreasing vascular volume) and cardiac output, thus initiating shock. IV fluids should be administered if shock is present. Oxygen should be available and administered if respiratory distress is evident.

The second step in the correction of the GDV is to decompress the stomach to allow gas to escape. The gas is most likely associated with one of the following: *aerophagia* (habitual swallowing of air), bacterial fermentation (with associated carbon dioxide production), or metabolic reactions. The gastric gas is unable to escape through normal physiologic means, such as vomiting or eructation, because the esophageal and pyloric sphincters are often twisted or rotated closed. The technician needs to choose an appropriately sized orogastric tube in correlation with the animal's size. The tube should be measured from the point of the nose to the xiphoid process. Tape can be applied to the tube to mark the appropriate length. A roll of tape placed between the upper and lower canine teeth can be used as a mouth gag to hold the patient's mouth open for placement of the stomach tube. Lubricant can be applied to the end of the tube for easier passage. The tube can be placed through the hole of the tape roll and down the esophagus (Figure 7-29). Sedation may be required to help keep the animal relaxed and manageable. Damage to the esophagus can occur if the tube is aggressively forced down the esophagus.

Once air has been removed from the stomach, the stomach should be lavaged with warm water to help remove any gastric contents. If attempts to pass the stomach tube are unsuccessful, percutaneous

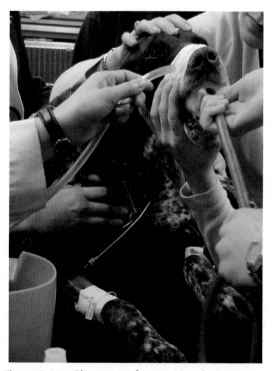

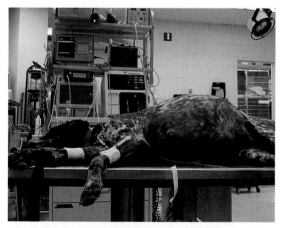

Figure 7-28 Nine-year-old German shorthair pointer with gastric dilatation and volvulus (GDV). Note the severely distended abdomen past the rib cage.

Figure 7-29 Placement of orogastric tube in German shorthair pointer with GDV. Note the roll of tape between the upper and lower jaws for easier placement of the tube.

decompression with a trochar can be attempted. A 14-, 16-, or 18-gauge needle or catheter can be inserted through a quickly clipped and prepped body wall and into the stomach. This allows the evacuation of gas and relieves pressure on the vessels.

The patient should be taken to surgery to correct the position of the stomach as soon as stabilization has been accomplished. The volvulus of the stomach hinders gastric blood flow and can cause necrosis of the stomach tissue. Timely treatment of a GDV can produce survival rates approaching 85%.

Special Instruments
A general-use soft tissue surgical pack should be sufficient for GDV surgery. A Balfour abdominal retractor should be available. An appropriately sized orogastric tube will be needed for decompression of the stomach intraoperatively.

Patient Positioning
The patient should be positioned in dorsal recumbency to perform a ventral midline incision.

Patient Draping
A four-quarter draping method should be considered for the GDV procedure.

Procedure for Treatment of Gastric Dilatation and Volvulus
The abdomen should be clipped from above the xiphoid process to the pubis. Adequate cranial clipping is important so that the surgeon can extend the incision as needed. Rotation of the stomach back to its normal position can be difficult if the proper exposure is not achieved. The entire abdomen should be clipped to allow a full abdominal exploratory surgery. The lateral aspects of the abdomen should be clipped as well, in the event that placement of a gastric feeding tube is warranted.

The surgeon makes a ventral midline incision from the xiphoid process to just caudal to the umbilicus. This incision can be extended for the exploratory procedure if necessary. Moistened laparotomy sponges should be placed on either side of the incision site and a Balfour retractor

positioned for better abdominal exposure. On entering the abdominal cavity, the first structure noted is the greater omentum, which usually covers the dilated stomach during a GDV. Blood may be evident in the abdomen, usually from rupture of the short gastric vessels. An orogastric tube should again be passed through the mouth, down the esophagus, and into the stomach to allow decompression of gas and the release of gastric contents. A warm gastric lavage should be performed until the contents from the stomach are emptied and the lavage water collected is clear.

The surgeon then attempts to rotate the stomach back to its original position. Most stomachs will twist or rotate in a clockwise direction and can rotate 90 to 360 degrees (Figure 7-30). To correct the malpositioned stomach, it will usually need to be rotated in a counterclockwise direction. The surgeon grasps the stomach at the pylorus region with the right hand and the greater

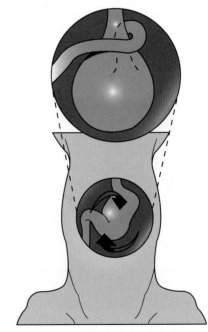

Figure 7-30 Stomach of dog with GDV generally rotates in a clockwise direction. (From Fossum TW: *Small animal surgery*, ed 2, St Louis, 2002, Mosby.)

curvature of the stomach with the left hand. The greater curvature should be pushed downward toward the floor while lifting up on the pylorus. This procedure should position the stomach back to its original placement. The stomach should then be explored for necrosis. If necrosis is evident, a partial gastrectomy may need to be performed. A full exploratory laparotomy should be conducted to be sure no damage has occurred to other abdominal organs. Often the spleen will follow the path of the stomach, and a splenic torsion may be apparent. The spleen should be observed for damage and a splenectomy performed, if warranted. A gastropexy procedure must be done to prevent a future GDV.

Permanent Gastropexy Procedures

A gastropexy ("pexy") procedure permanently affixes the stomach to the body wall and prevents further GDVs. Many educated owners of large-breed dogs may decide to have an elective gastropexy performed on their pet. This procedure can be done, for example, when a large-breed pet is admitted for an OHE. If available, a less invasive gastropexy procedure can be done laparoscopically. A variety of pexy procedures can be performed, although they vary on rates of dependability as well as frequency of surgical complications. The goal of all these procedures is to create a permanent adhesion between the gastric serosa and the peritoneal surface of the abdominal wall. To form a permanent adhesion, the gastric muscle must be in contact with the body wall muscle. Gastropexy procedures include the following types:

- Tube gastropexy
- Circumcostal gastropexy
- Muscular flap gastropexy
- Belt-loop gastropexy
- Incisional gastropexy

The term *incisional gastropexy* is a general term and is not necessarily specific to one particular technique. For example, some surgery textbooks refer to a *muscular flap gastropexy* as an "incisional gastropexy." There is also an incisional gastropexy technique that involves tacking the stomach to the ventral midline abdominal incision by incorporating the sutures of the gastropexy into the sutures used to close the abdomen. This particular incisional gastropexy has the major disadvantage of potential problems should the abdomen need to be opened again later. The surgeon may be more likely to incise through the stomach inadvertently while making the midline incision. A third type of incisional gastropexy is probably the most common procedure for tacking the stomach to the abdominal wall. An internal incision is made into the right ventrolateral body wall, exposing the abdominal muscles. A second incision is made into the seromuscular layer of the stomach antrum. The edges of the gastric incision are sutured to the internal abdominal wall incision. This connection will form a permanent adhesion. This particular type of incisional gastropexy is considered simple and effective has less potential for complications than other methods of gastropexy (Figure 7-31).

Postoperative Considerations and Instructions

One goal postoperatively for a GDV patient is to correct any fluid or electrolyte imbalances. Vomiting should be monitored and can be treated with antiemetics. If no vomiting is reported, water can be offered 1 day after surgery, and food can be introduced in small quantities 24 to 48 hours after surgery. Cardiac arrhythmias are common in GDV patients and generally occur 12 to 36 hours after the onset of GDV. The arrhythmias are usually ventricular in origin, have been reported in 30% to 50% of GDV patients, and may require treatment.

Complications from GDVs can include peritonitis and sepsis. Devitalized stomach tissue must be resected to avoid a possible septic peritonitis. Gastric viability at surgery is subjective, and postoperative necrosis and perforation can occur postoperatively despite careful assessment. Timely correction of a GDV is imperative for a good prognosis. The prognosis may be considered "guarded" if gastric necrosis was evident. On discharge of the patient, postoperative instructions for the client should include those listed in Chapter 11. Box 7-7 shows an example of a surgery report for GDV repair.

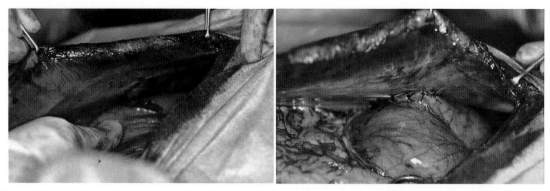

Figure 7-31   Incisional gastropexy. **A,** Incision is made into seromuscular layer of stomach antrum and is lined up with an incision in ventrolateral abdominal muscle wall. **B,** Completed gastropexy showing the incision in the stomach sutured to the incision in the abdominal muscle wall. (Courtesy Dr. David Holt.)

Cystotomy

Definition: Cystotomy refers to a surgical incision into the bladder. Related terms include the following:

- **Cystectomy:** Excision or resection of the urinary bladder
- **Cystostomy:** Surgical formation of an opening into the bladder
- **Uroabdomen:** Presence of urine in the abdominal cavity; generally associated with a ruptured bladder
- **Crystalluria:** Presence of crystals in the urine
- **Urolith:** Calculus or stone found in the urine or urinary system
- **Urolithiasis:** Formation of calculi in the urinary tract

Indications: A primary indication for performing a cystotomy is to remove cystic calculi. Removal of bladder stones is probably the most common bladder surgery performed in small animal surgery. In the dog the most frequent urolith observed is the *struvite* (45%-50% of all calculi). Other uroliths found in the dog include calcium oxalate, urate, silicate, and cystine crystals. Uroliths are most frequently noted in middle-aged dogs, although they can occur at any age.

Clinical signs associated with bladder stones include *hematuria* (blood in urine), *stranguria* (slow and painful discharge of urine), *dysuria* (difficulty urinating), and *pollakiuria* (abnormally frequent passage of urine). Stones may also become wedged in the urethra of male dogs and cause obstructions of the urethra. Animals with suspected cystic calculi should have radiographs. Abdominal radiographs of animals with calculi frequently reveal radiopaque densities in the urinary system. Obstruction of the urethra can lead to a buildup of urine in the bladder and can cause bladder distention. Bladder distention can lead to a rupture if left untreated. Rupture of the bladder can also result from trauma (e.g., hit by car) or from improper placement of a urinary catheter or forceful bladder expression. Most abdominal surgeries require expression of the bladder before transport into surgery. **The bladder of a trauma patient should not be expressed before surgery.** The condition of the bladder may be in question, and attempts to express a traumatic bladder may lead to a bladder rupture. Clinical signs of bladder rupture can include shock, fever, hematuria, anuria, and abdominal pain. Urine in the abdominal cavity can cause uremia and dehydration. A bladder rupture can lead to death if identification of the rupture is delayed. A uroabdomen can be diagnosed by performing

BOX 7-7   Surgery Report: Gastric Dilatation and Volvulus

Animal Hospital Name

Owner: John Doe

Address: 555 Sterling Lane

Jupiter, NY 55555

Phone number: 555-5555

Animal Name: Sasha

Animal #: 65656501

Species: Canine

Breed: Labrador

DOB: 01/05/02

Date of Surgery: 12/03/2005

Primary Surgeon: Dr. Vet

Assistant: Nurse Scrub

Diagnosis or Preoperative Signs: One-day history of retching, abdominal distention; gastric dilatation and volvulus

Surgical Procedure: Gastric dilatation and volvulus (GDV) correction and incisional gastropexy

Description of Surgical Procedure

Surgical Approach: The patient was placed in dorsal recumbency. A skin incision approximately 25 cm long was made from the xiphoid process to the pubis. The incision was continued through the fascia and linea alba, and the abdomen was entered. A large amount of falciform fat was resected.

Surgical Pathology: The stomach was rotated 270 degrees, grossly distended, and hypermotile. The pylorus was located ventrally and to the left of the fundus. There was no evidence of devitalized tissues. There was minimal hemorrhage in the abdomen.

Surgical Procedure: Moist laparotomy sponges were placed along the incision, and a Balfour retractor was placed. On entering the abdomen, the omentum was seen covering a gas-distended stomach that was rotated 270 degrees clockwise. The stomach was decompressed with an 18-gauge needle and suction. The stomach was then repositioned by pulling up on the pylorus to rotate the stomach counterclockwise back to its correct anatomic position. A stomach tube was passed and relieved a moderate amount of brown, malodorous fluid. The stomach was lavaged with warm water until the fluid leaving the stomach was clear. The entire surface of the stomach was inspected and appeared healthy. The abdomen was explored routinely. Next, an incisional gastropexy was performed; an incision was made into the seromuscular layer of the stomach in the region of the pyloric antrum. A second incision was made into the right ventrolateral abdominal wall, exposing the abdominal muscles. The edges of the gastric incision were sutured to the abdominal wall incision using two suture lines and a simple continuous pattern. The abdomen was lavaged with 2 liters of sterile saline, and the body wall was closed routinely.

Closure:
Incisional gastropexy: 2-0 PDS in two lines of simple continuous patterns.
Linea alba: 0 PDS in simple continuous pattern.
Subcutaneous tissue: 2-0 PDS in simple continuous pattern.
Subcuticular tissue: 2-0 Monocryl in continuous suture pattern.
Skin: skin staples.

an abdominocentesis. Creatinine and urea measurements of the abdominal cavity fluid are compared to blood serum levels. If the levels of creatinine and urea in the abdominal fluid are greater than the blood serum levels, a uroabdomen can be diagnosed. A contrast cystourethrogram can also be performed to diagnose the exact region of the bladder leakage.

Other indications to perform cystotomy include neoplasia and congenital abnormalities. The most common neoplasia associated with the bladder in dogs and cats is transitional cell carcinoma. In the dog, bladder cancer makes up less than 1% of all canine cancers. The incidence of bladder cancer in cats is much lower.

Table 7-1 lists treatment options and preventive measures for different types of canine urolithiasis. Box 7-8 lists canine predispositions for urinary calculi.

Special Instruments

A general-use soft tissue surgery pack will be sufficient for cystotomy. A bladder spoon should be available (Figure 7-32). Bladder spoons can aid in the retrieval of cystic calculi, especially those located in the neck of the bladder. A Balfour abdominal retractor should also be available.

Patient Positioning

The patient should be positioned in dorsal recumbency to perform a ventral midline incision.

Patient Draping

A four-quarter draping method should be considered for cystotomy.

Cystotomy Procedure

The entire abdomen should be clipped from xiphoid process to the pubis. The patient should be prepped from the xiphoid process to the pubis in the event an unexpected finding requires an extended incision. This additional clipping and prepping will allow the surgeon to extend the incision cranially if desired. A ventral midline incision beginning at the umbilicus and extending caudally to the pubis should be sufficient

TABLE 7-1	Treatment and Prevention of Canine Urolithiasis	
UROLITH TYPE	**TREATMENT OPTIONS**	**PREVENTIVE MEASURES**
Struvite	Surgical removal or dissolution Hill's s/d diet Control infection. Urease inhibitor? Keep urine pH <6.5, BUN <10 mg/dl, and urine specific gravity <1.020.	Hill's c/d diet Monitor urine pH and urine sediment; eliminate infections quickly and appropriately.
Calcium oxalate	Surgical removal	Hill's u/d diet or Hill's w/d diet plus potassium citrate
Urate	Surgical removal or dissolution Hill's u/d diet Allopurinol Control infection.	Hill's u/d diet Allopurinol if necessary Correct congenital portosystemic shunts.
Silicate	Surgical removal	Hill's u/d diet Prevent consumption of dirt.
Cystine	Surgical removal or dissolution Hill's u/d diet D-Penicillamine N-(2-Mercaptopropionyl)-glycine (MPG)	Hill's u/d diet Thiol-containing drugs if necessary

From Fossum TW et al: *Small animal surgery,* ed 2, St Louis, 2002, Mosby.
BUN, Blood urea nitrogen.

for cystotomy. The subcutaneous tissues and linea alba should be incised on the midline. Moistened lap sponges should be placed on either side of the incision and a Balfour retractor positioned for better exposure of the abdomen. The bladder should be isolated and lap sponges positioned beneath the bladder to segregate it from the rest of the abdomen. Stay sutures should be placed at the apex of the bladder to assist in manipulation as well as to prevent spillage of urine into the abdomen (Figure 7-33). The scrub nurse should grasp the stay sutures and gently lift upward to avoid spillage of urine.

The surgeon makes a stab incision on the ventral aspect of the bladder in a hypovascular region. The technician should have suction ready to place into the stab incision to remove the urine from the bladder before leakage occurs. The stab incision can then be extended with Metzenbaum scissors. A bladder spoon can be used to aid in the removal of cystic calculi, especially at the neck region of the bladder (Figure 7-34). A red rubber catheter can be passed through the urethra, and sterile saline should be flushed through the catheter to confirm the urethral passage is clear of cystic calculi and patent. Cystic calculi should be flushed back into the bladder if possible to avoid having to perform a urethrotomy (incision into the urethra).

BOX 7-8   Breed, Gender, Age, and Other Predispositions for Urinary Calculi in Dogs

Struvite Uroliths
- Miniature schnauzers, bichons frises, cocker spaniels
- Female more than male dogs; middle-aged dogs
- Urinary tract infection (UTI)

Calcium Oxalate Uroliths
- Miniature schnauzers, Lhasa apsos, Yorkshire terriers
- Male dogs, middle-aged to older dogs

Calcium Phosphate Uroliths
- Yorkshire terriers

Urate Uroliths
- Dalmatians, English bulldogs
- Dogs with portosystemic shunts

Silicate Uroliths
- German shepherds, golden retrievers, Labradors
- Male dogs, middle-aged dogs

Cystine Uroliths
- Dachshunds, English bulldogs (possibly basset hounds and rottweilers)
- Male dogs, middle-aged dogs

Modified from Fossum TW et al: *Small animal surgery,* ed 2, St Louis, 2002, Mosby.

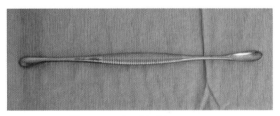

Figure 7-32   Bladder spoon.

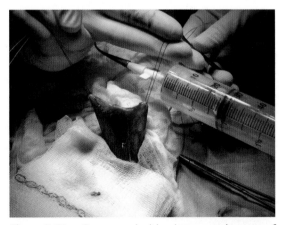

Figure 7-33   Cystotomy incision into ventral aspect of bladder. Note that stay sutures are used to lift gently upward on the bladder to avoid leakage of urine. A red rubber catheter is placed to flush any stones in the ure-thra back into the bladder.

Cultures of the bladder should be obtained. Some surgeons may also prefer to take a sample of the bladder for biopsy or culture. The bladder should be examined for deficiencies and closed according to the surgeon's preference. Closure of the bladder can consist of a two-layer or three-layer continuous closure or a simple interrupted suture pattern (Figure 7-35). The stay sutures can be removed, and the abdomen should be lavaged with warm saline. The abdomen should be closed routinely. Bladder stones retrieved from the bladder should be submitted for analysis.

Box 7-9 shows an example of a surgery report for a cystotomy.

ORTHOPEDICS

Definition: Orthopedic surgery is a branch of surgery dealing with the preservation and restoration of the function of the skeletal system and its articulation and association with its related structures (Figure 7-36).

Technician's Responsibilities

The purpose of this section is to familiarize the surgical technician with the basic presentation of fractures, with fracture evaluation, and with the types of repair available for the stabilization of different fractures. Understanding fracture management and repair will make the technician an asset to any veterinary practice. Being able to triage, evaluate, and either refer or prepare the patient for orthopedic surgery are all responsibilities that may fall on the technician.

Orthopedic fracture repair is a broad and highly specialized subject; readers wanting more in-depth coverage can supplement this chapter's discussion with additional reading (see Bibliography). Orthopedic surgery requires expensive specialized instruments and equipment along with an experienced orthopedic surgeon.

Orthopedic cases are usually not life-threatening situations. These cases can be considered life-threatening emergencies, however, if the skull or spine is involved or if the patient has lost large amounts of blood due to a long-bone fracture. Other cases that can be considered nonelective but are not life threatening are open fracture or open dislocation repairs. All these cases need to be fully evaluated, and the patient should be stabilized (e.g., open airway, controlled bleeding, stable vital signs, and managed pain) before further evaluation or surgery can occur. Elective orthopedic surgical cases that may present to the hospital include

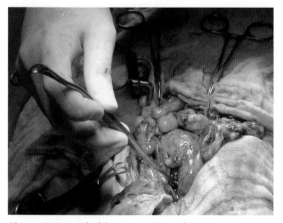

Figure 7-34 Bladder spoon is used to remove stones from neck of bladder.

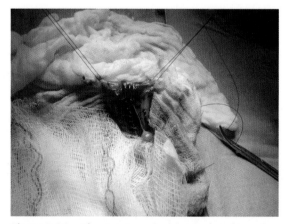

Figure 7-35 The cystotomy incision is closed in a simple interrupted suture pattern using an absorbable suture.

BOX 7-9   Surgery Report: Cystotomy

Animal Hospital Name

Owner: John Doe

Address: 555 Sterling Lane

Jupiter, NY 55555

Phone number: 555-5555

Animal Name: Sasha

Animal #: 65656501

Species: Canine

Breed: Labrador

DOB: 05/05/00

Date of Surgery: 01/03/2005

Primary Surgeon: Dr. Vet

Assistant: Nurse Scrub

Diagnosis or Preoperative Signs: Cystic calculi

Surgical Procedure: Cystotomy

Description of Surgical Procedure

Surgical Approach: The patient was placed in dorsal recumbency. A ventral midline incision was made from the umbilicus, extending caudally for 10 cm to the brim of the pelvis. The skin, the subcutaneous layer, and the linea alba were incised.

Surgical Pathology: Multiple calculi varying in size from 1 to 3 mm in diameter were removed from the bladder. On gross appearance, the bladder was red and inflamed.

Surgical Procedures: Stay sutures of 3-0 PDS were placed in the ventral aspects of the bladder to aid in retraction and manipulation. A stab incision was made in the ventral surface of the bladder. The urine in the bladder was suctioned out, and Metzenbaum scissors were used to extend the bladder incision. A bladder spoon was used to remove the calculi from the neck of the bladder. A #5 French red rubber catheter was placed in normograde fashion to flush out any remaining calculi using sterile saline. The bladder was then closed in a full-thickness, single-layer, interrupted suture pattern using 3-0 PDS. The abdomen was lavaged with sterile saline and closed routinely.

Closure:
Linea alba: 2-0 Prolene in simple interrupted suture pattern.
Subcutaneous tissue: 3-0 PDS in simple continuous suture pattern.
Subcuticular: 3-0 PDS in simple continuous suture pattern.
Skin: 3-0 nylon in simple continuous suture pattern.

Surgical Samples Collected: The cystic calculi were submitted for culture and sensitivity as well as stone analysis.

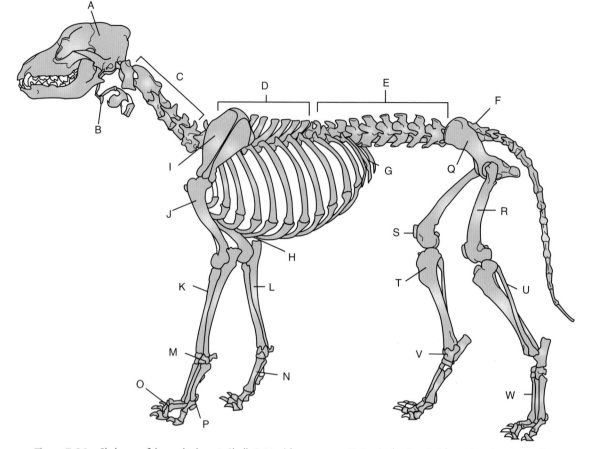

Figure 7-36   Skeleton of the male dog. *A,* Skull. *B,* Hyoid apparatus. *C,* Cervical spine. *D,* Thoracic spine. *E,* Lumbar spine. *F,* Sacrum. *G,* Ribs. *H,* Sternum. *I,* Scapula. *J,* Humerus. *K,* Radius. *L,* Ulna. *M,* Carpal bones. *N,* Metacarpal bones. *O,* Phalanges. *P,* Sesamoid bone. *Q,* Pelvis. *R,* Femur. *S,* Patella. *T,* Tibia. *U,* Fibula. *V,* Tarsal bones. *W,* Metatarsal bones. (From Evans H, deLahunta A: *Guide to the dissection of the dog,* ed 6, Philadelphia, 2004, Saunders.)

cranial cruciate or anterior cruciate ligament rupture, medial or lateral patellar luxation, hip dysplasia, or osteochondritis dissecans. These cases also need to be properly evaluated before surgery, but they are considered elective surgeries.

Patients that present with fractures can be assumed to be in significant pain and will need strong analgesics. As with any emergency case, however, under no circumstances should the technician administer any drugs without the approval of the attending veterinarian. It is the technician's responsibility to see that the fracture patient receives adequate pain management. Any fracture noted on examination should be immobilized and bandaged accordingly. External *coaptation*

(application of external appliance, such as a splint or cast) is important to reduce further disruption or damage to the fracture or fragments and the surrounding soft tissue and to prevent further blood loss at the fracture site. Stabilization of fractures also greatly enhances pain management and the animal's comfort level.

Types of bandages used to stabilize a fracture include the Robert Jones bandage (any long-bone fracture) and modified Robert Jones with metal or plastic splint (carpal, metacarpal, tarsal, metatarsal, and phalangeal fractures). A fiberglass cast with adequate padding can also be used for these same types of fractures. Fiberglass applied as a cast and not as a splint can make maintenance and changes technically difficult. Other bandages used for preoperative and postoperative support are the Ehmer sling (hip luxation), spica splint (humeral or femoral fractures), and Velpeau sling (scapular fractures). All these bandages, except for the Robert Jones, can be used as external coaptation if surgery is not an option.

Owners must always be informed of bandage and fracture complications associated with splinting or slinging. A bandage should be checked three or four times a day for signs of swelling, slippage, moisture, or soiling. If any of these scenarios occurs, the bandage should be changed.

Orthopedic Terms and Abbreviations

Nonelective: Referring to surgical cases that cannot wait for later scheduling.

Elective: Referring to surgical cases that can wait for later scheduling.

CCL: Cranial cruciate ligament.

ACL: Anterior cruciate ligament.

MPL: Medial patellar luxation.

HOD: Hypertrophic osteodystrophy; developmental disease that causes disruption of metaphyseal trabeculae in long bones of young, rapidly growing dogs.

OCD: Osteochondritis dissecans; inflammation of bone and cartilage that results in the splitting of cartilage pieces into the affected joint.

IVDD: Intervertebral disc disease associated with disc degeneration and extrusion, causing spinal cord compression and nerve root entrapment.

A-O: *Arbeitsgemeinshaft für Osteosynthesefragen,* Swiss for the Association for the Study of Internal Fixation (ASIF). These abbreviations are frequently seen together but separated by a slash: AO/ASIF. The AO is involved in research and development of medical devices used in orthopedic surgery. Their devices are available through a company called Synthes.

ASIF: Association for the Study of Internal Fixation.

Hip dysplasia: Abnormal development of coxofemoral joint characterized by subluxation or complete luxation of femoral head in younger patients and mild to severe degenerative joint disease in older patients.

Subluxation: Partial or incomplete separation of a joint.

Luxation: Complete separation of a bone from its articulation.

Dislocation: Complete separation of the articular surfaces of a joint.

Articular: Pertaining to a joint.

Reducible: Able to restore to the normal place or relation of parts, as to reduce a fracture.

Nonreducible: Unable to restore to the normal place or position.

Callus: Unorganized network of woven bone formed about ends of a broken bone, which is reabsorbed as healing is completed.

Interfragmentary: Refers to bone fragments of a fracture that may or may not be able to be reconstructed and stabilized.

Non-union: Failure of the fractured bone ends to unite.

Malunion: Faulty union and alignment of the fractured bone.

Delayed union: Delayed renewal of continuity in a broken bone or between the edges of a wound.

Aseptic loosening: Breakdown of bone and loosening of prosthesis in the absence of microorganisms.

Open reduction: Surgically opening and exposing to realign a fracture or joint.

Closed reduction: Nonsurgical realignment of fracture or joint.

Preoperative Considerations for Fractures

The patient history can provide pertinent information to help determine whether a patient is a good candidate for surgery and what type of fixation is best suited for a positive outcome. How old is the patient? How large and active is the animal? What is the overall health status of the patient? What is the temperament of the patient?

The patient's age is significant in terms of how much more the bones need to grow and how active the animal is. Generally, the younger the patient, the faster is the healing time; however, there is also a greater risk of angular limb deformities if the growth plates are still open and have been traumatized. Also, younger patients are more active and are more difficult to confine for long periods. The older the patient, the slower is the healing time. This can contribute to an increased chance of complications because of the longer recovery time. Older patients tend to be more sedentary and to have more difficulty recovering after long periods of inactivity and muscle loss.

The animal's size and weight affect recovery times and success as well. Any animal that is overweight has an increased risk of failure for any type of orthopedic repair. Too much force placed on any orthopedic repair too soon can cause premature loosening of the fixation and possible failure of the repair. Some large-breed dogs and overweight dogs and cats are often too weak after orthopedic surgery to lift or support their own weight and may need assistance to rise and walk.

The importance of the orthopedic surgery patient's overall health should never be underestimated. Any preexisting conditions that would put the patient at an increased risk for anesthesia or delayed healing need to be considered preoperatively. Problems with other joints or bones can contribute to poor comfort levels and increase the length of recovery.

Owner compliance is a major consideration in any orthopedic case. The animal's temperament influences how successful owners can be at following postoperative care instructions at home. Owner compliance is probably the most underestimated component of any orthopedic patient's recovery and outcome. If the animal is aggressive, difficult to handle, or difficult for the owner to treat, the chances for a successful recovery will be less than for the easily handled, stoic animal. If the owners are incapable of handling and treating the patient correctly postoperatively or cannot return for follow-up examinations, the consequences can be catastrophic.

Fracture Assessment

Fractures can be classified or described by the following factors:

1. Bone location (e.g., humerus, femur, tibia)
2. Open or closed fracture (open fractures have penetrated through the skin; the skin is intact in closed fractures)
3. Location of fracture on the bone (e.g., midshaft, articular)
4. Type of fracture (e.g., oblique, spiral, transverse)
5. Reducible or nonreducible fracture

To assess any fracture completely, after a thorough physical examination, radiographs should be taken. Some sedation is usually necessary to achieve complete relaxation and compliance of the patient for the radiographic views needed. In animals that are a sedation risk, radiographs can be taken through the bandage or splint. When taking radiographs of any long-bone fracture, the joint above and below the fracture site should be included on the film. Articular fractures should be centered on the film using the least amount of manipulation necessary. Standard anteriorposterior (anteroposterior, AP) **and** ventral-dorsal (ventrodorsal, VD) views are suggested for proper fracture evaluation. Radiographs should also be taken postoperatively to confirm proper alignment and repair. X-ray films also serve as a point of reference for follow-up radiographs.

Radiographs and a thorough physical examination should suffice in determining whether the fracture or fractures are open or closed. An *open fracture* is a fracture in which the skin and the soft tissue covering the bone were punctured, usually by the sharp ends of the fractured bone, creating a path for external contaminants to come in contact with the bone. The fracture is then considered to be "open" to the external environment; it is no longer closed to the external environment. If possible, open fractures should be cultured before cleaning and antibiotic therapy. Open fractures can be classified or labeled according to the mechanism of puncture and the severity of the soft tissue damage, as follows:

- *Grade I* open fractures have a small puncture hole in the skin around the location of the fracture. The bone broke through the skin and was exposed to external factors but is no longer visible. Soft tissue damage is minimal.
- *Grade II* open fractures have a larger puncture or tear in the skin around the location of the fracture, and more soft tissue damage

associated with the external trauma is evident.

• *Grade III* open fractures have large tears and in some cases, loss of skin at the area of impact. Soft tissue damage is extensive and usually caused by severe bone fragmentation along with the force of the external impact. Grade III open fractures can also be described as *shearing* injuries. These patients usually have lost so much soft tissue that the bone is exposed, and in some cases the bone is sheared away or even missing.

Complications tend to be worse and more life threatening with open fractures than with closed fractures. Complications associated with open fractures include skin necrosis and infection leading to bone death. With both open and closed fractures, bleeding, soft tissue damage, and swelling are concerns. With any open fracture, contamination and vascular compromise are of great concern and play a large part in choosing what type of repair is best suited for the condition.

A *closed fracture* is a fracture that at the time of impact did not puncture or tear the skin at or around the location of the fracture. Soft tissue damage and swelling can range from mild to severe. Figure 7-37 shows the anatomy of a long bone, and Figure 7-38 illustrates bone planes of a femur.

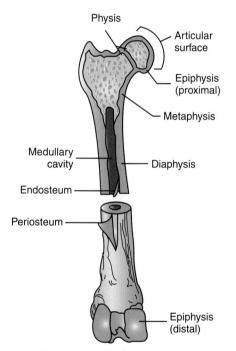

Figure 7-37   Anatomy of a long bone (femur). Diaphysis: long shaft or body of bone. Epiphysis (proximal/distal): ends of bone, usually wider than shaft, and either entirely cartilaginous or separated from shaft by cartilaginous disk. Metaphysis: wider end of shaft of the bone adjacent to epiphysis. Periosteum: fibrous covering around bone that is not covered by articular cartilage. This layer is important for bone growth, repair, nutrition, and attachment for ligaments and tendons. Articular surface: smooth layer of hyaline cartilage covering epiphysis where one bone forms a joint with another bone. Medullary cavity: space in diaphysis containing bone marrow. Endosteum: fibrous tissue lining medullary cavity of bone. Physis: growth plate.

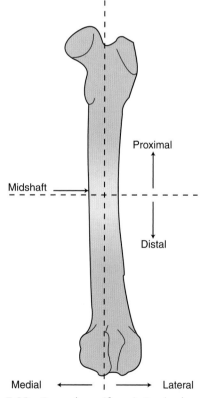

Figure 7-38   Bone planes (femur). Proximal: area closest to the body or point of origin. Distal: area farthest from the body or point of origin. Midshaft: center of shaft, or toward median plane. Lateral: farther from medial plane. Medial: toward median plane (inside or middle).

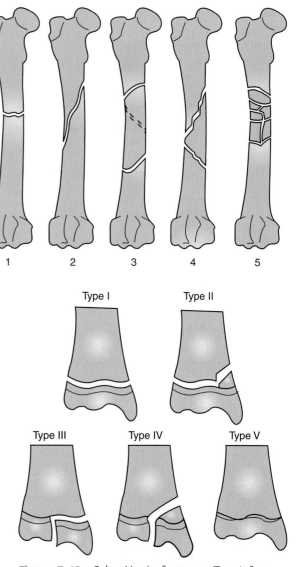

Figure 7-39 Types of fractures. *1,* Transverse: extending from side to side at right angle to long axis. *2,* Oblique: being on an incline or slanting. *3,* Spiral: curving around a center point or axis. *4,* Comminuted reducible: broken or crushed into numerous fragments but able to be placed or aligned with opposite end of fracture. *5,* Comminuted nonreducible: broken or crushed into numerous fragments and unable to be placed or aligned together with opposite end of fracture.

Types of Fractures

Five types of common fractures are shown in Figure 7-39.

Articular Fractures

Articular fractures, better known as *physeal fractures,* always involve the joint. These fractures are frequently seen in young, growing animals and are referred to as *Salter-Harris fractures.* Any fracture involving the physis or growth plate in early stages of bone development can be detrimental to development and may cause angular limb deformities. Physeal fractures can involve the physis itself or the physis and the bone above and below it. Salter-Harris fractures are identified according to the location of the fracture line and what areas of the bone are involved (Figure 7-40).

Y fractures and T fractures are types of articular fractures that involve the distal aspect of the humerus (Figure 7-41). The fracture lines run ventrodorsally through the humeral condyle and run in transverse or oblique configurations through the medial and lateral epicondyles.

Figure 7-40 Salter-Harris fractures. *Type I* fracture runs through physis. *Type II* fracture runs through metaphysis and physis. *Type III* fracture runs through physis and epiphysis. *Type IV* fracture runs through metaphysis, physis, and epiphysis. *Type V* fracture is crushing injury to physis; may not always be detected initially by radiographs.

Surgical Options for Fracture Repair

Surgical options for fracture repair are initially basic but can become very detailed. In general, the purpose for any fracture fixation is to bring the opposing ends of the fracture and joints back into alignment. After reduction of the fracture, the bone is restabilized and supported by internal or external fixation. Once the bone has been properly immobilized, the healing process and callus formation begin. *Internal fixation* is a form of rigid

Articular fractures

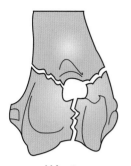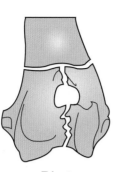

Y fracture   T fracture

Figure 7-41   Y and T articular fractures.

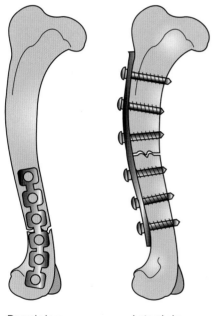

Dorsal view   Lateral view

Figure 7-42   Internal fixation (bone plate and screws).

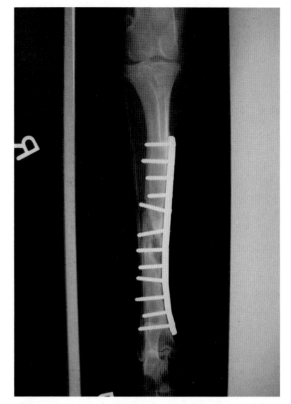

Figure 7-43   Radiograph (dorsal view) of a tibial fracture repair. An internal plate and screws were used for fixation.

Bone is the deepest tissue within the limb and therefore is afforded poor drainage in the event of infection. Bone infections *(osteomyelitis)* are serious and difficult to treat. Great care must be taken when preparing any patient for orthopedic surgery. A broad-spectrum antibacterial, antimicrobial, and antifungal scrub and final prep should be used before surgery, with adherence to strict sterile technique throughout surgery to prevent contamination.

Internal Fixation
Internal fixation devices include bone plates and screws (Figures 7-42 to 7-45), interlocking nails, intramedullary pins, Kirschner wires, and cerclage wire.

Bone plates come in a variety of shapes, sizes, and lengths. They are designed to be used with various sizes of screw. The plates are made of titanium

fixation placed under the skin and muscle directly on or in the bone surface or medullary cavity to regain stability. *External fixation* is a form of fixation applied through the exterior surface (skin and muscle) of the limb to the interior area (bone and medullary cavity) to help with stability.

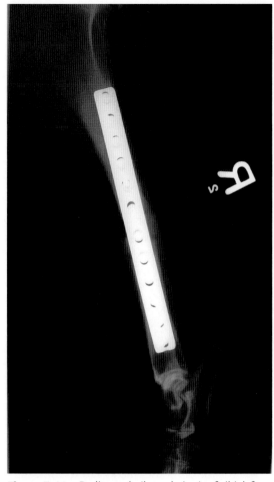

Figure 7-44   Radiograph (lateral view) of tibial fracture repair. An internal plate and screws were used for fixation.

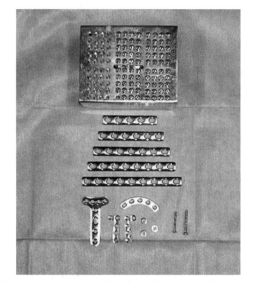

Figure 7-45   Internal orthopedic plate and screw set.

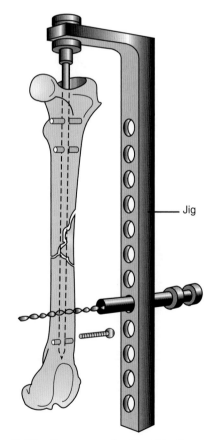

Jig

Figure 7-46   Placement of nail within the medullary cavity using an interlocking nail jig.

or stainless steel and are used with screws of the same material. Soft tissue and muscle dissection is necessary to gain adequate exposure of the fracture and to afford successful reduction of the fracture.

Interlocking nails are driven into the medullary cavity and secured in position by screws that engage the bone and the nail at its proximal and distal aspects. This type of fixation provides stabilization without extensive soft tissue dissection and muscle manipulation to expose and reconstruct the fracture (Figures 7-46 to 7-48).

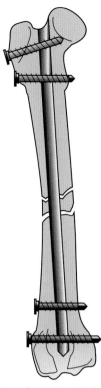

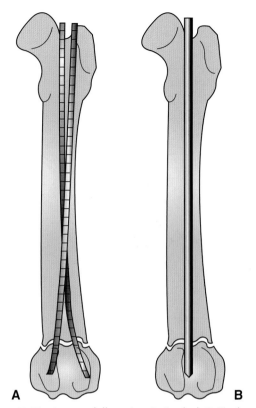

Figure 7-47 Completed interlocking nail fracture repair. Note two screws at proximal and distal ends of the bone used for securing the nail.

A **B**

Figure 7-49 Intramedullary pins. **A,** Stacked. **B,** Single.

Intramedullary (IM) pins are driven through the bone and into the medullary cavity with Jacob's chuck and can be approached as an open surgical technique or a closed pinning technique (Figures 7-49 and 7-50). IM pins can be used alone (single IM pin driven into medullary canal) or stacked (multiple IM pins driven into medullary canal). Intramedullary pinning is inexpensive compared to all other types of internal fixation but does not provide very rigid stability. Pins tend to migrate, and removal of the implant may become necessary.

Orthopedic wires (Kirschner or cerclage) can be used alone or combined with other fixation devices to achieve proper fixation. *Cerclage wire* comes in different diameters ranging from 0.4 to 1.5 mm and is used in fracture fixation for the reduction of fragments and the protection of fissures. Cerclage wires can be applied by passing them completely around the bone (full cerclage;

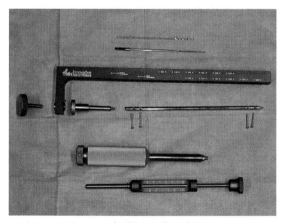

Figure 7-48 Interlocking nail and instrument set.

Figure 7-51) or by passing the wire through a predrilled hole placed through the bone (hemicerclage; Figure 7-52).

Kirschner wires, or *K-wires,* are small sections of precut wire that have pointed ends (trocar) for drilling through the bone. They come in multiple diameters for stiffness and can be used in combination with cerclage wire for interfragmentary reduction.

Postoperative Care

Postoperative care for internal fixation is strict confinement for 6 to 8 weeks. The patient is rechecked at suture removal, usually 10 to 14 days after surgery. Follow-up radiographs are taken every 4 to 6 weeks postoperatively to monitor bone healing. Young animals may need to be followed more closely because of the rate of bone healing and increased risk of angular complications. Internal fixation is not routinely removed unless the complications involve the implant.

External Fixation

External fixation used as primary repair includes casts, rigid splints, SK fixation, Kirschner-Ehmer (KE) fixation, and ring fixation (Figures 7-53 to 7-56). As with internal fixation, external fixation requires specialized equipment and has many more applications beyond the scope of this chapter.

External fixation devices stabilize the bones or fracture from the exterior of the limb. These devices use threaded cross-pins that are drilled

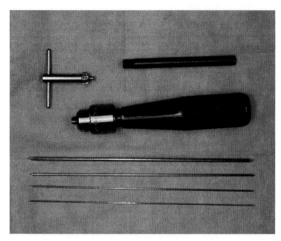

Figure 7-50   Jacob's chuck (used to drive pins through bone) and intramedullary pins.

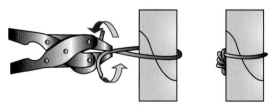

Figure 7-51   Full-cerclage wire application for fracture stabilization.

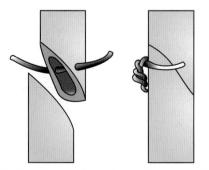

Figure 7-52   Hemicerclage wire application for fracture stabilization.

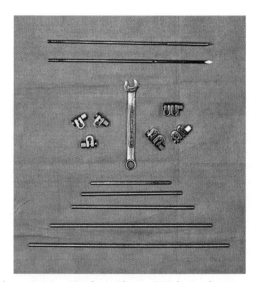

Figure 7-53   Kirschner-Ehmer (KE) bars, clamps, and wrench (for adjustment of clamps) used for external fixation.

into the bone, then attached to bars with clamps, nuts and bolts, or aluminum rings to make an external tension device. This will provide rigid stability until the fracture has time to heal. Once the fracture has closed, external fixation is removed. With any external fixation device, weekly to biweekly appointments are needed for fixator adjustments, cleaning of pin tracks, and bandage changes. External fixators are an affordable treatment option for long-bone fractures or temporary joint immobilization. They are not appropriate for fractures that may involve the pelvis or pelvic joints. External fixation devices can be created that best suits the fracture type and location. The devices can be continually modified or changed throughout the healing period.

The *ring fixator,* or *circular fixator,* is a type of external fixator that uses different-sized rings (usually three or four) and various types of pins (Figures 7-57 and 7-58). These pins are drilled through the bone and attached to the ring using clamps. The pin is then put under tension to pull the fracture back into alignment and is secured to the ring frame. Ring fixators have many uses in orthopedic surgery (see other texts).

Postoperative Care

Postoperative care for external fixators and ring fixators includes periodic visits for cleaning of pin tracts and tightening of clamps. In most cases the external bars or rings need to be padded and wrapped to prevent trauma to the patient and to reduce the risk of the fixator getting caught on objects (e.g., bedding material, crate, furniture). Radiographs should be taken postoperatively and then every 4 weeks until the fixator is removed. Activity should be restricted for the first 4 weeks, then left to the veterinarian's discretion.

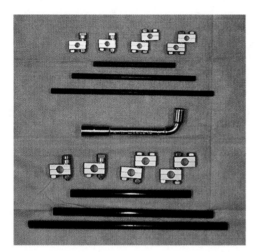

Figure 7-54   SK rods, clamps, and wrench (for adjustment of clamps) used for external fixation.

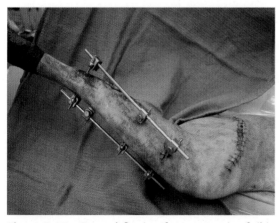

Figure 7-55   External fixation fracture repair of tibia and fibula in a dog.

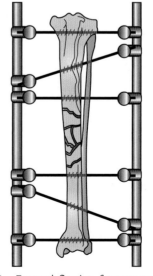

Figure 7-56   External fixation fracture repair of tibia and fibula.

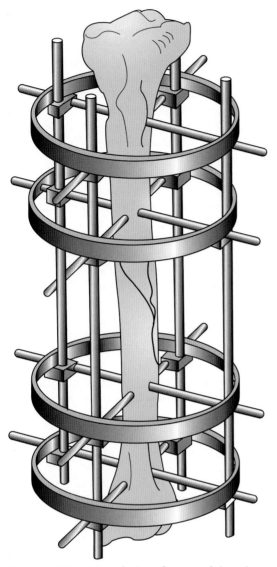

Figure 7-57   External ring fixator of long-bone fracture.

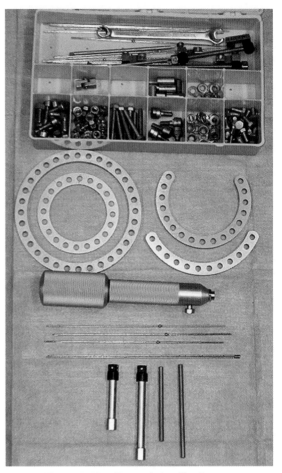

Figure 7-58   External ring fixation set.

Casts and Splints

Casts and splints are other external coaptation devices available for closed reduction of fractures at low cost and requiring no surgery. Anesthesia is necessary to sedate and relax the animal so that the fracture can be reduced, then splinted or cast. A radiograph is essential to ensure proper alignment before and after coaptation is applied. Splints work well on small, young, fast-healing animals. Splints are best suited for injuries that are distal to the elbow or stifle.

When using fiberglass or plaster cast material, periodic changes can be difficult. A cast cutter or oscillating saw is needed to cut the cast, and specialized cast spreaders are needed to remove the cast easily from the limb. Most patients require

Complications with Fixation

The following complications may occur with internal or external fixation:

- Non-union
- Malunion
- Delayed union
- Aseptic loosening
- Infection

sedation for cast and splint changes. They need to be still and pain free during the procedure. A sedated or anesthetized animal is less likely to react to the loud noises associated with the oscillating saw. Most casts require additional support (walking bar) to prevent the normal damage to the cast from walking. Casts need to be checked at least every 1 to 2 weeks.

Splints used as primary coaptation devices are easier to manage and change than casts. As with casts, however, splints are only suited for fractures that are distal to the elbow and stifle. Any animal with a splint should have the bandage changed and the fracture rechecked once a week.

Both casts and splints require similar care. They must be kept clean and dry and checked for slippage and mutilation by the animal. Any swelling in the toes or signs of malodor should also be noted. If observed, these changes need to be addressed immediately. Radiographs must be taken more often to confirm that fracture alignment and orientation have not changed. Any animal with a cast or splint must be confined to a crate or small room, with no opportunity to run, jump, play, climb stairs, or have free access to the outside until the fracture is healed.

Complications with Casts and Splints
The following complications may occur with casts or splints:

- Skin irritation
- Skin ulcers
- Non-union
- Malunion
- Delayed union
- Infection

Amputation

Amputation involves the complete removal of a limb from the body. Common indications for amputation include trauma resulting in severe soft tissue damage or irreparable fractures and neurologic injuries (e.g., brachial plexus avulsion). Other indications include neoplasia, ischemic necrosis, unmanageable arthritis, and severe congenital deformities. Both hindlimb and forelimb amputations are considered major surgeries and

should only be performed with a thorough knowledge of the patient's physical status. Preanesthetic blood tests, including complete blood count (CBC), chemistry panel, electrolyte status, and blood type and crossmatch, should be obtained before surgery whenever possible. The patient's preoperative condition is extremely important because a large amount of fluid, electrolytes, and blood is lost when the limb is removed. Patients should be stabilized before surgery with appropriate fluid, electrolyte, and blood replacement therapy. A balanced electrolyte solution should also be administered throughout the procedure to help maintain hydration and blood pressure.

A variety of techniques exist for removal of the forelimb and hindlimb. Forelimb amputation can be achieved by disarticulation of the shoulder joint or by removal of the scapula. Scapular removal is faster and easier and allows for a more cosmetically favorable result compared with shoulder disarticulation. Hindlimb amputation involves either midshaft femoral amputation or disarticulation of the coxofemoral joint. Midshaft amputation is considerably easier to perform than hip disarticulation. All techniques involve severing the muscles at their origins or insertions or directly through the muscle belly (Figure 7-59). Major nerves are then isolated and directly injected with a local anesthetic (Figure 7-60) before they are transected (Figure 7-61). Local nerve blocks

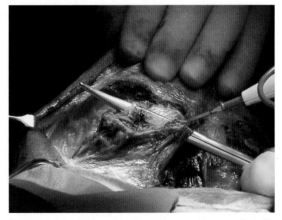

Figure 7-59 Dissection through sartorius muscle belly of medial hindlimb using electrocautery during a hindlimb amputation.

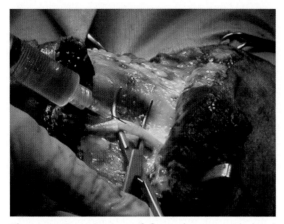

Figure 7-60   Injection of femoral nerve with local anesthetic before transection.

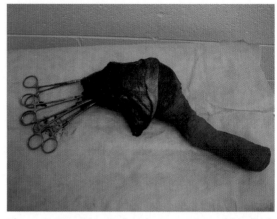

Figure 7-62   Disarticulated amputation of hindlimb postoperatively.

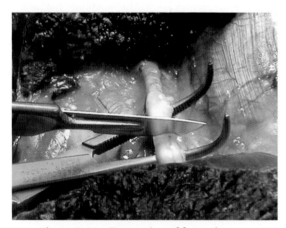

Figure 7-61   Transection of femoral nerve.

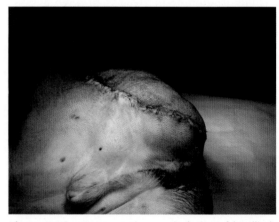

Figure 7-63   Postoperative surgical site of hindlimb amputation (disarticulated).

contribute significantly to postoperative pain control. Arteries and veins are isolated from surrounding tissues. Arteries are usually ligated first, thus allowing blood to drain through the venous system. In patients with neoplasia, however, veins are ligated first to limit the dissemination of tumor cells. Figures 7-62 and 7-63 show an amputated limb and the appearance of a disarticulated coxofemoral joint postoperatively.

Pain management is critical for amputation patients. A variety of analgesic protocols are currently available and are often used in combination for effective prevention of postoperative discomfort.

Epidural anesthesia should be performed preoperatively and can be achieved with various drugs; morphine is often used in forelimb amputations, and an opioid and local anesthetic are frequently used in hindlimb amputations. Epidural anesthesia with both an opioid and a local anesthetic is extremely effective in controlling postoperative pain. As mentioned, intraoperative visualization of the nerves allows direct injection of local anesthetic before transection. Systemic injections of opioids and nonsteroidal anti-inflammatory drugs (NSAIDs) are often administered postoperatively. Transdermal fentanyl patches are also recommended as part of the postoperative pain management program. These patches allow a slow, continuous administration of fentanyl over 72 hours. The patch is applied to a clipped area of the animal's skin immediately after surgery.

Cranial Cruciate Repair

Indications: Cranial cruciate ligament (CCL) ruptures are also referred to as *anterior cruciate ligament* (ACL) injury or "football player's knee" in human patients. CCL surgical repair should be performed for a partial or complete rupture of the ligament. Both the cranial and the caudal cruciate ligaments act as major stabilizing structures in the knee. The cruciate ligaments originate on either side of the femoral condyle, then course across the intercondylar fossa and attach on opposite sides of the tibia (Figure 7-64). These ligaments function as the primary check against hyperextension of the stifle joint and limit internal rotation of the tibia. Rupture of the CCL causes instability of the stifle, which leads to degenerative changes in the joint, including synovitis, degeneration of articular cartilage, osteophyte formation, and capsular fibrosis. The medial meniscus usually is also damaged in dogs with CCL rupture. The meniscus is a fibrocartilaginous structure between the femur and tibia that functions to cushion and center the joint. CCL rupture most often causes a bucket-handle type of tear in the medial meniscus.

Rupture of the CCL is the most common cause of hindlimb lameness in the dog. Ligament failure can result from both traumatic (acute) and degenerative (chronic) causes. Currently, degenerative causes are the most common reason for CCL rupture. Osteoarthritic changes act as a precursor to CCL weakening and rupture. Reports also indicate that 37% of dogs with a unilateral CCL tear will rupture the contralateral ligament within 2 years, indicating that degenerative processes often occur in both stifle joints.

Traumatic rupture results from hyperextension of the stifle joint or excessive internal rotation of the tibia. The CCL becomes tightly twisted, and the excessive mechanical forces cause the ligament to tear. Dogs often present with a history of running and catching their leg in a hole or trapping their leg in a fence or gate, or jumping to catch an object (e.g., Frisbee). Traumatic injuries account for approximately 20% of CCL ruptures.

Dogs that have sustained an acute rupture present with significant hindlimb lameness. However, the degree of lameness varies widely with the increasing chronicity of the injury. The hind leg is usually carried in flexion, and occasionally at rest the toe may touch the ground. Dogs may resist manipulation of the stifle joint because of the pain from acute inflammation. Joint effusion may also be palpable adjacent to the patellar tendon.

The major diagnostic tests for CCL injury include palpation, the tibial compression test, and the cranial drawer test (Figure 7-65). Palpation of the affected leg often reveals muscle atrophy,

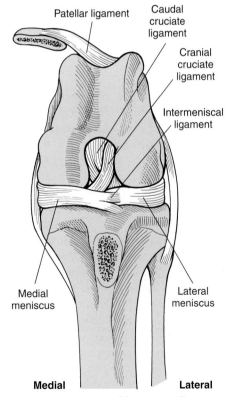

Figure 7-64 Orientation of the cruciate ligaments and menisci. (From Fossum TW: *Small animal surgery*, ed 2, St Louis, 2002, Mosby.)

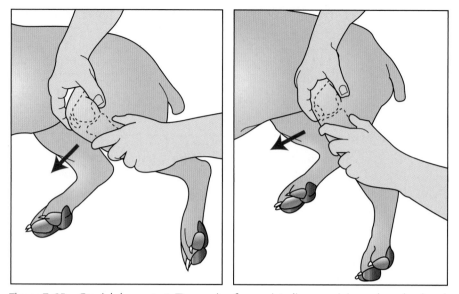

Figure 7-65   Cranial drawer test. To examine for cruciate ligament injury, place the thumb of one hand over the lateral fabella and the index finger over the patella. Stabilize the femur with this hand. Place the thumb of the opposite hand caudal to the fibular head with the index finger on the tibial tuberosity. With the stifle flexed and then extended, attempt to move the tibia cranially and distally to the femur. (From Fossum TW: *Small animal surgery,* ed 2, St Louis, 2002, Mosby.)

pain, joint effusion, and asymmetry. Flexion and extension of the stifle joint may result in an audible click associated with displacement of the medial meniscus. Examination of the affected joint reveals a positive cranial drawer sign (cranial displacement of the tibia) and increased internal rotation of the tibia with joint flexion.

Special Instruments
A variety of retractors are typically used for CCL surgery. Hohmann retractors allow inspection of the internal surfaces of the joint (Figure 7-66). Steinmann pins and a Jacob's chuck are used to drill holes in the tibia. Cruciate needles allow the passage of suture through dense tendons and tissues. Securos currently offers a crimping system that is used for extracapsular repairs (Figure 7-67). Both 40- and 80-lb-test nylon is available. A distractor is used to place tension on the suture loop and can be locked to check cranial drawer. Crimp tubes are then placed and crimped (with a special crimping tool) to hold the suture in place.

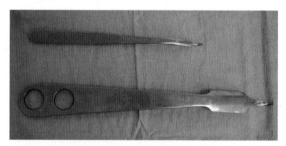

Figure 7-66   Hohmann retractors.

Patient Positioning
The patient may be placed in dorsal or lateral recumbency with the affected leg up for CCL repair. The leg should be clipped from the hip to the tarsus. An examination glove should be placed on the foot to cover the unshaven area. The leg should be suspended while it is scrubbed to ensure complete and circumferential sterility. It is important to prepare the limb in this suspended position to allow the greatest amount of manipulation during surgery (Figure 7-68).

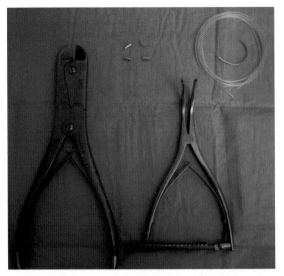

Figure 7-67   Securos Cruciate Repair System. *Left to right,* Crimper, crimp tubes, distractor, 80-lb fishing line and needle.

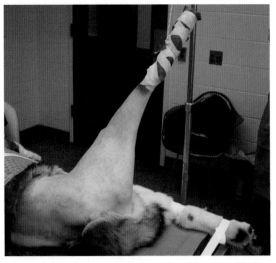

Figure 7-68   Lateral recumbency positioning with suspended leg is usually appropriate for orthopedic surgical preparation of a limb.

Patient Draping

The surgeon should grasp the suspended leg in a sterile manner, and the foot and tarsus should be covered with an appropriately sized stockinette. The leg is held suspended, and a three-cornered draping technique is used at the hip.

Cranial Cruciate Ligament Repair

A variety of surgical techniques have been designed to restore stability to the stifle and limit secondary degenerative joint disease. It is recommended that the joint capsule be opened with each technique to allow visualization and removal of the damaged ligament and menisci.

Intracapsular techniques involve replacement or reconstruction of the CCL using various materials, including biologic tissues (patellar tendon and fascia lata) and synthetic suture material. The joint is approached laterally (Figure 7-69), and a graft of tissue is isolated. A tunnel is then drilled through the cranial surface of the tibia. The graft is fed through the tunnel and over the top of the lateral condyle, thereby reconstructing the CCL.

Extracapsular techniques are usually faster and easier to perform than intracapsular repairs. Extracapsular repairs involve placement of sutures outside the stifle joint. The joint is approached laterally, and the appropriate suture (e.g., monofilament nylon, nylon fishing line) is loaded onto a properly sized cruciate needle. The needle is passed around the fabella, then through the patellar ligament. A hole is drilled through the tibial crest with a Steinmann pin, and the suture is passed through the hole (Figure 7-70). The stifle is then flexed into a normal standing position, and cranial drawer is tested. Once the suture is under the appropriate tension, it is tied or crimped into place. The retinaculum should be closed with a vertical mattress pattern to provide appropriate imbrication of the joint capsule.

Both intracapsular and extracapsular reconstruction techniques rely on a re-creation of the passive constraints of the stifle joint. In recent years a technique has been developed that re-creates joint stability by altering the active constraints of the joint. CCL rupture causes the tibia to slide forward and the femur to fall back, creating a shear force referred to as *cranial tibial thrust.* The tibial plateau–leveling osteotomy (TPLO) functions to change the angle of the tibia, thereby directly altering joint mechanics and creating a new plateau that eliminates cranial tibial thrust. Currently, surgeons must be certified to perform the TPLO technique.

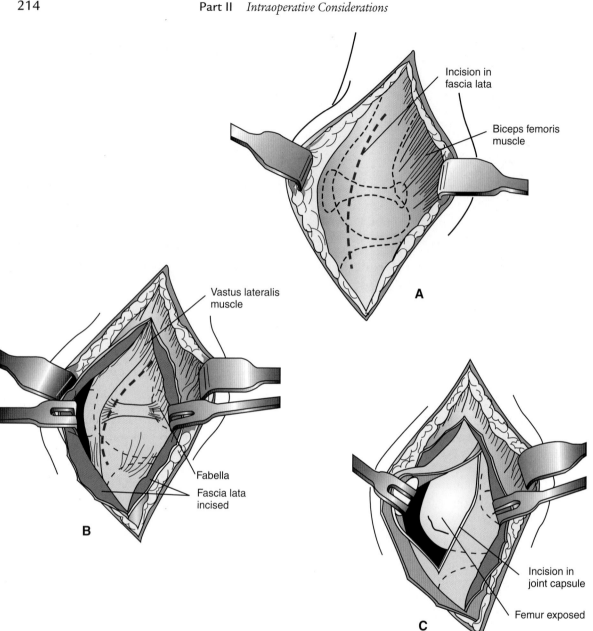

Figure 7-69   Lateral approach to stifle joint. **A,** Make a craniolateral skin incision centered over the patella. Incise the subcutaneous tissues along the same line to visualize the septum between the superficial leaf of the fascia lata and the biceps femoris muscle proximally and then the lateral retinaculum distally. **B,** Make an incision through the fascia lata proximally, and carry the incision through the fascia lata and lateral retinaculum distally. **C,** Incise the joint capsule and continue the incision proximally, adjacent to the patellar tendon. Then incise along the border of the vastus lateralis toward the fabella. Displace the patella medially to expose the cranial surface of the joint. (From Fossum TW: *Small animal surgery,* ed 2, St Louis, 2002, Mosby.)

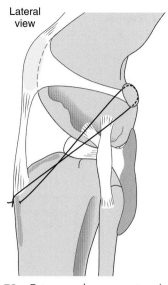

Lateral view

Figure 7-70 Extracapsular reconstruction using a heavy, nonabsorbable suture. The suture passes through deep fascia surrounding the fabella and through a predrilled hole in the tibial crest. Tying or crimping the suture eliminates the cranial drawer. (From Fossum TW: *Small animal surgery*, ed 2, St Louis, 2002, Mosby.)

Postoperative Considerations and Instructions

A soft bandage should be placed on the limb for 48 hours after CCL repair to protect the surgical site and reduce swelling. The patient should return in 14 days for a recheck and suture removal.

The most important postoperative consideration is exercise restriction. Dogs should be restricted to short leash walks for at least 6 weeks after surgery. Activity can then be gradually increased over a 12-week period. Owners are discouraged from allowing their animals to run free, jump, climb stairs, and play rambunctiously with other animals. Failure to comply with strict exercise restriction may result in repair failure and the need for a second surgery.

Because CCL repairs are considered moderately painful, pain management is a major focus during the recovery period. Perioperative pain control involves injection of a local anesthetic directly into the joint. Animals are often treated immediately postoperatively with a variety of injectable pain medications, including opioids and NSAIDs. Animals are then often sent home with instructions for the owner to administer an oral NSAID (e.g., carprofen) for several days after surgery.

In recent years a rigorous rehabilitation program has been advocated as part of the standard postoperative care for patients with CCL repair. Rehabilitation programs promote wound healing and decrease muscle spasm, adhesion formation, and edema while increasing muscle strength and joint range of motion (ROM). Typical programs include low-impact exercises (e.g., swimming), passive ROM exercises, heat, and whirlpool therapy.

Box 7-10 shows an example of a surgery report for a cranial cruciate ligament repair.

BIOPSY AND MASS REMOVAL

Biopsy and removal of a mass are important procedures in veterinary medicine. A biopsy is often recommended before mass removal. The biopsy is used to gather important information on the biologic and clinical behavior of the mass, allowing the formulation of an appropriate plan and prognosis. Current biopsy techniques include fine-needle aspiration, impression smear, punch, bone, excisional, and incisional biopsies.

Fine-Needle Aspiration Biopsy

Fine-needle aspiration (FNA) represents one of the simplest methods for cytologic evaluation of a mass. The technique is easy to perform, has minimal morbidity, and usually does not require sedation; however, FNA biopsy typically has a low diagnostic yield.

Technique

1. Obtain a 22- or 20-gauge needle and 5-ml syringe. Place the needle into the mass.
2. Apply negative pressure by pulling back on the hub of the syringe.
3. Withdraw the needle and syringe from the mass, and remove the needle from the syringe.

BOX 7-10   Surgery Report: Cranial Cruciate Ligament Repair

Animal Hospital Name

Owner: John Doe

Address: 555 Sterling Lane

Jupiter, NY 55555

Phone number: 555-5555

Animal Name: Sasha

Animal #: 656565

Species: Canine

Breed: Labrador

DOB: 05/05/01

Date of Surgery: 12/03/2005

Primary Surgeon: Dr. Vet

Assistant: Nurse Scrub

Diagnosis or Preoperative Signs: Cranial cruciate ligament rupture

Surgical Procedure: Right stifle arthrotomy, extracapsular cranial cruciate repair

Implants: 80-lb-test fishing line, two Securos clamps

Description of Surgical Procedure

Surgical Approach: An 8- to 10-cm parapatellar skin incision was made at the right stifle, and the underlying subcutaneous tissues were incised. The retinaculum and the joint capsule of the stifle were incised, and the interior of the stifle joint was visualized.

Surgical Pathology: Complete rupture of the cranial cruciate ligament.

Surgical Procedure: The remnants of the torn cranial cruciate ligament were removed and the joint was explored. No meniscal damage was evident at this time. The joint was lavaged with sterile saline, and the joint capsule was closed with 2-0 PDS in an interrupted suture pattern. Bupivacaine (10 ml) was injected into the joint capsule. A hole was then made in the tibial tuberosity using a Steinmann pin. A wire passer was used to pass 80-lb fishing line behind the lateral femoral fabellar ligament. The fishing line was then passed (medial to lateral) through the hole in the tibial tuberosity and then under the patellar ligament. A Securos clamp was then placed at the end of each line. A distractor was used to tighten the lines until the joint was stable. The joint was checked for drawer as well as range of motion. A Securos crimper was then used to crimp each of the clamps three times. The surgical site was lavaged with sterile saline and closed routinely.

Closure:
Joint capsule: 2-0 PDS in interrupted cruciate pattern.
Retinaculum: 2-0 PDS in interrupted suture pattern.
Subcutaneous tissue: 3-0 Monocryl in continuous suture pattern.
Skin: 3-0 nylon in interrupted suture pattern, followed by some skin staples.

4. Fill the syringe with air, replace the needle, and gently blow the fluid and cells onto a glass slide.

This method is generally performed several times to obtain representative samples.

Impression Smears

Impression smears are as simple to perform as FNA biopsy. This technique is especially useful for ulcerated surface tumors and is often performed on freshly cut surfaces. Impression smears of excised masses can also be easily made before the samples are placed into formalin.

Technique

First, gently blot the surface of the mass with a paper towel to remove any excess blood and exudates. Then, gently touch the surface of the mass to several areas of a glass slide. Take care not to twist or rub the slide against the mass because this can crush cells and destroy the integrity of the sample.

Needle Punch Biopsy

Needle punch biopsy instruments are currently manufactured by a variety of companies. Instruments are equipped with either a cutting or a core biopsy needle and are available as manual and automatic devices (Figure 7-71). These devices take a small piece of tissue (approximately the size of pencil lead) for histologic examination. These procedures are minimally invasive and generally are performed on sedated patients. Ultrasound-guided needle punch biopsies of various internal organs, including the liver, spleen, and prostate, are also common procedures.

Technique

The area to be biopsied is clipped and aseptically scrubbed. The overlying skin and muscle are often blocked with a local anesthetic. The mass is held with one hand, and a small stab incision is made into the overlying skin. The end of the needle is inserted through the stab incision; the instrument is fired; and the inner needle is advanced into the mass. The entire instrument is withdrawn from the mass, and the sample is gently removed from the sample chamber with a cotton swab or needle (Figures 7-72 and 7-73).

Punch Biopsy

The punch biopsy technique is used primarily for external skin and oral masses. It has the advantage of providing a larger surface sample; however, it does not penetrate deeply into the mass. Patients are generally placed under general anesthesia to undergo this procedure.

Technique

The area to be biopsied is clipped and aseptically scrubbed. The punch is rotated back and forth over the mass until the punch sits deeply in the lesion. The punch is removed, and a scissors is used to detach the sample from its base (Figure 7-74).

Bone Biopsy

The most common instruments used to obtain bone biopsy samples are the Michele trephine (Figure 7-75) and Jamshidi bone biopsy needle (Figure 7-76). Bone biopsies are often painful and therefore are usually performed under general anesthesia. The Jamshidi needle biopsy is less invasive but provides a smaller sample size compared with other methods. The Michele trephine technique removes a larger sample of bone, increasing the diagnostic yield, but it also increases the likelihood of a pathologic fracture at the biopsy site.

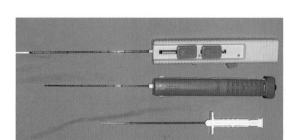

Figure 7-71 Three varieties of needle punch biopsy instruments.

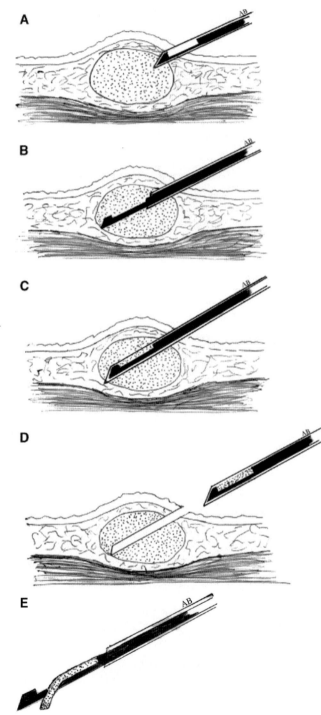

Figure 7-72   Use of the manual biopsy needle requires both hands and can be awkward. This can result in more discomfort for the patient and samples of lower quality. **A,** Tip of needle is inserted just into the tumor. **B,** Inner needle is advanced without advancing outer needle. **C,** Tissue from the tumor drops into trough of inner needle, and outer needle is advanced to cover inner needle, thereby cutting tissue within trough free from the main mass. **D,** With inner needle still completely within outer needle, thus protecting the sample, the entire unit is removed. **E,** Inner needle is advanced beyond end of outer needle to allow the sample to be removed from trough of inner needle. (From Mehler SJ, Bennet A: *Vet Clin Exotic Anim Pract,* 2005 [in press].)

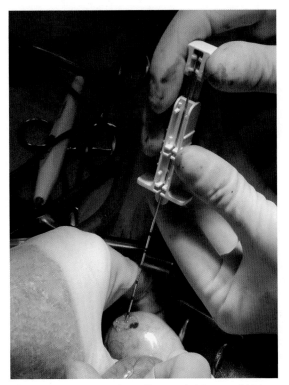

Figure 7-73 Manual needle punch biopsy of kidney during an exploratory laparotomy.

Technique

A small incision is made over the center of the lesion. The trephine or needle is pushed through the soft tissues until the bony cortex is reached. The stylet is removed, and the cannula or trephine is advanced through the bony cortex. Once an adequate sample has been obtained, the instrument is removed, and a wire is used to push the sample *out of the hub* of the needle (Figure 7-77). It is extremely important to avoid pushing the sample out of the tip of the needle, because this will destroy the architecture of the sample.

Incisional Biopsy

Incisional biopsies are generally used only after cytology or needle core biopsies have failed to provide a diagnostic sample. A small wedge of the tumor is removed from the mass and submitted for histopathology (Figure 7-78).

Excisional Biopsy

An excisional biopsy involves the complete removal of a mass (see Figure 7-78). Excisional biopsies are generally performed only on benign skin tumors or when the removal of the organ is indicated.

Biopsy Sample Handling and Fixation

It is imperative that tissue samples are handled gently at all times. Improper handling can ruin the diagnostic value of the sample. Impression smears should always be made before the sample is placed into fixative. It is often important to mark the margins of the surgical excision; this can be done by painting the outer edges of the excised mass with india ink or Alcian blue. The sample should then be allowed to dry for at least 20 minutes before it is placed into fixative.

All biopsy samples should be placed into a fixative before shipping. The most widely used fixative is 10% neutral buffered formalin. Proper fixation requires a ratio of 1 part tissue to 10 parts formalin. Tissue samples greater than 1 cm in thickness will not fix entirely; therefore, large masses should be sliced like a loaf of bread before they are placed into formalin. Multiple representative samples from a large mass can also be taken and preserved in the appropriate proportion of formalin. When multiple lesions or sites are biopsied, each sample should be placed into a separate and appropriately labeled container.

All sample containers must be properly labeled. Important identification information includes the date, the patient's last name (and hospital ID number if applicable), and the site from which the sample was obtained. All cytology slides should be properly labeled with pencil or ink that will not smear when the slide is moistened. All appropriate documentation must be completed and should include history, signalment, clinical findings, and tentative diagnosis.

EAR PROCEDURES

Aural Hematoma Repair

Definition: Aural hematoma refers to the formation of a hematoma within the auricular cartilage

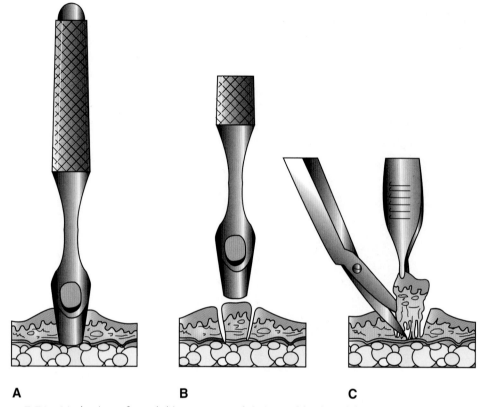

A   B   C

Figure 7-74   Mechanism of punch biopsy. **A,** Punch is rotated back and forth over suspect lesion until sufficient depth has been attained. **B,** Punch is removed or angled across base to sever deep attachments. **C,** Specimen may be gently grasped with thumb forceps and cut off deeply. (From Withrow SJ, MacEwen EG: *Small animal clinical oncology,* ed 3, Philadelphia, 2001, Saunders.)

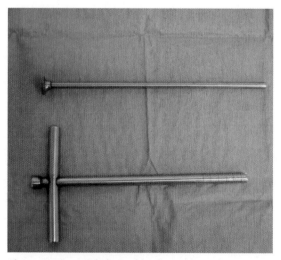

Figure 7-75   Michele trephine bone biopsy instrument.

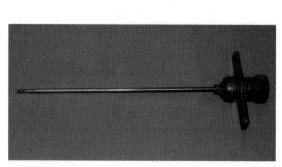

Figure 7-76   Jamshidi bone biopsy needle.

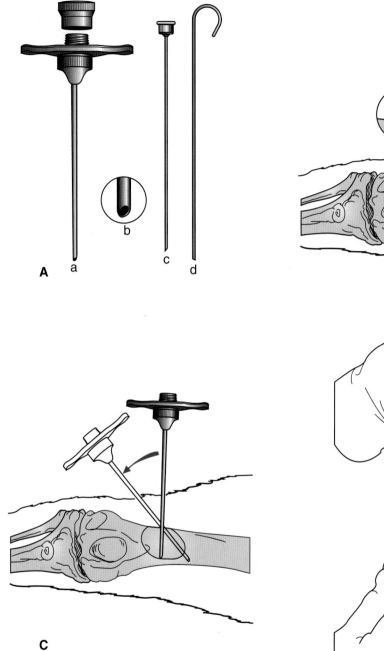
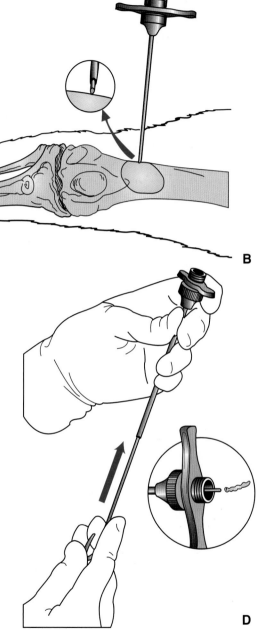

Figure 7-77   **A,** Jamshidi bone biopsy needle: cannula and screw-on cap *(a)*, tapered point *(b)*, pointed stylet to advance cannula through soft tissues *(c)*, and probe to expel specimen from cannula *(d)*. **B,** With stylet locked in place, cannula is advanced through the soft tissue until bone is reached. *Inset,* Close-up view showing stylet against bone cortex. **C,** Stylet is removed, and bone cortex is penetrated with cannula. Cannula is withdrawn, and procedure is repeated with redirection of the instrument to obtain multiple core samples. **D,** Probe is then inserted retrograde into tip of cannula to expel the specimen through the base *(inset).* (From Powers BE et al: *J Am Vet Med Assoc* 193:206, 1988.)

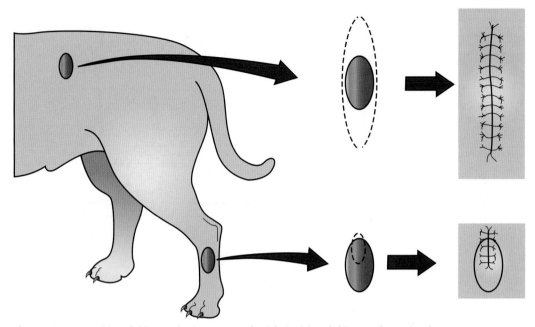

Figure 7-78   Excisional biopsy *(top)* contrasted with incisional biopsy *(bottom)*. The top tumor may be as easy to remove as to biopsy, and removal may not negatively influence other possible treatments (e.g., additional surgery, radiation). The bottom tumor, however, requires knowledge of the tumor type before excision, because inappropriate removal could compromise a subsequent aggressive excision (short of amputation). Note that the biopsy incision is in a plane that would be included in a subsequent resection. (From Withrow SJ, MacEwen EG: *Small animal clinical oncology,* ed 3, Philadelphia, 2001, Saunders.)

on the concave surface of the ear. The hematoma forms when the cartilage in the ear pinna fractures, usually from violent head shaking or scratching at the ears secondary to otitis, foreign bodies in the ear canal, atopy, and ear mites. It is important to treat the underlying cause of the aural hematoma to prevent further injury and recurrence. Auricular hematomas occur most frequently in pendulous-eared dogs, but they also occur in cats and erect-eared dogs.

Indications: Surgical correction of an aural hematoma should be performed as soon as possible to relieve the animal's pain and to prevent a permanently thickened, cauliflower-like ear.

Instrumentation

A soft tissue surgery pack will provide the surgeon with the necessary instruments for surgical correction of an aural hematoma.

Patient Positioning

Patients are usually placed in lateral recumbency with the affected ear dorsal.

Patient Draping

A single fenestrated drape should be sufficient for the aural hematoma procedure.

Treatment Options

A variety of treatment options exist for the repair of aural hematomas. The objectives of these treatments are to eliminate the hematoma and prevent reappearance of the condition. This section describes only one common treatment option.

Incision Drainage Procedure

Incision drainage is probably the most widely used procedure for the treatment of aural hematomas. Its purpose is to eliminate dead space between the layers of cartilage until scar tissue can form. An incision (S-shaped or straight) is made directly over the entire hematoma. Fibrin and blood clots are removed, and the area is lavaged. Several vertical mattress sutures are placed on the concave surface of the ear around the incision (Figure 7-79) to avoid pocket formation where fluid can collect. The incision itself should remain open to allow continual drainage.

Box 7-11 shows an example of a surgery report for incision drainage.

Lateral Ear Canal Resection

Definition: Resection of the lateral ear canal involves lateralization of the horizontal ear canal.

Indications: Lateral ear canal resection is indicated for animals with chronic otitis externa or neoplasia. Lateral wall resection allows drainage of the ear canal while affording ventilation of the canal. Bacteria thrive in moist and humid environments, so allowing ventilation reduces the risk of infection. Surgery improves the chronic condition in many patients, but it is not a cure. Appropriate medical management is usually required in conjunction with surgery.

Instrumentation
A soft tissue surgery pack should be sufficient for lateral ear canal resection.

Patient Positioning
The patient should be positioned in lateral recumbency with the affected ear upward and the head slightly elevated. A sandbag can be placed under the head for elevation.

Patient Draping
A four-quarter draping method should be used for lateral ear resection. The inner and outer aspects of the pinna should be aseptically prepared and can be left in the surgical field.

Lateral Ear Resection Procedure
The entire ear, including both sides of the pinna and the adjacent skin, should be clipped and aseptically prepared. The ear canal should be lavaged and cleaned before entering the OR. Once the animal is prepped and draped, the surgeon makes

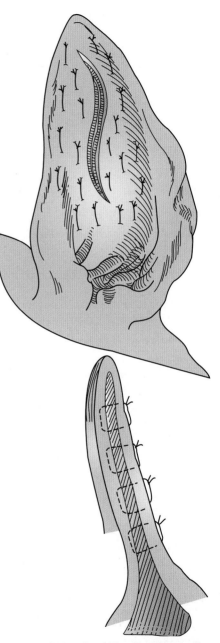

Figure 7-79   Sutures should be placed vertically rather than horizontally for aural hematoma repair. Sutures may be placed through the cartilage without incorporating the skin on the convex surface of the ear, or full-thickness sutures may be used. (From Fossum TW: *Small animal surgery,* ed 2, St Louis, 2002, Mosby.)

BOX 7-11   Surgery Report: Incision Drainage Procedure

Animal Hospital Name

Owner: John Doe

Address: 555 Sterling Lane

Jupiter, NY 55555

Phone number: 555-5555

Animal Name: Sasha

Animal #: 65656501

Species: Canine

Breed: Labrador

DOB: 05/05/01

Date of Surgery: 01/03/2002

Primary Surgeon: Dr. Vet

Assistant: Nurse Scrub

Diagnosis or Preoperative Signs: Aural hematoma right ear

Surgical Procedure: Incisional drainage of aural hematoma

Description of Surgical Procedure

Surgical Approach: An S-shaped incision was made directly over the aural hematoma on the concave region of the pinna of the right ear. Blood and clots were evacuated.

Surgical Pathology: Aural hematoma located on concave surface of right ear.

Surgical Procedure: An S-shaped incision was made with a scalpel over the fluctuant part of the hematoma. Blood was drained out of the cavity, and several small clots were removed with forceps and by blotting with sponges. Numerous simple mattress sutures of 3-0 nylon were placed in a vertical orientation in a staggered pattern through the skin on the concave side of the ear and the underlying cartilage. The S-shaped incision was left open to drain, and a bandage was placed covering the entire ear.

Closure: See above.

---

two parallel skin incisions from the tragus ventrally past the horizontal ear canal. The incision should extend past the region where the canal becomes horizontal. The skin flap is then excised at the proximal region. A vertical incision is made in the subcutaneous tissue over the vertical canal. The subcutaneous tissue is then reflected dorsally, exposing the auricular cartilage of the vertical canal. The cartilage of the vertical canal is then cut distally along the same incision line. The cartilage flap is reflected distally and the opening of the horizontal canal observed. The proximal two thirds of the cartilage flap are excised, and the remaining third is reflected ventrally to form a "drainboard," which is then sutured to the ventral skin incision. The drainboard technique was established by Zepp to maintain horizontal canal patency (Figure 7-80).

Postoperative Considerations and Instructions

A bandage may be placed over the ear after the lateral ear canal resection. The owner should be made aware of possible mutilation of the surgical site by the pet. An Elizabethan collar should be sent home with the owner to avoid self-mutilation complications. Although complications are uncommon, insufficient drainage and sustained ear infections may be seen postoperatively. Most lateral ear resections still require medical management by the owner. Before leaving the hospital, the owner should also be instructed on how to clean and administer medication into the hori-

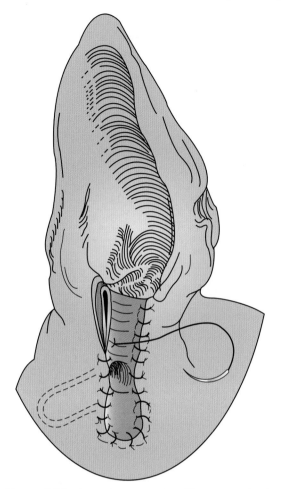

Figure 7-80 Lateral ear resection (Zepp procedure). (From Fossum TW: *Small animal surgery,* ed 2, St Louis, 2002, Mosby.)

zontal canal. Because the anatomy of the ear canal has changed, the tympanic membrane is more susceptible to damage. Analgesics should be sent home with the owner. Suture removal should be performed 10 to 14 days after surgery.

Box 7-12 shows an example of a surgery report for a lateral ear resection.

OPHTHALMIC PROCEDURES

Entropion Repair

Definition: Entropion refers to a "rolling in" of the eyelid. This can mean the upper lid only, lower lid only, or both lids. Different regions of the eyelid may be involved: the medial aspect, the lateral aspect, or the entire lid.

Indications: The primary indication for an entropion surgery is to alleviate ocular irritation caused by the eyelid or by the facial hairs adjacent to the lid, which come in contact with the conjunctiva and cornea.

Clinical Signs

Clinical signs of entropion may include lacrimation (tearing), *blepharospasm* (squinting, blinking), *photophobia* (sensitivity to light), *enophthalmos* (pulling back of the eye and a secondary, raised third eyelid), *conjunctivitis* (inflammation of the conjunctiva), *keratitis* (inflammation of the cornea) with or without corneal ulceration, and self-trauma (pawing at the eye). Decreased vision may also result from constant eyelid closure or from corneal scarring caused by the constant irritation.

Developmental entropion, or *conformational entropion,* is the most common form seen in small animals, mostly dogs. It is believed to be inherited. The most common breeds presenting with developmental entropion are the Chinese shar-pei, chow chow, Saint Bernard, rottweiler, Great Dane, bullmastiff, Labrador retriever, and English bulldog. Dogs with conformational entropion may have both eyes affected at the same time, but occasionally only one eye is affected.

Spastic entropion occurs secondary to ocular pain, which may result from a corneal foreign body, uveitis (intraocular inflammation), corneal ulceration, or chronic conjunctivitis. The painful eye is pulled back, causing the eyelid to roll inward. In cases of spastic entropion the primary problem must be addressed and resolved. Application of a topical anesthetic usually will temporarily resolve a spastic entropion. Dogs with developmental (conformational) entropion still have rolling in of the eyelid even after application of topical anesthetic.

Patient Positioning

The patient is placed in sternal or lateral recumbency for entropion surgery; several sandbags can be used to help position the head.

Patient Draping

Often a specialized eye drape is used for the patient undergoing entropion repair. An eye drape has a precut hole (fenestration) that is placed directly over the eye. The drape is secured with towel clamps.

Patient Preparation

Cleanliness and sterility of the surgical area are important in the patient with entropion. Shaving or clipping of the surgical area and the surrounding skin is done first. Baby shampoo diluted (1:3) with water is both effective and safe in cleansing the shaved area. Gauze squares soaked in the dilute baby shampoo are used to gently wipe away stray hairs and debris. Then, a very dilute (1:50) povidone-iodine (Betadine) solution is used in the same manner. To achieve asepsis, the dilute Betadine solution should be in contact with the skin for approximately 1 minute. The area is gently wiped with gauze squares soaked in sterile saline to remove the Betadine solution. If necessary, the eye is flushed with saline to remove any dirt, particles, or mucus that may be trapped under the lids or within the surrounding conjunctiva.

BOX 7-12   Surgery Report: Lateral Ear Canal Resection

Animal Hospital Name

Owner: John Doe

Address: 555 Sterling Lane

Jupiter, NY 55555

Phone number: 555-5555

Animal Name: Sasha

Animal #: 65656501

Species: Canine

Breed: Cocker Spaniel

DOB: 05/05/01

Date of Surgery: 01/03/2005

Primary Surgeon: Dr. Vet

Assistant: Nurse Scrub

Diagnosis or Preoperative Signs: Chronic otitis externa AU

Surgical Procedure: Lateral ear canal resection

Description of Surgical Procedure

Surgical Approach: Two parallel skin incisions were made from the tragus ventrally past the horizontal canal.

Surgical Pathology: The right and left ear canals were inflamed, with a marked amount of ceruminous discharge present.

Surgical Procedure: The skin incision was extended past the vertical canal, and the proximal skin flap was excised. A vertical incision was made in the subcutaneous tissue over the canal, and the tissue was reflected dorsally. The cartilage of the vertical canal was incised distally along the incision line. The proximal region of the cartilage flap was excised. The remaining cartilage flap was reflected ventrally and sutured to the ventral skin incision with 3-0 nylon. The same procedure was performed on the left ear.

Closure: See above.

AU, Both ears (Latin *aures unitas*).

Special Instruments

Because of the delicacy of eye surgeries such as entropion repair, specialized instruments are often required. Appropriate care and handling of the following ophthalmic instruments are important:

- **Bishop-Harmon forceps** is a straight tissue forceps typically used for handling eyelid and conjunctival tissues (Figure 7-81). These forceps come with delicate teeth (for grasping conjunctiva) or medium-sized teeth (for grasping eyelids).
- **Chalazion forceps** provides tissue stabilization and hemostasis (Figure 7-82).
- **Jaeger lid plate** resembles a shoehorn. It has flat, curved ends that are placed under the eyelid to provide a firm surface when making an incision (Figure 7-83).
- **Stevens tonotomy scissors** is a special ophthalmic scissors. These scissors have small, rounded tips, which make them efficient at undermining conjunctiva (Figure 7-84).
- **Needle holders** are used for handling delicate sutures; various types are available, such as the micropoint (Figure 7-85).

Surgical Options

Eyelid Tacking

Eyelid tacking is performed in young animals to roll out the eyelid temporarily (Figure 7-86). Young puppies (usually up to 16-20 weeks) with conformational entropion are candidates for temporary placement of sutures or staples. The Chinese shar-pei is a common breed to benefit from eyelid tacking. Even though eyelid tacking is a relatively simple procedure, standard postoperative care is important. An Elizabethan collar should be worn until the sutures or staples are removed. In some cases, a repeat surgery may be necessary. Permanent correction is usually delayed until the animal reaches its adult conformation.

In cases of spastic entropion, temporary eyelid tacking, in addition to treatment of the underlying cause, may result in resolution of the problem.

Hotz-Celsus Procedure

Several techniques are described to correct conformational entropion. The Hotz-Celsus procedure is a widely used approach that involves excision of a crescent-shaped section of skin and muscle (a "smile") from the affected portion of the eyelid (Figure 7-87). Eversion of the eyelid is accomplished by suturing the resulting skin defect.

A Jaeger lid plate is first inserted under the affected portion of the lid for stabilization. An incision is made approximately 2 to 3 mm from the eyelid margin using a No. 15 Bard Parker blade. The incision should be the same length as the rolled-in portion of the lid. A second incision

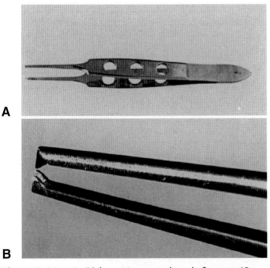

A

B

Figure 7-81   **A,** Bishop-Harmon thumb forceps (Storz Ophthalmics, St Louis). **B,** The 1 × 2 intermeshing teeth. (From Nasisse MP, Grevan VL, Constantinescu GM: *Vet Clin North Am* 27[5]:969, 1997.)

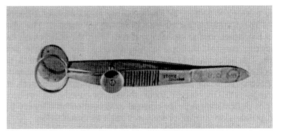

Figure 7-82   Desmarres chalazion forceps (Storz Ophthalmics, St Louis). (From Nasisse MP, Grevan VL, Constantinescu GM: *Vet Clin North Am* 27[5]:970, 1997.)

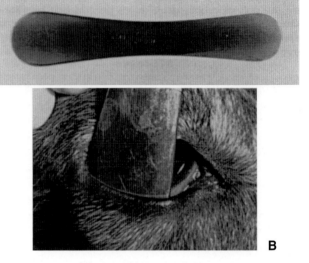

A

Figure 7-83 **A,** Jaeger lid plate (Storz Ophthalmics, St Louis). **B,** Plate positioned under the eyelid, illustrating how it would be used to perform a Hotz-Celsus procedure. (From Nasisse MP, Grevan VL, Constantinescu GM: *Vet Clin North Am* 27[5]:971, 1997.)

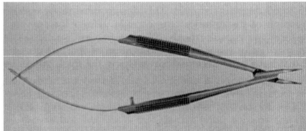

B

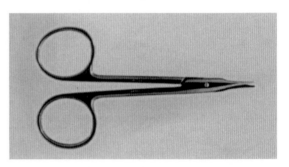

Figure 7-84 Stevens tenotomy scissors (Storz Ophthalmics, St Louis). (From Nasisse MP, Grevan VL, Constantinescu GM: *Vet Clin North Am* 27[5]:975, 1997.)

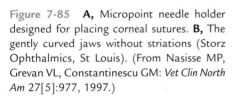

A

Figure 7-85 **A,** Micropoint needle holder designed for placing corneal sutures. **B,** The gently curved jaws without striations (Storz Ophthalmics, St Louis). (From Nasisse MP, Grevan VL, Constantinescu GM: *Vet Clin North Am* 27[5]:977, 1997.)

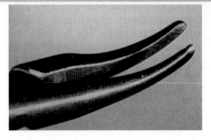

B

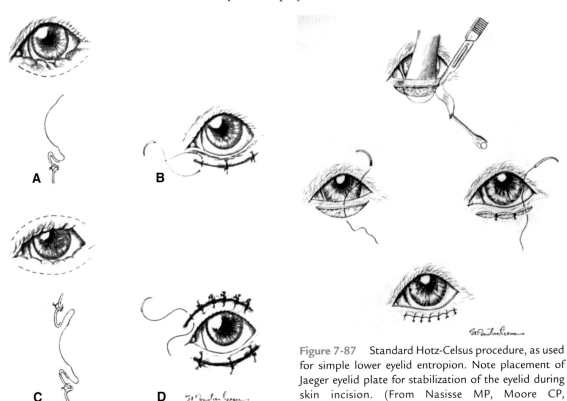

Figure 7-86   Eyelid tacking. Temporary eversion of lower eyelid (**A** and **B**) and both upper and lower eyelids (**C** and **D**). This procedure results in eversion of the eyelid margin while inverting a furrow of skin *(dashed line)* between bites of the vertical mattress sutures. (From Nasisse MP, Moore CP, Constantinescu GM: *Vet Clin North Am* 27[5]:1019, 1997.)

Figure 7-87   Standard Hotz-Celsus procedure, as used for simple lower eyelid entropion. Note placement of Jaeger eyelid plate for stabilization of the eyelid during skin incision. (From Nasisse MP, Moore CP, Constantinescu GM: *Vet Clin North Am* 27[5]:1020, 1997.)

is made distal to the first incision, creating a "smile" or crescent-shape. The outlined strip of skin and muscle is removed by sharp dissection.

Subcutaneous sutures are usually not necessary with the Hotz-Celsus procedure. Skin sutures are placed approximately 1 to 2 mm apart in a simple interrupted pattern. Common sutures used are silk, gut, and polyglactin 910 (Vicryl). Small sutures are preferred, usually 5-0 or 6-0, because they produce a better cosmetic effect.

Complications with the Hotz-Celsus procedure may result from making the initial incision too far from the eyelid margin or placing the sutures too far apart.

Postoperative Considerations

A patient is often discharged the day of entropion surgery. Tissue swelling may occur, although this should resolve within a few days. Warm compresses at home may be applied to the area to help with any swelling. Sutures are left in place for about 10 to 14 days. Nonabsorbable sutures are most frequently used. Absorbable sutures can also be used, especially if removing the sutures will be difficult because of an aggressive or uncooperative animal. A topical ophthalmic antibiotic is usually sent home with the owner to be used two or three times a day for 10 to 14 days after surgery.

An Elizabethan collar should be worn until the sutures are removed, to prevent the sutures from being rubbed out before healing has been completed. The awkwardness of the Elizabethan collar, especially in large dogs, often requires restriction of activity until the collar is removed.

A recheck examination is recommended 10 to 14 days after surgery, or sooner if there are any problems. Box 7-13 shows an example of a surgery report for entropion repair.

Eyelid Mass (Neoplasm) Removal

Eyelid Anatomy and Function

The eyelids are one of the main structures that protect the globe, specifically the cornea. Eyelids are composed of skin and accessory parts, including hair follicles and glandular structures. Dogs have eyelashes only on the upper lid; cats have no eyelashes. The inside of the eyelids are lined with a highly vascularized mucous membrane, the conjunctiva. Interposed between the surface skin of the eyelids and the conjunctiva are muscle and fibrous tissue. The eyelids contain glands that contribute to the ocular tear film. The *meibomian* (tarsal) *glands* run parallel to the upper and lower eyelid margins. These glands secrete the oily (lipid) component of the preocular tear film.

Besides protection, other functions of the eyelids include distributing the tear film across the

---

BOX 7-13   Surgery Report: Entropion Repair

Animal Hospital Name

Owner: John Doe

Address: 555 Sterling Lane

           Jupiter, NY 55555

Phone number: 555-5555

Animal Name: Fluffy

Animal #: 65656501

Species: Canine

Breed: Rottweiler

DOB: 05/05/04

Date of Surgery: 01/03/2005

Primary Surgeon: Dr. Vet

Assistant: Nurse Scrub

Diagnosis or Preoperative Signs: Entropion OU

Surgical Procedure: Hotz-Celsus entropion repair OU

Description of Surgical Procedure

Surgical Approach: The patient was placed in sternal recumbency and the head positioned with sandbags. Each eye was clipped, prepped, and covered with a sterile eye drape. Towel clamps were used to secure the drape in place.

Surgical Procedures: Ophthalmic scissors were used to make a "smile" incision into the skin and subcutaneous tissue of the ventral eyelid approximately 5 mm from this lid margin. The incision was wider laterally and tapered medially over a distance of approximately 1 cm. Minimal bleeding was encountered and effectively stopped using gentle pressure from a sterile cotton-tipped applicator. A simple interrupted 6-0 silk suture was first placed in the middle of this incision to re-appose the edges, followed by subsequent simple interrupted sutures approximately 2 mm apart to appose the skin edges.

Closure: See above.

OU, Each eye (Latin *oculus uterque*).

cornea and removing stray hairs or debris from the cornea.

Incidence and Differential Diagnosis

Eyelid masses are found in both dogs and cats. Breeds of dogs that are more predisposed to eyelid masses include poodles, Labrador retrievers, and mixed breeds. Generally, eyelid masses are seen in older dogs.

Canine eyelid masses are usually benign and *may* be differentiated based on their clinical appearance, but they should always be examined histologically as well.

Feline eyelid neoplasms are usually malignant and can rarely be differentiated from each other based solely on their clinical appearance.

Eyelid neoplasms may be raised, alopecic (having hair loss), pigmented or nonpigmented, and may or may not become ulcerated. Cytologic examination, specifically by fine-needle aspiration and biopsy samples of eyelid masses, may be helpful.

Canine Eyelid Neoplasms

A meibomian (sebaceous) adenoma is the most common eyelid neoplasm in dogs. It arises from the meibomian gland and is found near the meibomian orifice. Other, less common benign neoplastic masses include melanoma, papilloma, and histiocytoma. Malignant neoplastic masses occur less often in dogs and include mast cell tumors, adenocarcinomas, basal cell carcinomas, squamous cell carcinomas, hemangiosarcomas, and fibrosarcomas.

Feline Eyelid Neoplasms

Squamous cell carcinoma is the most common feline eyelid tumor and is often found in cats with white or pink eyelids. Other neoplasms include basal cell carcinoma, fibrosarcoma, and mast cell tumor.

Indications for Surgery

An eyelid mass should be removed if (1) the mass becomes too large, (2) there is concern about malignancy, (3) corneal or conjunctival irritation is present, or (4) the patient is traumatizing the mass, with or without bleeding. In some cases the owner may request removal of the mass to achieve an improved cosmetic appearance. Generally, the smaller the mass to be removed, the easier it is to reconstruct the lid, therefore preserving normal eyelid function. When the eyelid mass becomes too large (greater than one third of the length of the eyelid), skin flaps may be necessary for eyelid reconstruction. If the eyelid mass is not completely removed, it may recur.

Patient Positioning

The patient is placed in sternal or lateral recumbency for eyelid mass removal; several sandbags can be used to help position the head.

Patient Draping

Often a specialized eye drape is used. An eye drape has a precut hole that is placed directly over the eye. The drape is secured with towel clamps.

Patient Preparation

See previous section on patient preparation for entropion repair.

Special Instruments

See previous section on special instruments for ophthalmic procedures.

Surgical Options

Eyelid mass removal and subsequent eyelid repair involve careful apposition of the conjunctiva, eyelid margin, and the surrounding skin for cosmetic healing and optimal function of the eyelid. The alignment of the eyelid margin, both horizontally and vertically, is critical.

Wedge Resection

A wedge resection of the eyelid mass and adjacent eyelid is a simple, common procedure (Figure 7-88). A chalazion forceps or a Jaeger lid plate may be used for stabilization. A full-thickness "house-shaped" incision is made using sharp dissection. The incision is closed using two layers. Subcutaneous sutures are placed in a simple interrupted pattern using 5-0 Vicryl. Skin sutures are placed using a figure-8 pattern for apposition of the eyelid margin, and a few simple interrupted sutures are placed for the remainder of the incision using 6-0 Vicryl.

The mass is routinely biopsied and submitted for histopathology to confirm the diagnosis. Box 7-14 shows an example of a surgery report for wedge resection of eyelid mass.

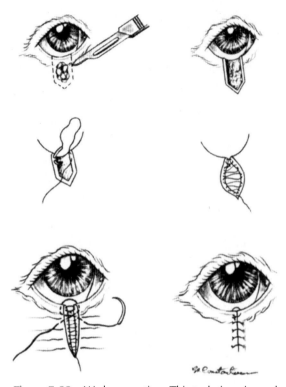

Figure 7-88   Wedge resection. This technique is used for full-thickness eyelid repair and applies to eyelid shortening (ectropion repair), mass excision, and eyelid laceration repair. This two-layer closure allows precise apposition of the eyelid margins and a stable repair with minimal chance of ocular irritation from suture knots. (From Nasisse MP, Moore CP, Constantinescu GM: *Vet Clin North Am* 27[5]:1038, 1997.)

Protrusion (Prolapse) of Gland of Third Eyelid

Protrusion of the gland of the third eyelid is also known as glandular hypertrophy, glandular hyperplasia, "cherry eye," and prolapse of third eyelid gland.

Third Eyelid Anatomy and Function

The *third eyelid,* also known as the "nictitating membrane," serves as added protection for the globe. It will rise up from the ventromedial aspect of the orbit (part closest to nose) and over the globe to protect it when the animal pulls its globe back into the orbit, for whatever reason.

Movement of the third eyelid also aids in removal of dirt and particles from the eye. On the underside of the third eyelid is a small gland that secretes and distributes approximately 30% of the tear production. Because the gland significantly contributes to the precorneal tear film, it should not be removed. Clinical studies have confirmed extensive clinical experience that *keratoconjunctivitis* (KCS, "dry eye") is frequently seen in such animals, often years later, especially in breeds susceptible to prolapse of the gland.

Mechanism of Prolapse

Prolapse of this third eyelid gland is the most common primary disorder of the third eyelid. A prolapse may result from a weakness in the connective tissue attachment between the ventral aspect of the third eyelid and the periorbital tissues; therefore the gland becomes everted while remaining attached to the cartilage of the third eyelid. This weakness allows the gland, which is normally found ventrally, to flip up dorsally, where it then becomes enlarged and inflamed because of chronic exposure. Abrasions and drying of the exposed gland may result in secondary inflammation and swelling. If the gland becomes severely infected, preoperative treatment with topical antibiotics is recommended.

Occasionally, in the early stages of prolapse, the gland will return to its normal position on its own or with manipulation. Unfortunately, the gland will usually reprolapse. Surgical intervention is the definitive treatment.

Clinical Signs

Common clinical signs of third eyelid gland prolapse include ocular discharge, conjunctivitis, and the pink, swollen mass on the third eyelid seen by owners. Tear production may be affected in some patients and may decrease.

Incidence

Protrusion of the gland of the third eyelid is usually seen in puppies and dogs less than 2 years of age. It can occur in one or both eyes. Breeds predisposed to this disorder are the cocker spaniel, English bulldog, Boston terrier, Great Dane, and pug.

BOX 7-14   **Surgery Report: Wedge Resection of Eyelid Mass**

Animal Hospital Name

Owner: John Doe   **Animal Name:** Fluffy

Address: 555 Sterling Lane   **Animal #:** 65656501

   Jupiter, NY 55555   **Species:** Canine

Phone number: 555-5555   **Breed:** Labrador

                                       DOB: 05/05/01

Date of Surgery: 01/03/2005

Primary Surgeon: Dr. Vet

Assistant: Nurse Scrub

Diagnosis or Preoperative Signs: Upper eyelid mass OS (3-4 mm in length)

Surgical Procedure: Eyelid mass resection

Description of Surgical Procedure

Surgical Approach: The patient was placed in sternal recumbency and the head positioned with sandbags. The left eye was clipped, prepped, and covered by a sterile eye drape. Towel clamps were used to secure the drape in place.

Surgical Pathology: A 3-mm mass on the eyelid margin at the meibomian glands.

Surgical Procedures/Correction: A chalazion forceps was placed around the eyelid mass to protect the globe, stabilize the tissue, and aid in hemostasis. Using a beaver blade, a wedge-shaped incision (5 mm wide × 15 mm tall) was made at the eyelid margin. The mass was incised using a blade and removed using ophthalmic scissors.

Closure:
Subcutaneous layer: using 5-0 Vicryl, two sutures were placed in simple interrupted suture pattern.
Skin layer: a figure-8 suture through the skin at the lid margin was placed using 6-0 silk. Three simple interrupted sutures using 6-0 silk were also placed.

Surgical Samples: The mass was resected and submitted for histopathology.

OS, Left eye (Latin *oculus sinister*).

Patient Positioning
The patient is placed in sternal or lateral recumbency for third eyelid gland surgery; several sandbags can be used to help position the head.

Patient Draping
Often a specialized eye drape is used. An eye drape has a precut hole that is placed directly over the eye. The drape is secured with towel clamps.

Patient Preparation
See previous section on patient preparation for entropion repair.

Special Instruments
Because of the delicacy of eye surgeries, specialized instruments are often required. Appropriate care and handling of ophthalmic instruments are important. In addition to those instruments

listed in the section on entropion repair, the following instrument is useful for surgical correction of third eyelid gland prolapse:

- **Barraquer lid speculum** is used to retract the eyelids without putting pressure on the eye itself (Figure 7-89).

Surgical Options

For years, surgical removal of the third eyelid gland was the treatment of choice for third eyelid protrusion. As the importance of the third eyelid gland in tear production became more apparent, however, surgical repositioning of the gland became widely recommended. Therefore, removing the third eyelid gland should be avoided, because this may and probably will predispose the eye to develop KCS (dry eye).

Numerous techniques are currently available for correcting prolapse of the third eyelid gland (Figures 7-90 and 7-91), with some providing greater success than others. The choice is usually the surgeon's preference. A simple, common procedure is discussed next.

Morgan Pocket Technique

The Morgan pocket technique involves creating a conjunctival pocket where the third eyelid gland is secured (see Figure 7-90). The third eyelid is grasped and suspended using forceps on the nasal and temporal sides. Two 1-cm parallel incisions are made on the posterior surface of the third eyelid. The incisions are arched toward each other, with one incision made above the third eyelid gland and the second made below it. Apposition of the two outermost incisions, with gentle

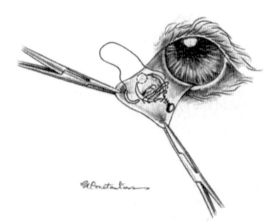

Figure 7-90   Morgan pocket technique for repair of prolapsed gland of third eyelid (TE). This method involves securing TE gland into a conjunctival pocket formed on posterior surface of TE. When suturing the conjunctival margins, openings are left on either end to allow drainage of secretions. Suturing begins by oversewing and burying the knot (subcutilcular pattern), then runs continuously through the conjunctiva from side to side, and finally is tied on anterior ventral surface of TE. This method of suturing prevents corneal irritation from the suture knots. (From Nasisse MP, Moore CP, Constantinescu GM: *Vet Clin North Am* 27[5]:1055, 1997.)

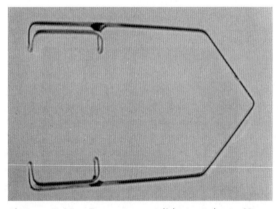

Figure   7-89   Barraquer eyelid speculum (Storz Ophthalmics, St Louis). (From Nasisse MP, Moore CP, Constantinescu GM: *Vet Clin North Am* 27[5]:972, 1997.)

Figure 7-91   (facing page) **A,** Typical appearance of prolapsed third eyelid gland. **B,** Elliptical incision. **C,** Initial anchor suture. **D,** Initial suture carried to opposite side of gland. **E,** Placement of a second suture. **F,** Initial suture is drawn together and tied. **G,** Inversion of prolapsed tissue. Dotted lines indicate that suture and knots lie under the conjunctiva. **H,** Appearance of third eyelid immediately after surgery. (From Bojrab MJ: *Current techniques in small animal surgery,* ed 2, Philadelphia, 1983, Lea & Febiger.)

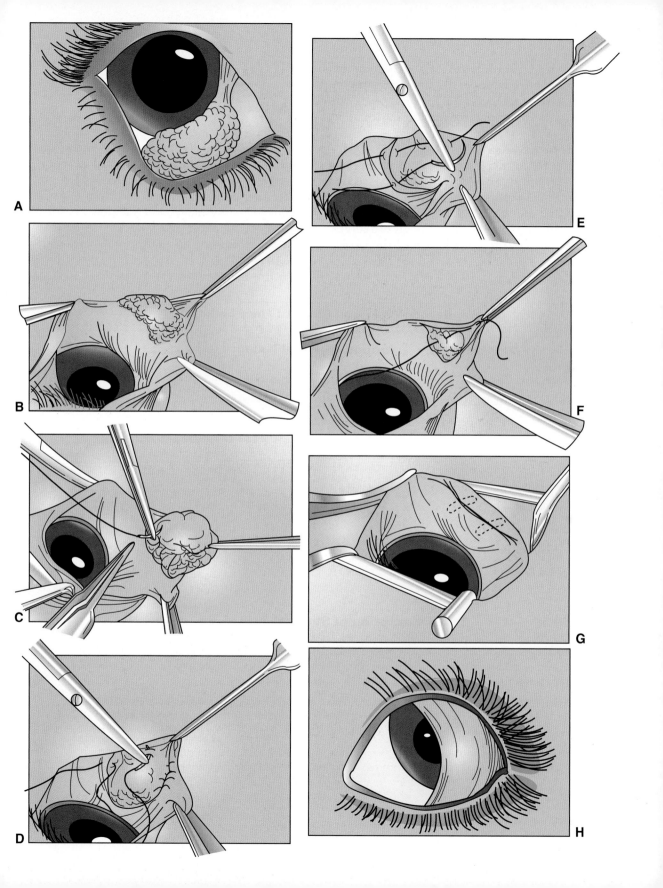

downward pressure applied to the gland, results in the gland being buried in the conjunctival pocket. Care must be taken to avoid the suture ends contacting the cornea and therefore causing irritation.

Postoperative Considerations

Inadequate positioning of the third eyelid gland may result in reprolapse. Usually a second attempt and possibly a third attempt to resecure the gland are made, typically using a different approach. Box 7-15 shows an example of a surgery report for correction of a prolapsed third eyelid gland.

MINIMALLY INVASIVE SURGERY

Laser Surgery

Laser surgery has been used in human medicine for many years but has only recently entered the field of veterinary medicine as a viable option to traditional surgery. More veterinarians are integrating laser surgery into their own practice because of its advantages over traditional surgery. Individual practices must decide about the cost-effectiveness of laser surgery compared with traditional surgery.

BOX 7-15   Surgery Report: Prolapsed Gland of Third Eyelid

Animal Hospital Name

Owner: John Doe

Address: 555 Sterling Lane

Jupiter, NY 55555

Phone number: 555-5555

Animal Name: Fluffy

Animal #: 65656501

Species: Canine

Breed: Pug

DOB: 05/05/01

Date of Surgery: 01/03/2005

Primary Surgeon: Dr. Vet

Assistant: Nurse Scrub

Diagnosis or Preoperative Signs: Prolapsed gland of the third eyelid, OD

Surgical Procedure: Morgan pocket technique

Description of Surgical Procedure

Surgical Approach: The patient was placed in left lateral recumbency to allow access to the right eye. The leading edge of the third eyelid was grasped with two small, noncrushing forceps and reflected away from its origin.

Surgical Procedures/Correction: With sharp dissection, two 1-cm incisions were made parallel to one another through the bulbar conjunctiva dorsal and ventral to the free margin of the gland. Blunt dissection was used to free up the conjunctiva for ease of suturing.

Closure (technique and suture): 6-0 Vicryl suture was used in a simple interrupted, buried pattern to appose the two incisions together, thus replacing the prolapsed gland within the third eyelid.

Surgical Samples: None.

OD, Right eye (Latin *oculus dexter*).

This section discusses the role of laser surgery in veterinary medicine, laser safety, and the advantages and disadvantages of using lasers as an alternative to traditional surgery.

How Does the Laser Work?

The word *laser* is short for **l**ight **a**mplification by **s**timulated **e**mission of **r**adiation. Lasers are able to create light at distinct wavelengths and distinct delivery parameters. Laser light wavelength and frequency determine the color of the laser light and the way the laser light interacts with its target surface. When laser light hits its target, it may be reflected, absorbed, scattered, or transmitted through the tissues, depending on the type of laser light being used. The types of lasers most often used in veterinary medicine are the carbon dioxide (CO_2) laser, diode laser, and neodymium:yttrium-aluminum-garnet (Nd:YAG) laser. The CO_2 and diode lasers are discussed here.

The clinical functions of the CO_2 and diode lasers consist of ablation, incision, and excision of soft tissue. Both the CO_2 and the diode lasers operate through photothermal laser-tissue interaction. This means that the laser light is absorbed and transformed into heat within the tissue. Water, hemoglobin, melanin, and some proteins absorb different wavelengths of light, which causes heating of the tissue. For example, the CO_2 laser is highly absorbed by water. The diode laser is highly absorbed by melanin and hemoglobin.

Heating of the tissue at different temperatures causes certain changes in the tissue. At 42° to 45° C, blood vessels are destroyed, resulting in necrosis of tissue. As tissue temperatures reach 50° to 100° C, proteins denature and coagulation occurs, causing irreversible tissue damage. Once tissue temperature surpasses 100° C, solid tissue becomes gaseous vapor and smoke plume. Increased heating of tissue can cause burning, resulting in carbonization of the tissue. This carbonization is called *char*. Charring occurs when tissue absorbs heat faster than it can be released. Heating to this extent results in damage to the surrounding tissue. Carbonization of the tissue also acts as a foreign substance and can hinder wound healing as well as cause inflammation at the site.

CO_2 Lasers versus Diode Lasers

CO_2 lasers are available at a wavelength of 10,600 nanometers (nm) (Figure 7-92). The CO_2 laser comes equipped with a selection of hand pieces and tips. Tips come in a variety of sizes (0.3-1.4 mm), and specific tips are used for specific surgical procedures. The CO_2 laser is considered a class IV laser system, as are most medical lasers. Lasers are separated into classes I to IV according to the degree of possible safety hazards to patients and users. The CO_2 laser is used predominantly to create surgical incisions, to excise after incision,

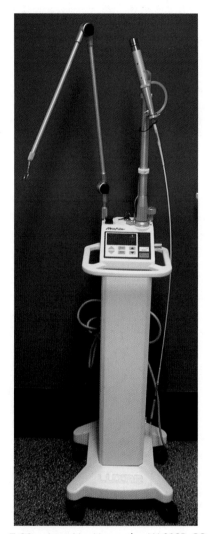

Figure 7-92   Accu Vet Novapulse LX-20SP CO_2 laser (Lumenis).

or for ablation of tissue. Most CO_2 lasers use a noncontact mode in which the laser tip never comes in contact with the tissue.

The 10,600-nm wavelength of the CO_2 laser is perfect for incising and vaporization because it is highly absorbed by water. Because most tissues have high water content, the laser energy is absorbed very close to the surface. The effect of the laser energy on tissue is determined by the laser wavelength, target tissue, spot size, power, and exposure (including exposure duration). Because laser wavelength (10,600 nm) and presumably the target tissue are known, the surgeon must decide the settings for the spot size, power, and exposure. *Spot size* refers to the diameter of the aperture. The distance of the tip from the tissue determines the exact spot size on the target tissue. Moving the tip away from the target tissue increases spot size. Moving the tip closer to the target tissue decreases spot size. The size of the tip also determines the spot size on the target tissue. Power settings are in watts (W), and the surgeon will select the appropriate wattage for a specific surgery. Power density depends on the set power, the spot size, and the distance of the tip from the tissue. The *exposure* refers to the duration of the laser beam, or how long the tissue is exposed to the laser beam. The clinician uses spot size, power, and exposure to control the interaction of the CO_2 laser beam and its effects on the tissue.

Available wavelengths for diode lasers in veterinary medicine range from 805 to 980 nm (Figure 7-93). The diode laser is also considered a class IV laser. Diode lasers are small, compact units that emit wavelengths that are easily transmitted through small, flexible optical fibers, allowing use with most flexible and rigid endoscopes. Diode lasers also come equipped with a variety of hand pieces and tips. The diode laser can reach its target tissue using a contact mode or a noncontact mode, whereas most CO_2 lasers use a noncontact mode of light transmission. Noncontact fibers are available in squared, cleaved, or polished tips and are more appropriate for ablation procedures. Contact fibers tend to be sculpted and are more appropriate for incisional purposes. Diode laser light has better absorption in hemoglobin and melanin, whereas the CO_2

laser light has better absorption in water. More collateral thermal damage may occur with the diode laser because of the deeper penetration, unlike the absorption of water closer to the surface with the CO_2 laser. Because of the enhanced absorption of hemoglobin, the diode laser may provide more proficient incisions and better hemostasis, especially of larger vessels.

The CO_2 and diode lasers can be used in a continuous mode or a pulse mode. The mode, tip size, and settings chosen by the clinician will vary depending on the type of procedure performed. When using either the CO_2 or the diode laser, the clinician should start with low power settings and a short duration of exposure until becoming familiar with the effects of the laser on the target tissue. Also, the laser energy should be delivered perpendicularly from the hand piece to the target tissue. When incising tissue, the clinician will apply lateral tension perpendicular to the incision. This will help reduce the formation of char. A record or log should be kept of each procedure performed as well as the power and duration settings. This task will most likely be the technician's responsibility. A log of procedures will aid the surgeon in deciding what settings to use for future procedures.

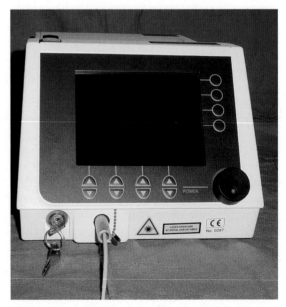

Figure 7-93 Accu Vet V25 fiber-coupled diode laser system (Lumenis).

Advantages and Disadvantages

The many advantages to using a laser device rather than a scalpel blade for specific surgical procedures include the following:

- More rapid healing time of tissue
- Cauterization of blood vessels during incision
- Sterilization of tissue during incision (less risk of postoperative infection)
- Minimal risk of damage to underlying healthy tissue (CO_2 laser specifically)
- Less need for suturing
- Reduced postoperative discomfort or pain
- Reduced postoperative swelling
- Decreased surgery time in many cases

The major disadvantages of laser surgery involve cost and safety. Laser machines may not be cost-effective for some small animal practices, and strict safety guidelines must be followed when using any laser device (see following section on laser safety).

Laser Procedures in Veterinary Medicine

Numerous procedures can be performed using the CO_2 and diode lasers. Lasers are often used with traditional surgeries. For example, the surgeon may prefer to use the laser to make an abdominal incision for a laparotomy because of decreased bleeding, decreased postoperative pain, and the decreased healing time that lasers afford the patient. Diode lasers may be used for endoscopic and laparoscopic procedures because of their fiber-directed laser energy. Lasers may be used for surgical procedures ranging from minor elective surgeries (e.g., feline declaw, lump removal) to more extensive procedures (e.g., celiotomy, thoracotomy). Other laser procedures include canine and feline castration, dewclaw removal, amputation, cystotomy, soft palate resection, oncologic procedures (e.g., neoplasia removal), and ophthalmic procedures. Whether to use laser energy or traditional surgery is ultimately the surgeon's decision.

Laser Safety

Laser safety may be the technician's most important responsibility when assisting with laser surgery.

It is imperative that precautions be taken to protect the clinical staff as well as the patient from the array of hazards associated with laser surgery. Many hospitals will assign a laser safety officer, often the nurse or technician. The safety officer is responsible for following safety guidelines established by the manufacturer of the laser machine or by the American National Standards Institute (Standards ANSI Z136.3-1988 and Z136.1-1993). These guidelines give specific instructions to follow for laser safety and laser use. Most laser companies also provide user and safety training when a hospital purchases a laser machine. Laser surgery should never be performed by anyone who has not had proper training or education about laser use and safety. The ANSI Standards recommend that prospective laser users become knowledgeable about policies and procedures, review clinical literature, attend courses for a certain number of hours, consult with an experienced operator of laser surgery, and receive training on specific equipment before operating laser machines.

Laser Hazards

Laser warning signs should be posted in the OR as well as on all doors entering the OR. Figure 7-94 shows the warning sign for class IV lasers.

Dangers associated with class IV lasers include eye, skin, fire, and smoke plume hazards.

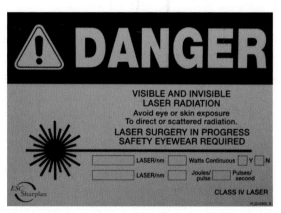

Figure 7-94 Laser warning signs should be posted on the doors to the operating room as well as within the OR.

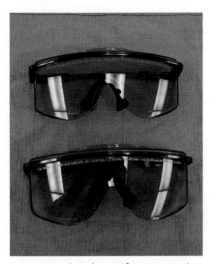

Figure 7-95 Wavelength-specific eye protection goggles for the diode laser.

Eye Hazards

Everyone in the laser OR must wear the eye protection goggles specific for the particular laser light (Figure 7-95). Different lasers emit different wavelengths, and the protection worn must coincide with the laser wavelength. Scattered reflections from the laser beam can cause serious corneal or retinal damage. The eyes of the patient should also be protected from scattered laser light. With the CO_2 laser, moistened sponges can be placed over the eyes for protection because the CO_2 laser beam is absorbed by water. Patient eye shields are also available.

Skin Hazards

Skin hazards may occur from direct or scattered laser beams. It may be in the clinician's best interest to wear gloves and a gown for added protection.

Fire Hazards

Possible fire hazards include the surgical drapes, anesthetic agents, oxygen, animal's fur, alcohol products used in surgical preparation, and methane from flatulence. With the CO_2 laser, wet sponges can be placed around the surgical area for protection of drapes. Any exposed fur around the surgical region can also be moistened with water. A nonalcohol surgical prep should always be used with all laser procedures (e.g., chlorhexidine or povidone-iodine preparation). The anesthetist

should always make sure the cuff of the endotracheal (ET) tube is inflated properly to decrease the chance of gaseous vapor or oxygen escaping. Standard polyvinyl chloride (PVC) tubes may be at risk for damage and ignition during a laser procedure. Laser-safe ET tubes can be purchased for procedures within the oral cavity. Another alternative is to lay moistened sponges around the standard ET tubes to prevent a possible fire hazard when working with CO_2 lasers. Because methane is considered another possible source for fire ignition, moistened sponges can be placed within the rectum of the patient when performing perianal surgical procedures (CO_2 laser). Fire extinguishers should be readily available in any laser OR in the event of unexpected ignition.

Smoke Plume Hazards

The smoke plume emitted from laser contact with tissue contains toxic and carcinogenic chemicals as well as bacteria and viral particles. An evacuator is usually purchased with the the laser machines. Laser surgeries should never be performed without an evacuation system. The smoke evacuator should be within 1 to 2 inches of the smoke's origin. Laser surgical masks are also available. Regular OR masks may not filter all toxic or infectious particles.

Feline Declaw Procedure (CO_2 Laser)

Feline declaw is also referred to as *feline onychectomy*. The CO_2 laser is ideal for performing this procedure (Figure 7-96). Traditional feline declaw surgeries have many potential complications, including pain, excessive hemorrhage, swelling, and infection. Laser declaw, if done correctly, should not have the complications associated with the traditional declaw methods. Remember that laser surgery affords the patient less pain postoperatively, cauterization of small vessels, decreased swelling, and sterilization of the tissue during excision. These positive aspects support the use of laser for feline onychectomy.

The surgeon will decide the wattage, mode, and tip size used for the procedure. The technician will ensure that the OR and its occupants are "laser safe." A hemostat can be positioned on the claw for manipulation and extension of the nail. A 360-degree circumferential incision is made

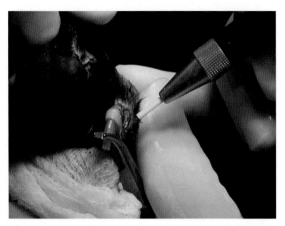

Figure 7-96   Feline onychectomy using CO_2 laser. A 360-degree circumferential incision is made through the skin and underlying fascia between second/third phalangeal articulation using 0.8-mm ceramic laser tip.

through the skin and the underlying fascia between the second and third phalanx. This incision exposes the common digital extensor tendon. The laser is then used to transect the common digital extensor tendon, as well as the deeper synovial layer at its insertion on the distal phalanx. Gentle distraction of the nail at this point will expose the collateral ligaments. The collateral ligaments are then incised bilaterally, and the joint (second/third phalanges) can be disarticulated. The third phalanx is further freed up by laser transection of the deep digital flexor tendon caudal to its ungual process. Care should be taken to avoid thermal damage to the digital pad and other soft tissue attachments caused by misdirection of the laser beam. This procedure should be repeated on each remaining claw.

At the end of the laser procedure, each digit should be meticulously examined. Any char noted on the digit should be removed with sterile gauze. Bandages can be placed for significant hemorrhage, but the laser declaw procedure is usually associated with minimal or no hemorrhage.

Postoperative Instructions
In addition to the general postoperative and discharge instructions for any declaw surgery described in Chapter 11, more specific recommendations exist for laser declaw surgery. As stated, postoperative pain tends to be decreased with

a laser declaw, but not absent. As with any procedure, appropriate analgesics should be administered postoperatively. Slight epithelial swelling is normal after surgery and may aid the redundant epithelium in covering the surgical site. Closure of the laser declaw site is usually not indicated. In most cases the patient will bear weight on the paws the same day or 1 day postoperatively.

Box 7-16 shows an example of a surgery report for a laser declaw procedure.

Laparoscopy

As with laser surgery, laparoscopy is also considered a minimally invasive procedure. Laparoscopy has been a beneficial diagnostic apparatus in human medicine for many years and is now being increasingly used in the veterinary field. The first clinical application of laparoscopy in dogs was in ovarian function studies performed in the early 1960s, and the first laparoscopic liver biopsy procedure in a dog was reported in 1972.

A laparoscopy is a minimally invasive abdominal procedure performed for the purpose of examining the peritoneal cavity and its viscera. A type of endoscope, called a *laparoscope,* is placed through a small midline incision or opening into the abdominal wall for inspection of the abdominal contents. Other incisions can be made into the abdominal wall (lateral to midline) for the insertion of laparoscopic instruments. These specialized instruments can be used for biopsy purposes as well as to perform specific procedures (e.g., spay, gastropexy) within the abdominal cavity. In many cases, laparoscopy can take the place of a full abdominal surgical procedure. In most cases, the procedure affords the patient a swift recovery with less potential for complications. This section describes the equipment and procedures associated with laparoscopy.

Advantages and Relative Contraindications
Advantages to performing laparoscopic procedures over traditional surgical laparotomies include the following:

- Improved patient recovery
- Smaller surgical incisions

BOX 7-16   Surgery Report: Laser Declaw

Animal Hospital Name

Owner: John Doe

Address: 555 Sterling Lane

　　　　　Jupiter, NY 55555

Phone number: 555-5555

Animal Name: Fluffy

Animal #: 65656501

Species: Feline

Breed: DSH

DOB: 05/05/04

Date of Surgery: 01/03/2005

Primary Surgeon: Dr. Vet

Assistant: Nurse Scrub

Diagnosis or Preoperative Signs: Normal healthy cat

Surgical Procedure: Front laser declaw

Description of Surgical Procedure

Surgical Approach: The patient was placed in left lateral recumbency. The distal forelimbs were scrubbed with chlorhexidine scrub.

Surgical Procedure: Each claw was extended by grasping the base of the nail with a hemostat. Using a CO_2 laser, a circumferential incision was made through the skin in the region of the second and third phalanx articulation. The laser was used to transect the common digital extensor. The collateral ligaments were incised bilaterally. The third phalanx (P3) was additionally freed following laser transection of the deep digital flexor tendon caudal to the ungual process of P3. Care was taken to avoid damage to the digital pad and other soft tissue attachments. The procedure was repeated for each claw.

Closure: No closure was necessary.

DSH, Domestic shorthair.

- Lower postoperative morbidity rate
- Lower postoperative infection rate
- Decreased postoperative pain
- Decreased hospitalization stay in most cases

There are few contraindications for laparoscopy because of its minimal invasiveness. Potential contraindications include ascites, abnormal clotting times, poor patient condition, obesity, and small body size. These are considered relative contraindications and are addressed according to the surgeon's discretion.

Laparoscopic Equipment

The necessary equipment to perform a laparoscopy includes the laparoscope or telescope, trocar-cannula units, fiberoptic light cable, light source, Veress insufflation needle, gas insufflator, and camera/video system (optional).

Laparoscopes

Laparoscopes for small animals range in size from 1.7 to 10 mm in diameter. The most common size tends to be the 5-mm-diameter scope for dogs and cats (Figure 7-97). Laparoscopes are also designed with varying telescope angles. The scope with a 0-degree field of view allows the surgeon to

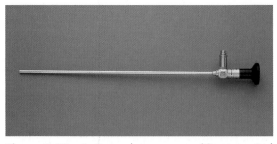

Figure 7-97 A 5-mm laparoscope. (Courtesy Karl Storz.)

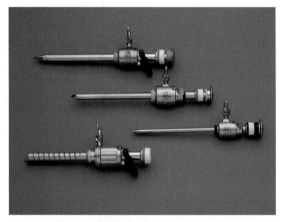

Figure 7-98 Smooth and threaded trocar-cannula units. (Courtesy Karl Storz.)

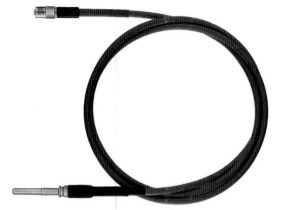

Figure 7-99 Fiberoptic light cable. (Courtesy Karl Storz.)

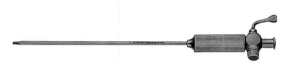

Figure 7-100 Veress insufflation needle. (Courtesy Karl Storz.)

observe the field precisely in front of the scope. Other angled scopes include the 30-degree and 45-degree fields of view. These angled telescopes enable the operator to look over the top of organs and examine small areas. Laparoscopes with an offset eyepiece that contains a channel for the introduction of accessory instruments are called *operating laparoscopes*. Trocar-cannula units are not needed with this type of scope.

Trocar-Cannula Units

Trocar-cannula units contain a trocar for puncturing through the abdominal wall and a cannula for the insertion of a telescope or laparoscopic instrument. These instruments are produced as threaded cannulas or smooth cannulas (Figure 7-98). The threaded cannulas screw into the abdominal wall, which allows for better gripping of the cannula. Threaded cannulas are less likely to slip or fall out

of the abdomen. Laparoscopic cannulas also contain a trumpet valve that thwarts the escape of gas from the abdomen.

Fiberoptic Light Cable and Light Source

A fiberoptic cable emits light from the light source to the scope (Figure 7-99). The light from the scope illuminates the abdomen so that the operator can see the organs clearly. Light cables come in an assortment of diameters. A 4- to 5.5-mm cable is recommended for general use in dogs and cats.

Many light sources are available (e.g., xenon 300 W). The light cable is attached to the light source for illumination of the abdomen.

Veress Insufflation Needle

The Veress insufflation needle is used for the original insufflation of the peritoneal cavity (Figure 7-100). This needle is composed of a sharp outer trocar and a blunt inner stylet. The stylet consists of a small opening to allow gas to insufflate into the abdomen. The outer trocar functions to puncture through the abdominal wall into the abdominal cavity. The trocar is then retracted, and the inner stylet with the small opening is exposed. Gas is then insufflated through the opening.

Gas Insufflator

Gas insufflators are also referred to as *laparoflators*. Tubing is connected from the gas insufflator to the Veress needle. The gas insufflator pushes gas through the tube to the needle to inflate the abdomen. This inflation lifts the abdominal wall away from the abdominal viscera. This allows the surgeon to view the abdominal organs as well as to perform biopsies or surgical procedures. Gas insufflators include CO_2, nitrous oxide, and room air. CO_2 is recommended because of its rapid rate of absorption. The laparoflators allow the operator to control the volume of gas being emitted and regulate the intra-abdominal pressure. Excessive intra-abdominal pressure decreases venous return to the heart and reduces the ability to ventilate. Excessive pressure can also interfere with excursions of the diaphragm. The abdominal pressures should not exceed 15 mm Hg.

Camera/Video System

A camera attached to a video system and monitor is mounted on top of the laparoscope (Figures 7-101 and 7-102). This system enables everyone in the OR to view the internal abdominal cavity on a monitor.

Special Instruments

A general-use soft tissue instrument pack should be available for laparoscopic procedures. The surgeon will require scalpel handles, blades, mosquito forceps, thumb forceps, needle holders, suture scissors, suture, and a bowl for saline. Laparoscopic instruments to have available include biopsy instruments, cutting instruments, and palpation probe (Figures 7-103 and 7-104). These instruments can be passed through cannulas of accessory ports to aid in biopsy retrieval or to perform surgical procedures. Most laparoscopic instruments are insulated so that they can be used with electrocoagulation units.

Instrument Care

Laparoscopic equipment is expensive and should be handled gently. The scopes and fiberoptic light

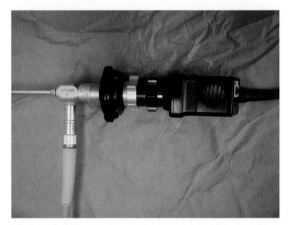

Figure 7-102   A 5-mm laparoscope with attached light cable. The camera is attached at the eyepiece of the laparoscope.

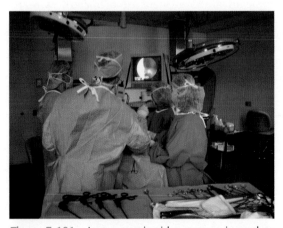

Figure 7-101   Laparoscopic video camera is used to allow viewing of the abdominal cavity on a monitor.

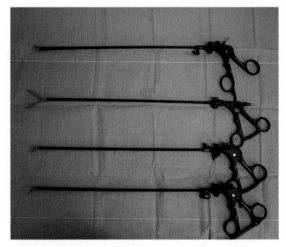

Figure 7-103   Various laparoscopic biopsy and grasping instruments.

cables can be easily damaged. These items can be cleaned with gauze and alcohol after each procedure and stored in their cases. The scopes and light cable can then be gas sterilized (ethylene oxide) or cold sterilized (also known as *high-level disinfection* [HLD]) before the procedure. Acceptable cold sterilization consists of 2% glutaraldehyde (Cidex).

A common alkylating agent approved by the Food and Drug administration (FDA) is 0.55% ortho-phthalaldehyde (Cidex-OPA). It has a strong mycobactericidal activity level and a strong stability over a wide pH range of 3 to 9 and requires no activation. Pentax and Olympus (two companies that manufacture laparoscopes) list OPA as a disinfectant compatible with flexible and rigid endoscopes for manual cleaning. The manufacturer states that 12-minute soaks are required to destroy all pathogenic organisms, but guidelines change and the manufacturer's instructions should be checked periodically. Gloves and eye protection should be worn when handling Cidex-OPA because it is a potential respiratory and dermal irritant. Cidex-OPA should be used in a well-ventilated area. The technician should refer to the manufacturer's detailed warnings and recommendations in the packet insert for further information. Once the instruments have been sterilized in Cidex, they should be rinsed thoroughly with sterile saline before entering the abdominal cavity. **Laparoscopes and light cables should never be autoclaved unless the manufacturer states they are "autoclave safe."** (See the section, Maintenance of Endoscope, on p. 255 for more information on HLD.)

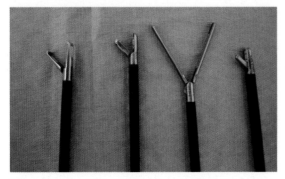

Figure 7-104   Various laparoscopic biopsy and grasping instrument tips. *Left to right,* Atraumatic grasping forceps, biopsy forceps with teeth, bowel grasper, and biopsy punch forceps.

Patient Draping

A four-quarter draping method should be considered for laparoscopic procedures. Single fenestrated drapes are specifically not appropriate for this procedure.

Laparoscopic Procedure

A patient undergoing a laparoscopy should be fasted for 12 hours to prevent regurgitation during anesthesia and to keep the stomach from being distended. The bladder should be expressed before entering the OR. An increased risk of traumatic puncture is present when these organs are distended. Distended organs can also make visualization of the target organs difficult. Most laparoscopic procedures are done with the patient under general anesthesia. The patient's abdomen should be clipped from the xiphoid process to the pubis as for any abdominal surgery. The clip should extend wide laterally for the placement of accessory ports. The animal may be placed in dorsal, left or right lateral recumbency. The positioning of the patient will depend on the procedure. For purposes of this discussion, assume the patient has been placed in dorsal recumbency. The abdomen should be prepared routinely.

Once the patient has been draped, the laparoscopic setup can begin. The surgeon should put on an extra pair of gloves for removing the scope and light cable from the Cidex. A nonsterile technician pours sterile saline over the scope and light cable for rinsing purposes. The items should be rinsed thoroughly to remove all the glutaraldehyde from the cable and scope. The items should then be dried with a sterile towel and the extra gloves removed. Next, a sterile sleeve is used to cover the camera, and the scope is placed on the head of the camera. The camera shows the images of the abdominal contents on a monitor to allow visualization of the abdomen by everyone in the OR. One end of the insufflation tubing is passed to a nonsterile technician and attached to the insufflator. The other end remains sterile and will be placed on the Veress needle.

The surgeon makes a 2- to 3-mm skin incision into the abdominal skin at midline for entry of the Veress needle. Once the Veress needle is placed, a drop of saline can be introduced at the hub of the needle. This will help the surgeon know when the abdominal cavity has been penetrated. Negative pressure in the abdominal cavity will draw the saline into the needle. Proper placement of the Veress needle is important. Subcutaneous emphysema can occur if the needle is placed between the muscle and subcutaneous tissue. Once proper placement is achieved, the outer trochar of the needle is retracted, and the blunt stylet with opening is uncovered. The insufflation tubing can then be connected to the needle, and insufflation can begin. Remember: insufflation of the abdomen should never exceed 15 mm Hg. The insufflator or laparoflator can be regulated to stop at 15 mm Hg. If pressure in the abdomen should decrease, the insufflator will increase the volume of gas being released.

Once insufflation of the abdomen has been achieved, a trocar-cannula can be placed. A skin incision is made through the skin in the region of the Veress needle. The trochar aspect of the unit will puncture through the abdominal wall for introduction of the cannula (Figure 7-105). Once the cannula has been sufficiently placed, the trochar is removed and the telescope (with camera) can be introduced through the cannula (Figure 7-106). The scrub team should now be able to view the abdominal contents on the monitor (see Figure 7-101). In many cases the picture will

appear foggy at first because of the heat from the abdomen. The scope can be removed and wiped with a warm, moistened, sterile gauze sponge. The scope can then reenter the abdominal cavity through the cannula port.

If a surgical procedure or biopsy is to be performed, the introduction of a second and a third cannula may be required for instrumentation purposes. The same technique can be used as for the telescope cannula. These cannulas will most likely be placed lateral to midline (Figure 7-107). Placement of the cannulas will depend on the

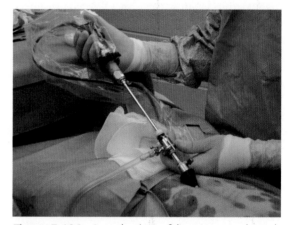

Figure 7-106 Introduction of laparoscope through 8-mm cannula.

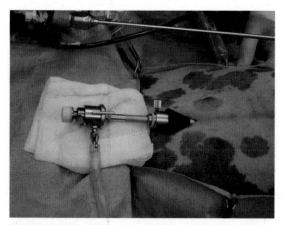

Figure 7-105 After removal of Veress needle, 8-mm trocar-cannula unit is introduced at midline. The laparoscope will be introduced into the abdomen through this cannula. Note the attached tubing for insufflation of the abdomen.

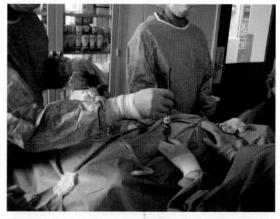

Figure 7-107 An accessory cannula has been introduced on the right side of this dog's abdomen. A blunt probing instrument has been inserted through the cannula to allow for manipulation of the abdominal organs.

location of the organ being biopsied; Figure 7-108 shows an intraoperative laparoscopic liver biopsy. When placing additional cannulas, the surgeon can view the placement into the abdominal cavity by directing the scope to the region of placement. This will ensure proper placement without causing damage to the abdominal viscera. The laparoscopic instruments can then be placed through the accessory ports for manipulation, biopsy, or surgical procedure.

Box 7-17 shows an example of a surgery report for a laparoscopic procedure.

Endoscopy

Endoscopy is the technique of examining internal body structures using specialized optical instruments. Endoscopy is generally considered a high-yield and noninvasive or minimally invasive procedure. It is high yield in that it often results in diagnostic and therapeutic benefits for the patient. The body is entered ("invaded"), usually through an orifice (e.g., mouth, anus), but no incision (noninvasive) or a small incision (minimally invasive) is required to enter the body. In the diagnostic workup of most cases, noninvasive tests (e.g., radiography, ultrasonography, some endoscopic procedures) are performed before minimally invasive procedures (e.g., other endoscopic procedures), which are performed before invasive procedures (e.g., exploratory celiotomy).

Endoscopic Procedures

Endoscopes can be used for the following noninvasive and minimally invasive procedures:

- **Cystoscopy,** to evaluate the bladder and lower urinary tract through the urethra.
- **Gastrointestinal (GI) endoscopy,** including:
  - **Esophagoscopy,** to examine the esophagus by way of the mouth.
  - **Gastroscopy,** to examine the stomach and upper small intestine (duodenoscopy) through the mouth.
  - **Colonoscopy,** to examine the colon by way of the anus.
- **Rhinoscopy,** to evaluate the nasal passages through the nares.
- **Tracheobronchoscopy,** to evaluate the trachea and bronchi by way of the mouth.

Endoscopes can also be used to examine the inside of joints (arthroscopy) and the abdominal cavity (laparoscopy), but these require incising the tissues, whereas the procedures listed above do not require incisions.

This discussion is limited to GI endoscopy. The other types of endoscopy listed are not common in private practice and are beyond the scope of this text.

Gastrointestinal endoscopy is indicated for the patient with chronic vomiting, diarrhea, or weight loss when other diagnostic tests (intestinal parasite

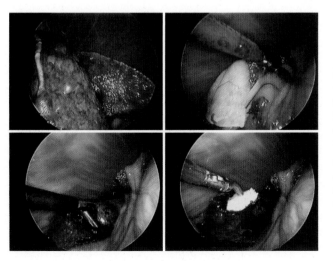

Figure 7-108 Intraoperative laparoscopic liver biopsy. *Top left,* Laparoscopic view of diseased liver lobes. Note the many diffuse nodules throughout the liver lobes. *Top right,* Grasping instrument is placed through an accessory port to remove omentum away from the proposed biopsy site. *Bottom left,* Biopsy forceps is used to biopsy a piece of liver for diagnostic purposes. *Bottom right,* Absorbable gelatin sponge is placed at the biopsy site to control hemorrhage. This will stay in place and be absorbed by the body.

| BOX 7-17 | Surgery Report: Laparoscopic Procedure |

Animal Hospital Name

Owner: John Doe

Address: 555 Sterling Lane

Jupiter, NY 55555

Phone number: 555-5555

Animal Name: Sasha

Animal #: 65656501

Species: Canine

Breed: Doberman pinscher

DOB: 05/05/01

Date of Surgery: 01/03/2005

Primary Surgeon: Dr. Vet

Assistant: Nurse Scrub

Diagnosis or Preoperative Signs: Liver disease

Surgical Procedure: Laparoscopy

Description of Surgical Procedure

Surgical Approach and Procedure: The patient was placed in dorsal recumbency, and a Veress needle was inserted at the level of the umbilicus. The abdomen was insufflated with CO_2 through this needle until the pressure was approximately 10 mm Hg. On conclusion of insufflation, a 5-mm laparoscopic cannula was inserted into the hole created by the Veress needle. The video laparoscope was directed into the abdomen through the cannula port, and the abdominal contents were examined. A second cannula was then placed approximately 7 cm lateral to the first site for the insertion of a laparoscopic biopsy instrument. A biopsy sample was retrieved from the left medial liver lobe. The region was observed for hemorrhage. Little hemorrhage occurred.

Surgical Pathology: All liver lobes were diffusely abnormal. Small nodules (1-2 mm in size) were observed throughout the liver lobes.

Closure:
3-0 PDS: Closure of the small incisions in the body wall and subcutaneous tissue in a simple interrupted suture pattern.
3-0 nylon: Closure of the skin incisions in a simple interrupted suture pattern.

---

tests, blood work, radiographs, ultrasound) have proved inconclusive. Other clinical signs that may warrant upper or lower GI endoscopy are anorexia, constipation, *dysphagia* (difficulty or inability to swallow), *hematemesis* (blood in vomitus), *hematochezia* (frank blood in stool), *melena* (black, tarry stool from digested blood), mucoid feces, regurgitation, retching, *ptyalism* (hypersalivation), and *tenesmus* (ineffectual straining to defecate).

In addition, if the patient swallowed a foreign body (e.g., coins, nuts, bolts), endoscopy offers an alternative to surgically opening the stomach to remove the foreign body.

Endoscopy allows the clinician to examine tissues directly, obtain biopsy samples, and perform therapeutic procedures, such as the retrieval of foreign bodies. General anesthesia and proper fasting are required for all endoscopic procedures.

For each procedure that requires passing the endoscope through the mouth, the patient should be intubated with an endotracheal (ET) tube, and a mouth speculum should be used to prevent any damage to the endoscope. The cuffed ET tube will aid in preventing aspiration of reflux or regurgitated material from the oropharynx during the procedure.

Endoscope Selection

Endoscopy equipment is now affordable for private practices and not only for referral centers and educational institutions. Manufacturers such as Pentax and Olympus now offer a variety of affordable, high-quality used instruments and endoscopes if new equipment is not an option. Supply and repair companies such as Endoscopy Support Services offer a variety of endoscopy equipment from these manufacturers. These three companies will meet the needs of most endoscopists.

When purchasing endoscopy equipment, veterinarians should primarily consider (1) the probable frequency of use and the equipment's versatility, (2) the quality of the optical system, and (3) the ease of maneuvering the endoscope. Purchase price is important with many veterinarians, but it can be a costly mistake if a cheaper, low-quality endoscope is purchased instead of a higher quality scope; a thorough examination may be compromised, and a definitive diagnosis may not be achieved. High-quality endoscopes will benefit hospitals because their cost can usually be covered after 2 years, and if maintained properly, the endoscopes will provide many more years of service.

A standard flexible endoscope with a diameter of 8 to 11 mm and a working length of 100 cm is usually adequate for feline and canine upper GI examinations and colonoscopies (Figure 7-109). A new endoscope should have these features and capabilities: (1) a four-way distal tip deflection with at least 180 degrees of upward deflection (for retroflexion), (2) water flushing, (3) air insufflation, (4) suctioning, (5) locking deflection controls, (6) an accessory channel with a diameter of 1.8 to 2.4 mm, and (7) forward-viewing optics. Some endoscopes are now manufactured with a working length of 140 to 150 cm for large-breed

dogs so that the duodenum and ileum can be entered. Endoscopes with two-way tip deflection are available but are not recommended, especially for upper and lower GI examinations.

Flexible Endoscopes

Because they are long and pliable, flexible endoscopes are better than rigid endoscopes for procedures that require bending or flexibility to examine areas such as the stomach, duodenum, and colon. Flexible endoscopes are used for noninvasive procedures and are available with either a two-way (up/down) or a four-way (up/down and left/right) distal tip deflection. The deflections are controlled by an angulation knob mounted on the control section of the endoscope. Older endoscopes have a maximum upward tip deflection of 180 degrees, whereas newer endoscopes have an upward tip deflection of 210 degrees (Figure 7-110). Endoscopes range in length from 50 to 170 cm, with insertion tube diameters ranging from 1 to 15 mm.

There are two types of flexible endoscopes: fiberoptic (Figure 7-111) and video (Figure 7-112). *Fiberoptic Endoscope*
With a fiberoptic endoscope, a light cable carries light by fiberoptic bundles from an external light source through the control section and to the insertion tube. The control section is protected by

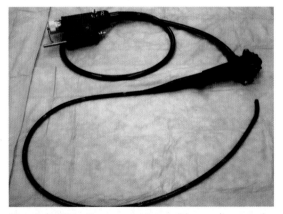

Figure 7-109 Pentax veterinary video endoscope for small animal procedures with insertion tube length of 100 cm and diameter of 11 mm. (Courtesy MJR-VHUP, Philadelphia.)

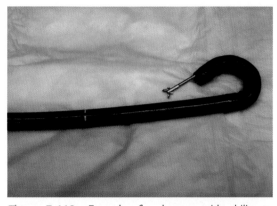

Figure 7-110   Example of endoscope with ability to retroflex 210 degrees. (Courtesy MJR-VHUP, Philadelphia.)

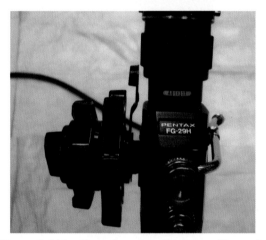

Figure 7-111   Control section for Pentax fiberoptic endoscope. The angulation system is on the right side of the endoscope (right side of endoscope appears on left side of figure). The large inner knob deflects up and down, and the small outer knob deflects right and left. The top valve is for suctioning, and the bottom valve is for air insufflation and flushing water to clean a dirty lens. If any images are to be taken, a camera head can be attached from the eyepiece on the endoscope to the endoscopy unit. (Courtesy MJR-VHUP, Philadelphia.)

hard plastic and contains the viewing lens, angulation control knobs, biopsy ports, white balance, and camera controls. The control section also has an eyepiece. The insertion tube houses the fiberoptic light strands and channels for air insufflation and water flushing, biopsy and retrieval instruments, and suction. When the air/water valve is compressed, water flushes and rinses the

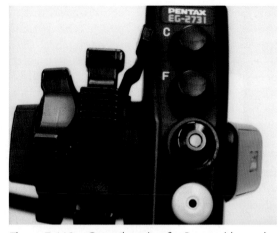

Figure 7-112   Control section for Pentax video endoscope. The angulation knobs and valves are the same as for the fiberoptic endoscope except images can be directly taken from the endoscope. The "F" button is to freeze an image, and the "C" button is to capture an image so it can be printed and stored in a computer. (Courtesy MJR-VHUP, Philadelphia.)

lens on the distal tip of the endoscope. When the air/water valve port is covered, insufflation occurs and can be regulated (Figure 7-113).

The biopsy channel port is located at the base of the control section at the junction with the insertion tube. The insertion tube itself is protected by a waterproof sleeve. Although the endoscope has three distinct sections (light guide plug, umbilical or universal cord, and control section), it is a one-piece unit that is sealed and watertight.

The distal tip of the insertion tube can bend more easily than the rest of the endoscope because a rubber insert covers the last few inches. Tip deflections can be fixed in any position by using the lock mechanisms situated next to the angulation knobs. This construction allows the endoscopist to control and maneuver the endoscope with ease. The umbilical cable or universal cord connects the light guide plug to the control section of the endoscope. The light guide plug inserts into the light source. The plug has ports for the air/water and suction channels.

The fiberoptic endoscope is a direct viewing system. Fiberoptic bundles composed of thousands of individual fibers transmit light from the

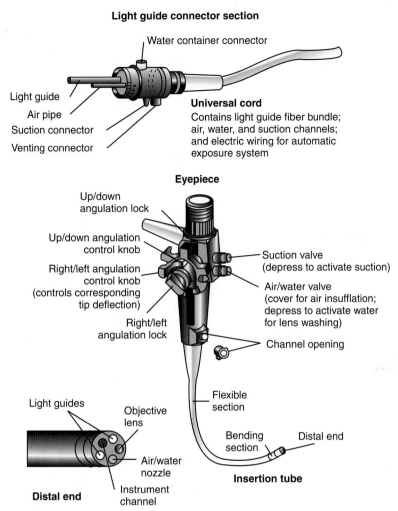

Figure 7-113   Components of typical fiberoptic endoscope. (From Stasi K, Melendez L: *Vet Clin North Am Small Anim Pract* 31:592, 2001.)

light guide plug to the distal tip of the insertion tube. The fibers' flexibility allows light to bend around corners and curves. Fiberoptic endoscopes also use a fiber bundle to transmit images from the objective lens at the distal tip, through the eyepiece, and to the endoscopist's eyes. The image guide bundles are set up so that each fiber will carry a portion of the image and will be in the same place at both ends of the bundle. Video cameras can be attached to the eyepiece of fiberoptic endoscopes to display images on a monitor. The final image is made up of the many small pieces of the whole image, so if a fiber breaks, it will result in a black or gray dot on the image.

The automatic brightness system in some fiberoptic endoscopes controls the light level. Illumination decreases as the object in view draws closer, and brightness increases as the object recedes farther away. The color, texture, and reflectivity of the tissue in view all affect the intensity of brightness. The auto-brightness control will compensate for these differences.

Video Endoscope

Video endoscopes are similar in construction to fiberoptic endoscopes except they do not have a direct viewing lens aided by an eyepiece. Images are seen on a video screen. The image bundle in a fiberoptic endoscope is replaced in a video endoscope with a camera unit consisting of a lens assembly and an electronic chip known as a "charged coupled device" (CCD). The CCD chip is housed in the distal end of the insertion tube. The CCD chip is connected to an external video processor by approximately 16 small wires. The external video processor assembles the image and transmits it to a video monitor (Figure 7-114).

The automatic brightness system can control the light level in all video endoscopes as in some fiberoptic endoscopes. Video endoscope systems have the capability to freeze and capture images from recording-device buttons in the control section. Other media, such as videotapes, computer files, and prints, can aid in capturing information. The light guide plug in a video endoscope is heavier than that in a fiberoptic endoscope and needs to be handled with care. The terminals in the light guide plug are not waterproof and must be covered by soaking caps (supplied with the endoscope) before immersion in solutions for cleaning.

Rigid Endoscopes

Rigid endoscopes are better than flexible endoscopes for procedures involving a direct pathway that are better viewed with a straight or a direct line of sight. Such areas include the ears, nose, urinary bladder, joint spaces, and abdominal or thoracic viscera. Rigid endoscopes are used for noninvasive to moderately invasive procedures that involve tissues that lie relatively close to the body surface and can be visualized with a straight line of sight. Procedures using rigid endoscopes include otoscopy and rhinoscopy. Some procedures, such as arthroscopy, laparoscopy, and thoracoscopy, require small incisions to allow access of the object lens into the specific area to be examined. (For more information on rigid endoscopy, see Bibliography and previous section on laparoscopy.)

Endoscopy Preparation

Endoscopy should be restricted to veterinarians, whether in a private practice or an educational institution, who have had the necessary training and expertise to use all endoscopy equipment safely and effectively. If possible, a technician who

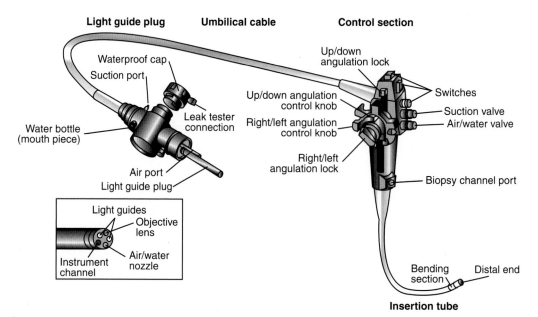

Figure 7-114   Components of typical video endoscope. (From Schumway R, Broussard J: *Clin Tech Small Anim Pract* 18:255, 2003.)

works with the veterinarian performing endoscopy should also have the necessary training to assist with patient preparation, equipment setup, patient monitoring, obtaining biopsies, freezing/capturing and storing images, equipment breakdown, equipment cleaning, performing file backups, maintaining order of the endoscopy room, and ordering supplies.

The endoscopy assistant is responsible for preparing and setting up the procedures. The endoscope of choice should be hooked up to the endoscopy machine with appropriate valves and biopsy channel covers. Before the procedure, have the patient data ready in the computer. Turn on the machine when the endoscope is attached, and make sure the light source is on. The endoscope should be tested while the machine is warming up. First, confirm that an adequate amount of distilled water is available for flushing; the water valve can then be depressed to confirm water comes out of the distal end. Water flushing is done to rinse off a soiled lens on the distal tip of the endoscope. Second, gently cover the air/water valve, and submerge the distal end of the insertion tube in a bowl of water to check for bubbles; this is a test for insufflation. Third, leave the tip submerged in a bowl of water and test for suctioning. Any necessary accessory instruments or items, such as biopsy forceps, oral speculum, pathology request forms, water-soluble lubricant gel, gauze pads, and formalin cups or slides, should all be available and ready for use.

Endoscopy Work Area

The endoscopy room should be large enough to accommodate the cart or tower for the endoscopy unit (light source/suction unit, video printer/monitor, computer, keyboard), the patient, anesthesia machine, endoscopy equipment (endoscopes, accessory instruments), a designated area to clean the endoscopy equipment, shelves and cabinets for miscellaneous storage needs, counter space, and a sink. Having the endoscope unit on a cart is convenient and allows portability to different areas of a hospital (Figures 7-115 and 7-116).

Ideally, a well-ventilated storage cabinet will be available in the endoscopy room to protect and store the endoscopes (Figure 7-117). If a cabinet is

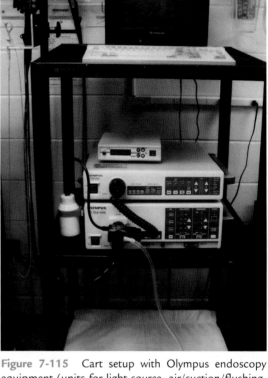

Figure 7-115 Cart setup with Olympus endoscopy equipment (units for light source, air/suction/flushing, and brightness control), water bottle, TV monitor, biopsy forceps, and video endoscope (hanging on cart pole mount), with appropriate valves and biopsy channel cover. (Courtesy MJR-VHUP, Philadelphia.)

not available, wall mounts or cart pole mounts are acceptable (Figure 7-118). Storing endoscopes in their original custom-padded cases is not recommended; the hanging position rather than the coiled position is strongly advised. Also, endoscopes should never be placed on a flat surface (not even temporarily) because they could fall off or be knocked onto the floor, resulting in costly repair. After cleaning, endoscopes should be hung to dry either in a hanging storage cabinet or on a wall or cart pole mount, where they remain until required for another procedure. Hanging endoscopes allows any residual droplets of moisture in the insertion tube to drain. Residual moisture in the accessory channel may promote growth of bacteria and fungi and clogging of the air/water channel.

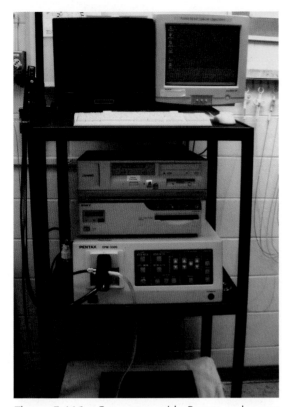

Figure 7-116 Cart setup with Pentax endoscopy equipment (units for light source, air/suction/flushing, and brightness control), water bottle, TV monitor, computer (to store patient data and images), digital printer, biopsy forceps, and video endoscope (hanging on cart pole mount), with appropriate valves and biopsy channel cover. (Courtesy MJR-VHUP, Philadelphia.)

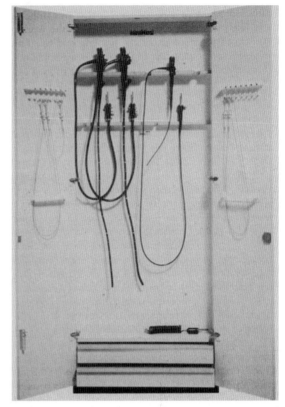

Figure 7-117   Cabinet for storage of endoscopes and accessory instruments. (From Tams T: *Small animal endoscopy*, ed 2, St Louis, 1999, Mosby.)

This is why endoscopes should not be stored in their custom-padded case; being encased in a coiled fashion does not allow air movement to circulate through the channels, and problems are more likely to develop.

Handling the Endoscope

The control section of a flexible endoscope is the only area designed to bear its weight. When transporting an endoscope, one hand should hold the control section while the other hand holds the ends of the insertion tube and umbilical cable. The optics at the tip of the insertion tube are delicate, so extra care should be taken to protect them from damage.

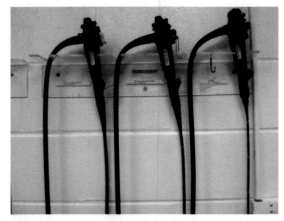

Figure 7-118   Typical wall mount for multiple endoscopes provides appropriate hanging position especially after cleaning and disinfecting. (Courtesy MJR-VHUP, Philadelphia.)

Currently, flexible endoscopes are designed for left-hand holding and manipulation of the control section. The right hand is used to advance or "drive" the insertion tube. Also, torque can be applied as necessary to maneuver the endoscope. The use of the right hand can be helpful in aiding the movement of the angulation control knobs and operating the control knob locking devices. When activated, the locking devices, one for each control knob, will hold the endoscope tip in a specified locked position. This allows the endoscopist to perform other functions, such as using an accessory instrument, applying torque to the insertion tube, and freezing and capturing images.

There are basically two ways to hold the control section during endoscopy, described as the "two-finger grip" (Figure 7-119) and the "three-finger grip" (Figure 7-120). The straighter the endoscope can be maintained throughout a procedure, the more precisely it can be controlled and maneuvered. Practice and patience are required to obtain efficient and valuable endoscopic capabilities.

Maintenance of Endoscope

Properly maintaining endoscopes and their accessory instruments is extremely important. Failure to adequately clean and disinfect endoscopes and their accessory instruments could lead to iatrogenic transmission of infection between patients. There are a variety of methods for cleaning and disinfecting endoscopes and instruments. Referring to the manufacturer's recommendations will help establish the cleaning protocol. This section covers the authors' preferred method for cleaning and disinfecting endoscopic equipment.

Endoscopes should be cleaned and disinfected immediately after the completion of any procedure. If this is not possible, abundant amounts of clean tap water should be suctioned to remove as much gross debris as possible. This practice prevents the adherence of large pieces of organic material to the channels and allows for easier cleaning once time permits.

To maximize the effect of the water moving through the suction channel, (1) place the insertion tube in a bowl of water, (2) depress the suction button for approximately 5 seconds while aspirating up the water, and (3) release the suction button, which breaks the suction and causes the water to "jump" or swish back and forth in the channel (like water being agitated in a washing machine). Afterward, the outer sheath should be

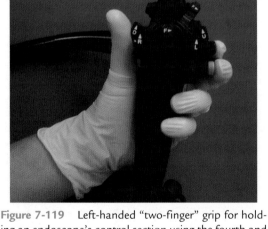

Figure 7-119 Left-handed "two-finger" grip for holding an endoscope's control section using the fourth and fifth fingers. The index and middle fingers operate the suction and air/water valves, respectively. The thumb operates the angulation knobs. (Courtesy MJR-VHUP, Philadelphia.)

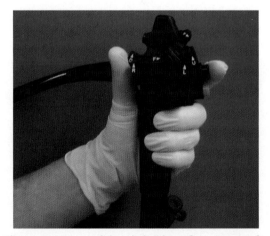

Figure 7-120 Left-handed "three-finger" grip for holding an endoscope's control section using the third, fourth, and fifth fingers. The index finger operates the suction and air/water valves, and the thumb operates the angulation knobs. (Courtesy MJR-VHUP, Philadelphia.)

gently wiped down with wet gauze sponges to remove gross debris.

Endoscopes should be inspected for damage before being submerged in solutions that may damage parts not designed for exposure. A leak test should be performed to ensure that the internal and external parts of the endoscope did not incur damage during a procedure.

Because of the GI endoscope's delicate design, holes and tears of the inner lumen of the scope make it possible for water and other debris to contact otherwise impermeable areas of the scope. If the endoscope fails the leak test, it should not be submerged or used, and the manufacturer should be contacted immediately for inspection and repair. To leak-test, the appropriate soaking caps are placed, and the leak tester is attached and tested according to the manufacturer (Figure 7-121). The cleaning and disinfecting protocol then can be completed.

The most important step in prevention of infection during endoscopy is manual cleaning. Organic soil (blood, feces) may contribute to the failure of disinfection by harboring embedded microbes and preventing the penetration of germicides. Also, some disinfectants are inactivated by organic material. The endoscope, after being disassembled and passing the leak test, should have the following channels cleaned with a cleaning brush: suction: air/water and biopsy, including

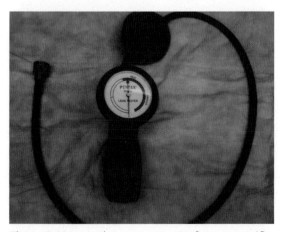

Figure 7-121   Leak testers are manufacturer specific. This Pentax leak tester is compatible with all Pentax endoscopes. (Courtesy MJR-VHUP, Philadelphia.)

the detachable suction and air/water valves; the biopsy channel cover; and the whole exterior of the endoscope. This cleaning process should take place in an enzymatic cleaner designed to clean organic material by breaking down proteins and enhancing the efficacy of brushing and flushing. Endozime, a bacteriostatic enzymatic cleaner, is a unique formulation of protease and amylase enzymes, digesters, and buffers that can clean in 2 to 3 minutes. Allowing the endoscope to be submerged in Endozime for at least 10 minutes after precleaning is sufficient. Endozime needs to be diluted, and with any enzymatic solution, dilution protocols should be followed according to the manufacturer's instructions.

After the appropriate time has elapsed with the endoscope submerged in the enzymatic cleaner, the exterior should be rinsed off with water, including the appropriate channels that do not need soaking caps, and then purged with air before being exposed to the disinfectant. The endoscope should be purged with water, followed by air, before disinfection. This will help prevent contamination of the disinfectant with the enzymatic solution and dilution of the disinfectant itself.

High-level disinfection (HLD) is recommended for endoscopes because they cannot withstand available sterilization methods. HLD is a cleaning process that kills all microorganisms except large numbers of bacterial spores. Because they are not rendered sterile, endoscopes cleaned using HLD are considered semi-critical items. These endoscopes may contact broken skin or mucous membranes, which are usually resistant to common spores, but they should not contact vascular or other sterile body tissue. The FDA-approved alkylating agent Cidex-OPA is often used, as discussed earlier for laparoscopes. Submerging an endoscope in Cidex-OPA for 40 minutes is sufficient, and it should not be submerged for longer than 60 minutes. After being removed from Cidex-OPA, the interior and exterior portions of the endoscope should be thoroughly rinsed and flushed with sterile or filtered water. If using tap water, 70% alcohol should be the final rinse because tap water may contain microbes (e.g., *Pseudomonas, Mycobacterium*). The endoscope can then be purged with air and allowed to hang to dry either on a wall mount or in a well-ventilated storage cabinet.

As with the endoscope, failure to adequately clean the biopsy and retrieval instruments can spread disease. With inadequate cleaning, instruments also may not open or may break when opened. Not only should instruments be pre-cleaned with water, followed by an enzymatic cleaner with a brush, but detachable parts (e.g., valves, biopsy channel covers) should be cleaned as well. The same cleaning protocol used on the endoscope can be used on the biopsy instruments. Cleaning brushes are usually disposable, but if they are thoroughly cleaned by HLD, they can be reused. Water bottles and tubes used for endoscopic irrigation are difficult to clean and disinfect, so sterile water should be used rather than tap water.

NOTE: Reported iatrogenic infections from endoscopes not thoroughly disinfected include *Escherichia coli, Pseudomonas, Klebsiella, Serratia,* and *Salmonella.* Other organisms of concern in gastroenterology settings include *Campylobacter, Clostridium difficile,* and *Helicobacter pylori,* as well as many viral pathogens.

Biopsy Sampling

Endoscopic biopsy samples are obtained with flexible forceps. Samples obtained using forceps with a 1.8-mm cup are usually sufficient for diagnostic histopathology, but cups of 2.4 mm or larger are always better because samples retrieved are substantially larger and deeper. The correct cup size is determined by the size of the endoscope's biopsy channel. Biopsy tissue samples obtained with flexible endoscopes may not always be deep enough to allow diagnosis of submucosal lesions, whereas using rigid endoscopes usually yields diagnostically sufficient amounts of tissue. It is ideal, but not always possible, to visualize the biopsy site. Depending on the difficulty in advancing the endoscope through areas of narrowing, such as the pyloric sphincter and ileocolic junction to obtain biopsies of the duodenum and ileum, respectively, the clinician may blindly lead the tip of the insertion tube to the site and carefully obtain "blind" tissue samples.

Any biopsy sample, especially intestinal and gastric mucosa samples, must be handled carefully to minimize artifacts and distortion. If possible, tissue samples should be carefully removed from the biopsy forceps using a 25-gauge needle (Figure 7-122). Cytology can assist in making or confirming a diagnosis, but unremarkable cytology findings do not rule out specific disorders.

It is important that tissue samples from different locations be placed in different vials of formalin and properly labeled so the pathologist can correctly identify the area sampled. Tissue samples should not be allowed to dry out or be damaged before placement in formalin.

Tissue samples that are too small and samples that have excessive artifact are common problems with endoscopy. For example, a lymphoma can be submucosal, and a superficial biopsy sample may only contain reactive cells above the tumor and may miss the neoplastic cells from the tumor. This could be misinterpreted as a diagnosis for inflammatory bowel disease. When obtaining biopsy samples, three to five full-thickness biopsy samples are usually sufficient, but obtaining six to eight may be more helpful, especially with both mucosal and submucosal samples. Clinicians should follow up with the pathologist to determine whether the quality of the tissue samples was adequate and if the histologic findings are consistent with the patient's clinical signs.

Even though endoscopy is considered a minimally invasive procedure, one rare but significant

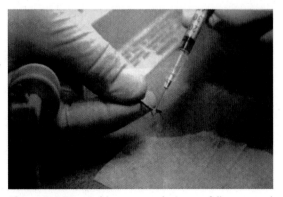

Figure 7-122 A biopsy sample is carefully removed with a small-gauge needle. (From Tams T: *Small animal endoscopy,* ed 2, St Louis, 1999, Mosby.)

complication is perforation. Therefore, when biopsy samples are obtained from diseased areas, extra caution and care should be taken to avoid applying too much force against mucosal walls.

Instrumentation

Many flexible instruments are available for use with endoscopes that have an accessory channel. Both flexible and rigid endoscopes can accommodate flexible instruments. Basic instrumentation includes biopsy forceps (e.g., oval/ellipsoid cups, serrated cups, alligator cups, serrated/nonserrated bayonets), instruments for grasping foreign bodies (e.g., "rat tooth" forceps, wired snares, wired baskets, meshed nets, two- or three-pronged grasping forceps), cytology brushes, aspiration tubes, injection needles, and coagulating electrodes (Figure 7-123).

Foreign bodies should not be retrieved through the accessory channel. Once the object has been visualized and firmly secured, the entire endoscope should be removed from the patient. Following this recommendation will prevent costly damage to the accessory channel of the flexible endoscope. When retrieved, foreign bodies should be cleaned off as well as possible and placed in a secure bag or container for the animal's owner.

Biopsy forceps cups tend to lock in the position in which they dry after cleaning, which will require releasing any tension before use. If locked in a closed position, cups can be soaked in warm water or mineral oil for several seconds, then gently separated with a small-gauge needle. Once the biopsy forceps cup is open, the finger control at the top of the instrument is used to open and close the cup several times to ensure free movement. If locked in an open position, cups can be soaked for several seconds in warm water, and then gentle digital pressure can be applied to the cups to work them closed. Again, the finger control is used to ensure that the cups are moving freely.

Disposable sheathed cytology brushes are recommended for obtaining brush samples, such as a gastric or duodenal mass or intestinal mucus. One cytology brush should be used per patient because cells from one sample may be transferred

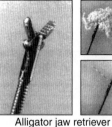

Short oval cup

Alligator jaw retriever

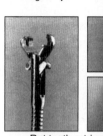

Long ellipsoid cup

Rat tooth retriever

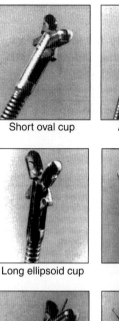

Long ellipsoid cup with needle

Three-pronged grasper

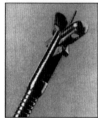

Serrated cup

Forked jaw grasper

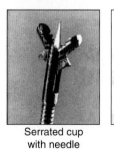

Serrated cup with needle

Three-pronged forked jaw grasper

Figure 7-123 Examples of biopsy forceps graspers and retrievers. (Courtesy Endoscopy Support Services, Brewster, NY.)

to the cytologic sample of another patient if the brush is used on more than one patient. This can happen because cytology brushes are difficult to clean thoroughly. Polyethylene tubing can be used to perform a duodenal wash through the endoscope to examine for evidence of giardiasis or to collect intestinal fluid for identification or quantification of bacteria.

Esophagoscopy

Esophagoscopy is the endoscopic technique of examining the esophagus. Esophagoscopy is a useful tool in the diagnosis and treatment of esophageal disease and is indicated for the evaluation of animals with signs of esophageal disease. These signs may include (but are not limited to) regurgitation, dysphagia, odynophagia, ptyalism, change in appetite, and weight loss. Esophagoscopy is the method of choice for diagnosing disorders that affect the mucosa or alterations affecting the lumen of the esophagus (Figure 7-124).

Esophageal foreign bodies, inflammation (esophagitis; Figures 7-125 and 7-126), esophageal strictures, ulcers, and neoplasia are conditions affecting the esophageal mucosa or lumen that can be definitively diagnosed by esophagoscopy.

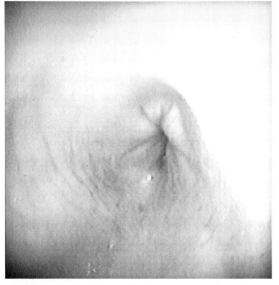

Figure 7-124 Normal-appearing canine lower esophageal sphincter. (Courtesy MJR-VHUP, Philadelphia.)

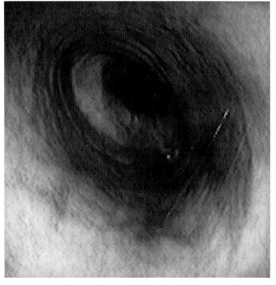

Figure 7-125 Inflamed canine lower esophageal sphincter. (Courtesy MJR-VHUP, Philadelphia.)

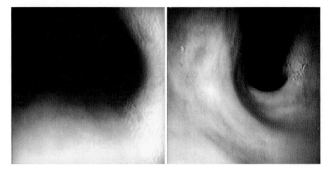

Figure 7-126 *Left,* Mild reflux esophagitis in 10-year-old male German shepherd. *Right,* Retroflexed view of gastroesophageal sphincter and cardia. (Courtesy MJR-VHUP, Philadelphia.)

However, contrast radiography is more useful than esophagoscopy in diagnosing megaesophagus, hiatal hernias, vascular ring anomalies, and gastroesophageal intussusception. Whenever an esophagoscopy is performed, it is important to enter the stomach and retroflex the scope's tip to view the gastroesophageal sphincter area to detect leiomyomas or other easily missed lesions.

Instrumentation

The endoscope of choice for cats and dogs is a flexible scope (fiberoptic or video).

Endoscopes used for esophagoscopies generally have an insertion diameter of 7.8 to 10 mm, a four-way tip deflection, and a 1.8- to 2.8-mm biopsy channel. Utilizing the larger biopsy channel will allow larger biopsy forceps to be used so larger samples can be obtained. The presence of a mass or suspected esophagitis is a primary indication for esophageal biopsies. The accessory instruments that may be needed include biopsy forceps, grasping forceps, cytology brushes, and balloon dilation catheters.

Cytology brushes are used to obtain brush cytology samples. A sheathed cytology brush is preferred to prevent contamination and loss of specimen material when the brush is withdrawn through the accessory channel of the endoscope. The area to be sampled is carefully brushed. The bristles of the cytology brush are then gently rolled on a clean microscope slide for evaluation.

Esophagoscopy Technique

1. The anesthetized and intubated patient should be placed in left lateral recumbency with a secured oral speculum.
2. The insertion tube should be prelubricated with a water-soluble gel to aid easy passage. The endoscope is then directed centrally through the oropharynx and guided dorsal to the ET tube and larynx so that the cranial esophageal sphincter (CES) comes into view.
3. The CES is the entrance to the esophagus and is normally closed, which appears as a star-shaped area of folded mucosa dorsal to the larynx. The endoscope should meet minimal or no resistance as it is being advanced within the esophagus.
4. With insufflation, the scope should advance in a slow, continuous motion, using only

minor adjustments in tip deflection and torque to maintain a full view of the lumen and mucosal surfaces.
5. At the lumen of the thoracic esophagus, pulsations of the aorta can be seen at the level of the base of the heart.
6. When advancing the endoscope through the gastroesophageal sphincter (GES), little or no resistance should be encountered.
7. To move the endoscope into the stomach, the tip of the insertion tube should be deflected approximately 30 degrees to the left (see note below) while applying slight upward deflection as the tip is advanced through the slitlike opening of the GES.
8. To examine the GES, the endoscope should be retroflexed. This is also known as the "J maneuver." The extent of retroflexion can be 180 or 210 degrees.

NOTE: When referring to directional technique (i.e., left or right), the patient's orientation is the point of reference. Therefore, when instructed to turn the tip of the endoscope to the left, this refers to the patient's left. This applies to every endoscopic technique described in this chapter.

Canine mucosa differs from feline esophageal mucosa. A dog's esophageal mucosa is normally pale pink or grayish, and the surface is smooth and glistening. In dog breeds such as the chow chow and shar-pei, patches of pigmented mucosa may be observed. A cat's esophageal mucosa differs from that of a dog because of the presence of submucosal vessels and circular rings formed by circumferential mucosal folds, creating a characteristic pattern in the distal third of the cat's esophagus (Figures 7-127 and 7-128).

Gastroscopy

Gastroscopy is the endoscopic technique of examining the stomach. Gastroscopy is indicated for the evaluation of animals with signs of gastric disease. The signs may include (but are not limited to) nausea, salivation, vomiting, hematemesis, melena, unexplained abnormal changes in breathing, and anorexia. Gastroscopy identifies abnormalities of the mucosa and reveals distortion of the stomach's normal anatomic relationship to other abdominal organs by displacement or extrinsic compression. Many consider gastroscopy to be a more valuable diagnostic tool than radiography for disorders affecting the stomach.

The following conditions can be definitively diagnosed by gastroscopy or a combination of gastroscopy and associated diagnostic tests (cytology, histology): chronic inflammation (with or without overgrowth of *Helicobacter* organisms), superficial erosions, foreign bodies, motility disorders, ulcerations, and neoplasia. Gastroscopy can also be a therapeutic intervention when used to remove foreign bodies (Figures 7-129 to 7-131) and place feeding tubes (gastrostomy tubes and percutaneous endoscopy-guided [PEG] gastrostomy tubes).

Gastric biopsy is currently required for a diagnosis of *Helicobacter* infection. The bacteria are not uniformly distributed throughout the stomach; therefore, obtaining samples from various areas (body, fundus, antrum) is recommended. *Helicobacter* may be diagnosed by cytologic evaluation of the gastric mucosa or by examination for gastric mucosal urease activity.

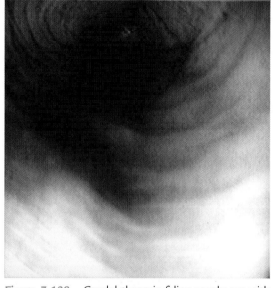

Figure 7-128   Caudal thoracic feline esophagus with herringbone pattern not seen in canine esophagus. This esophagus is mildly inflamed. (Courtesy MJR-VHUP, Philadelphia.)

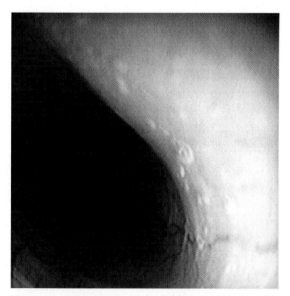

Figure 7-127   Distal third of feline esophagus with distinctive circular ring formation (herringbone pattern). This esophagus is mildly inflamed. (Courtesy MJR-VHUP, Philadelphia.)

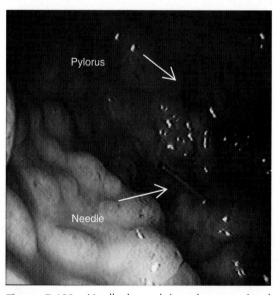

Figure 7-129   Needle located in pylorus; retrieved without complications in 3½-year-old male Labrador. (Courtesy MJR-VHUP, Philadelphia.)

Instrumentation

The endoscope of choice for cats and dogs is a flexible scope (fiberoptic or video) with the same specifications as for esophagoscopy. Accessory instruments that may be needed for gastroscopy include biopsy forceps, grasping forceps, cytology brushes, and PEG tubes. Biopsy forceps (1.8 or 2.4 mm) with serrated edges or bayonets will usually obtain full-thickness samples. Standard pinch biopsy forceps can be used, but sample size may be smaller, which is why larger biopsy forceps cups are preferred. The same grasping forceps used for esophagoscopies can also be used for retrieval of gastric foreign bodies. Cytology brushes can be helpful to obtain cells from the surface of a lesion for tentative diagnosis, such as gastric lymphosarcoma. A sheathed cytology brush is preferred over an unsheathed brush in order to prevent contamination.

Gastroscopy Technique

1. Fasting a patient for 12 to 18 hours and withholding water for 4 or more hours before a gastroscopy may be the key to a successful and a thorough examination.
2. The anesthetized and intubated patient should be placed in left lateral recumbency (LLR) with a secured oral speculum. With the patient in LLR, the antrum and pylorus are away from the tabletop, which improves the ability of the scope to traverse these structures more readily, allowing the endoscopist to examine the stomach completely.
3. Because the esophagus is in a posterior plane in relation to the stomach, the tip of the insertion tube needs to be deflected in the distal esophagus before it can be advanced to the stomach.
4. The endoscope tip should be centered at the gastroesophageal (GE) orifice, and as the scope is advanced, the tip should be deflected to the left approximately 30 degrees with simultaneous slight upward deflection as the GE junction is passed. No resistance should be encountered as the scope advances to the stomach, if the tip was properly directed.
5. The endoscope tip should be positioned just through the GE junction to obtain an overview of the gastric lumen. As the tip enters the stomach, the rugal folds are seen, and the stomach is often partially or completely collapsed.

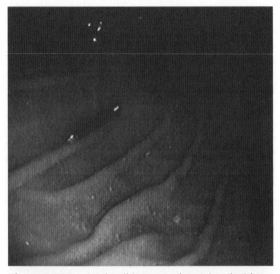

Figure 7-130   Steel nail in stomach; retrieved without complications in 6-month-old male vizsla. (Courtesy MJR-VHUP, Philadelphia.)

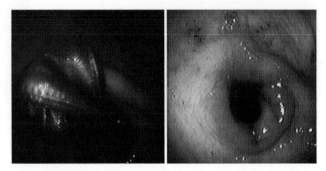

Figure 7-131   *Left,* Article of clothing wedged in pyloric sphincter. *Right,* Inflammation and swelling after minor complications in retrieving object in 9-year-old female malamute. (Courtesy MJR-VHUP, Philadelphia.)

6. Gastric distention is required using insufflation to the point that the rugal folds begin to separate. This allows for spatial orientation and the identification of most gross abnormalities. In cats and small dogs, insufflation can be achieved within seconds, whereas large-breed dogs may require 30 to 120 seconds of constant insufflation for adequate distention.

7. The initial examination of the stomach should note the presence/absence of fluid or ingesta, the ease/difficulty with which the gastric walls distend with insufflation, and the gross appearance of the rugal folds and the mucosa.

8. The stomach should be empty in a properly fasted patient; however, a small pool of fluid in the fundus or at the proximal aspect of the greater curvature is considered normal. Aspiration should be performed, but with great care if a large pool of fluid is present and obscuring the rugal folds.

9. As the scope is gradually advanced through the proximal stomach, the gastric body can be evaluated by using the control knobs to deflect the tip.

10. With the patient in LLR, the smooth lesser curvature is on the endoscopist's right and the rugal folds of the greater curvature are seen below and to the left. The endoscope is then advanced along the greater curvature until the angulus, which extends from the lesser curvature, is identified.

11. The angulus separates the body of the stomach from the antrum. The insertion tube must be maneuvered around the angulus to the antrum in order to advance to the pylorus through the pyloric sphincter and enter the duodenum.

12. During a gastroscopy, the cardia and fundus can only be visualized if the insertion tube is retroflexed (J maneuver).

13. The retroflexion maneuver allows a "face view" of the angulus, cardia, and fundus. This maneuver must be initiated at a point proximal to or opposite the angulus to provide a face view of the angulus.

14. The scope is advanced along the greater curvature to the level of the distal body.

15. The tip of the insertion tube is then deflected upward as far as possible as the scope advances farther. An upward tip deflection between 180 and 210 degrees is required to visualize the cardia.

16. Panoramic examination of the proximal stomach is completed by rotating the insertion tube. The retroflexed scope tip should be reversed gradually to allow further examination of the gastric mucosa.

NOTE: Gastroscopies should follow esophagoscopies for a thorough upper GI examination, with the duodenum examined last and gastric biopsies usually obtained after duodenal biopsies.

Biopsy Sampling

Six to 10 gastric biopsies should be taken even if the gastric mucosa appears normal (Figure 7-132). This is important because some patients with a histologic diagnosis of mild to moderate gastritis have no gross mucosal lesions; and patients with gastric motility disorders may have mucosal erythema but no histologic abnormalities. The gastric rugal folds are the best areas from which to

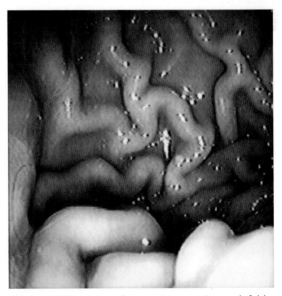

Figure 7-132   Normal-appearing gastric rugal folds. (Courtesy MJR-VHUP, Philadelphia.)

obtain biopsy samples because they are easy to grasp with forceps.

With any biopsy sampling, the forceps are extended beyond the endoscope tip and advanced to the desired area. The biopsy forceps should be advanced directly into the mucosal folds at a 45- to 90-degree angle. If forceps cups are being used and run parallel to the folds, they will tend to slide along the mucosal wall. Serrated-edge or bayonet-type forceps will prevent this and are more effective in obtaining adequate samples. Forceps should remain closed until the actual site is visualized, then opened and firmly placed into the tissue until resistance is met. The forceps then can be closed and withdrawn in the accessory channel. Biopsies should be taken at various sites of the stomach, including the cardia, fundus, angulus, antrum, and pylorus (Figures 7-133 to 7-136).

If erosive or ulcerative lesions are present in the stomach, the biopsy samples should be collected from the upper wall where the lesions merge with the normal-appearing mucosa (Figures 7-137 and 7-138). Caution should be used when maneuvering the endoscope around the pit of an ulcer because perforation could result. Obtaining biopsy samples of superficial erosions is usually safer.

Biopsy samples from gastric masses should be taken as deeply as possible (Figure 7-139). If the samples are too superficial, fibrous or granulomatous tissue may be retrieved. Lymphosarcoma and benign gastric polyps can usually be diagnosed on biopsy. However, to diagnose adenocarcinoma and other neoplastic masses, deeper tissue samples are required.

Duodenoscopy

Duodenoscopy is the endoscopic technique of examining the duodenum. Duodenoscopy aids in the diagnosis and treatment of small intestine disease. Clinical signs may include (but are not limited to) vomiting, hematemesis, diarrhea, melena, change in appetite, and weight loss. Duodenoscopy identifies abnormalities of the mucosa and reveals distortion of the small intestine's normal anatomic relationships by displacement or extrinsic compression.

The following diagnoses and conditions can be identified with the use of duodenoscopy: intestinal parasites, inflammation (inflammatory bowel disease; Figures 7-140 to 7-142), lymphangiectasia, ulcerations, and neoplasia. Intestinal parasites (generally ascarids) are occasionally encountered on direct examination. These parasites can be easily removed, but biopsies should still be obtained. If *Giardia* is suspected, a saline lavage can be performed to retrieve trophozoites. Partial-thickness biopsies obtained by duodenoscopy may be preferable to full-thickness biopsies obtained by abdominal exploratory surgery for patients with a protein-losing enteropathy. Duodenoscopy is preferred in hypoproteinemic patients, especially if the total protein is 3.5 g/dl or less, because rate of healing is delayed once total protein falls to that level. The most common causes of protein-losing enteropathy in dogs are

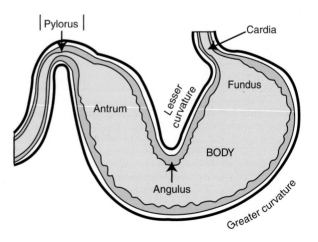

Figure 7-133 Five basic regions of the stomach. The areas indicated with an arrow are the three most important landmarks for a gastroscopy. (From Tams T: *Small animal endoscopy*, ed 2, St Louis, 1999, Mosby.)

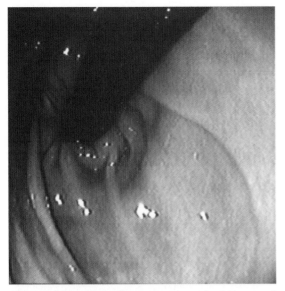

Figure 7-134 View of gastroesophageal sphincter and cardia via retroflexion ("J maneuver") of endoscope. (Courtesy MJR-VHUP, Philadelphia.)

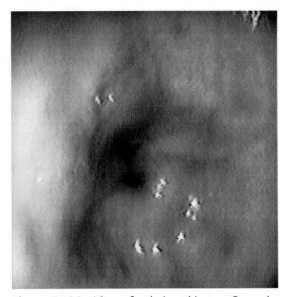

Figure 7-136 View of pyloric sphincter. Once the sphincter opens, the duodenum can then be entered by the endoscope. (Courtesy MJR-VHUP, Philadelphia.)

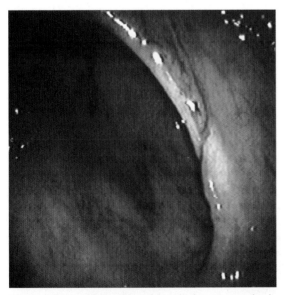

Figure 7-135 View of angulus, which separates body of stomach from antrum. (Courtesy MJR-VHUP, Philadelphia.)

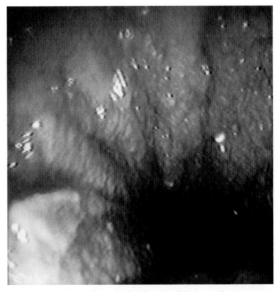

Figure 7-137 Ulcerated pylorus with irregular mucosa from 9-year-old male Labrador. This dog was diagnosed with chronic gastritis and chronic duodenitis. (Courtesy MJR-VHUP, Philadelphia.)

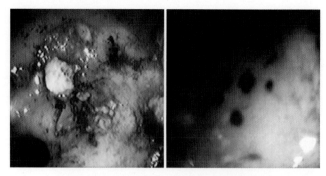

Figure 7-138 Small gastric erosions from 3-year-old female Australian cattle dog. (Courtesy MJR-VHUP, Philadelphia.)

inflammatory bowel disease, lymphoma, and lymphangiectasia. Lymphoma is the most common intestinal neoplasia and is believed to be more common in cats than in dogs.

Instrumentation

The endoscope of choice for performing duodenoscopy in cats and dogs is a flexible scope with a four-way tip deflection with the same insertion tube diameters and biopsy channel diameters used for esophagoscopies and gastroscopies. Use of a larger scope will allow larger biopsy samples, but attempting to advance through the pyloric sphincter may be more challenging in smaller patients.

Flexible biopsy forceps are primarily the accessory instruments for duodenoscopies. Forceps cups tend to slide along the wall of the intestinal lumen. To prevent this, bayonet-type forceps that contain a central needle may be helpful. However, to obtain adequately sized tissue samples, standard alligator jaw forceps should be used and are the best forceps for duodenoscopies. After obtaining

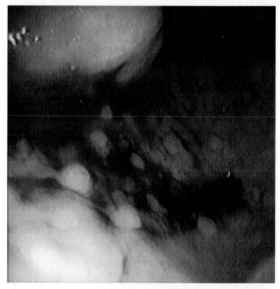

Figure 7-139 Multifocal and diffuse, raised, pale circular lesions throughout regions of gastric mucosa from 12-year-old male domestic shorthair cat. This cat was diagnosed with gastric and duodenal lymphosarcoma. (Courtesy MJR-VHUP, Philadelphia.)

Figure 7-140 Significant duodenal inflammation with mild ulceration from 2-year-old female German shepherd. This dog was diagnosed with moderate form of chronic lymphoplasmacytic and neutrophilic enteritis. (Courtesy MJR-VHUP, Philadelphia.)

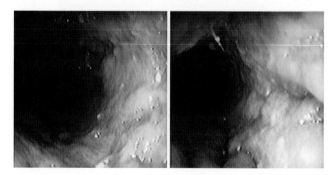

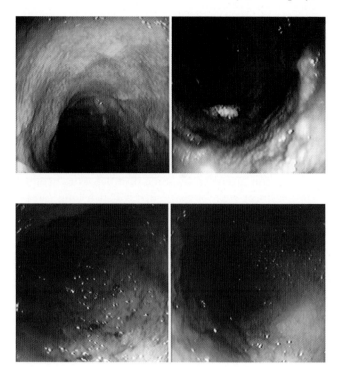

Figure 7-141 Edematous duodenum with dilated lacteals and pinpoint ulcerations from 8½-year-old bichon frise. This dog was diagnosed with chronic duodenitis. (Courtesy MJR-VHUP, Philadelphia.)

Figure 7-142 Friable, "cobblestone" duodenum with small, ulcerated areas from 4-year-old male domestic short-hair cat. This cat was diagnosed with severe, chronic duodenitis. (Courtesy MJR-VHUP, Philadelphia.)

biopsy samples, some bleeding will be observed. However, even with samples collected from abnormal intestinal sites that tend to bleed more than normal sites, the amount of blood lost from biopsy sampling is generally not enough to be clinically significant.

Duodenoscopy Technique

1. Fasting a patient for 12 to 18 hours and withholding water for 4 or more hours before a duodenoscopy may be the key to a successful and a thorough examination, as with gastroscopy.
2. The anesthetized and intubated patient should be placed in LLR with a secured oral speculum.
3. As the endoscope advances through the stomach until it reaches the pylorus, minor tip adjustments may be necessary to maintain the pyloric orifice in the center of the field of view.
4. Minimal forward pressure can be applied to advance the tip directly through the open pyloric orifice to reach the first segment of the duodenum; however, if the pyloric orifice is closed or slightly open, variable resistance may be encountered.
5. The insertion tube tip can be guided into the pyloric canal by applying leftward tip deflection alone or with slight to moderate upward tip deflection while advancing the scope.
6. A blurred image will be seen once the insertion tube tip is in the pyloric canal because the pyloric walls are usually pressed in around the tip of the insertion tube.
7. Turning both inner and outer control knobs on the endoscope in a clockwise direction as the scope advances will provide a downward and rightward tip deflection that will aid entry into the proximal duodenum.
8. The color of the gastric mucosa is usually cream, and on entering the duodenum, the color of the mucosa will become pinkish red.
9. The tip of the insertion tube should then be directed into the descending duodenal lumen, without using excessive force.

10. As the tip of the insertion tube lies against the superior wall of the proximal duodenum, it should be angled acutely upward and sometimes also to the left. This maneuver with gentle advancement will provide a tunneling view of the descending duodenum.
11. Air insufflation should be maintained to allow distention of the duodenal walls.
12. At times, minor forward or backward movements of the insertion tube may aid in freeing the endoscope tip.

NOTE: Air insufflation should be monitored carefully because excessive air may reflux into the stomach and cause unnecessary gastric distention. If this occurs, the endoscope should be withdrawn into the stomach and then air-suctioned.

Biopsy Sampling

It is best to obtain biopsy samples when the sites to be sampled can be visualized at the end of the endoscope. However, this may not be possible when collecting biopsies from the small intestine, and samples may need to be collected "blindly." It is also important to note that the intestinal mucosa is more friable than the gastric mucosa. There are ways to obtain "blind" intestinal biopsy samples from the farthest regions of the small intestine (i.e., jejunum). However, some veterinarians are not comfortable with obtaining blind biopsy samples and will attempt the same technique used for gastric biopsies.

One technique is to advance the endoscope as far as possible, then feed the biopsy instrument of choice through the accessory channel and along the lumen until resistance is met. The view of the forceps cups will be obstructed. When resistance is met, the forceps should be retracted slightly so that the forceps cups can be opened. The forceps can then be firmly readvanced into the mucosal wall, and the sample can be obtained, usually with minimal resistance.

Another technique is to have the forceps cups opened as soon as the instrument is fed beyond the endoscope tip. The forceps should then be advanced until true resistance is met, because this may help to seat the forceps cups more deeply and to obtain a larger sample consisting of the submucosa. If the endoscope cannot be advanced

through the pylorus to the duodenum, for whatever reason, blind biopsies of the proximal descending duodenum can usually be obtained. This requires special care because there is a risk of damaging the duodenal papilla. To avoid the papilla, the forceps should be advanced as far along the duodenal lumen as possible.

Small intestinal biopsy samples can vary in size. Biopsy samples tend to be small with normal mucosa but invariably larger when the mucosa is compromised by some disorder. For example, a linear strip of tissue up to 1 inch long can be obtained with marked inflammatory disease because the mucosal and submucosal integrity is altered.

Colonoscopy

Colonoscopy is the endoscopic technique used to examine the rectum, large intestine, and cecum. Colonoscopy aids in the diagnosis and treatment of large bowel disease. Clinical signs may include (but are not limited to) diarrhea, hematochezia, fecal mucus, tenesmus, dyschezia, constipation, and chronic vomiting (especially in cats). Hematochezia, fecal mucus, and tenesmus are signs of diarrhea in large bowel disease, and patients with these signs usually have self-limiting disease or a disorder that can be resolved with symptomatic treatment and supportive care. Chronic vomiting is usually more common in upper GI disease, although in cats this may indicate inflammation of the ascending colon or ileum, which is why every attempt should be made to enter the ileum during colonoscopy.

Colonoscopy should be performed when clinical or laboratory findings (e.g., significant weight loss, hypoalbuminemia) suggest that a patient has a serious disorder (e.g., intussusception, histoplasmosis, adenocarcinoma) or when the clinical signs and symptoms of colonic disease do not respond to specific therapeutic trials. However, patients who have diarrhea with large bowel disease but are otherwise healthy should be tested for parasitic disease, dietary allergy or intolerance, fiber-responsive diarrhea, and clostridial colitis before colonoscopy is considered.

The most frequently diagnosed disorders include a variety of mucosal inflammatory disorders, with lymphocytic plasmacytic colitis the most common (Figures 7-143 and 7-144), and rectal polyps. Colonoscopy is much more accurate than contrast radiography in diagnosing large intestine disorders. Most patients with idiopathic colitis have grossly normal mucosa, so it is imperative that the colon be properly prepared for obtaining high-quality biopsy samples at various levels of the colon.

Strictured areas with relatively normal mucosa usually result from a submucosal lesion. In these cases, biopsying must be aggressive enough to ensure that submucosal tissue is obtained. Cytologic studies are sensitive in detecting histoplasmosis (*Histoplasma capsulatum* infection) and protothecosis (*Prototheca* infection) and may be useful in detecting some neoplasms and eosinophilic colitis.

Instrumentation

A patient with generalized colonic disease or with an affected descending colon would benefit from rigid colonoscopy and sometimes proctoscopy to obtain a diagnosis. Rigid techniques are better for the evaluation of dense, infiltrative lesions involving submucosal tissue and allow the collection of larger tissue samples containing the submucosa.

Rigid proctoscopy is limited in regard to the length of the colon that can be examined, but it is still useful. The rigid proctoscope can be used to evaluate the rectal area, which is the primary site for neoplasms in the colon. Proctoscopy can also help remove polyps and biopsy deep submucosal masses or strictures.

Flexible endoscopes allow examination of the entire colon plus the cecum, ileocolic valve, and ileum. A four-way tip deflection with the same insertion tube diameters and biopsy channel diameters used for upper GI endoscopies is best. As for all endoscopic procedures, an endoscope with a larger biopsy channel (2.4-2.8 mm) is ideal, but the insertion tube diameter in relation to the size of the patient also is a factor; in small dogs and cats a compromise may be necessary with a smaller biopsy channel (1.8 mm). Also, when using endoscopes with a larger diameter, it may be more difficult to enter the ileum, as with the pyloric sphincter.

Flexible biopsy forceps are primarily the accessory instruments for colonoscopies. Serrated ellipsoid forceps with or without fenestrations are

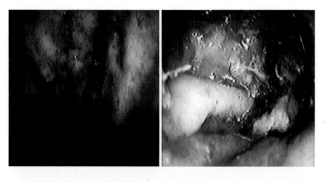

Figure 7-143 *Left,* Moderately to severely inflamed duodenum with mild ulcerative areas. *Right,* Moderately inflamed ileocolic valve from 2-year-old female German shepherd. This dog was diagnosed with moderate to severe lymphoplasmacytic, neutrophilic, and erosive colitis. This dog was also diagnosed with enteritis (see Figure 7-140). (Courtesy MJR-VHUP, Philadelphia.)

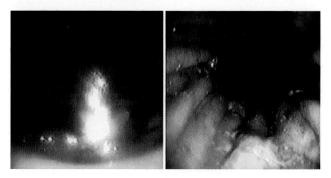

Figure 7-144 *Left,* Rectal mass from 2-year-old male Brittany spaniel. *Right,* Moderately inflamed colon from same patient. This dog was diagnosed with rectal papillary adenocarcinoma and moderate lymphoplasmacytic colitis. (Courtesy MJR-VHUP, Philadelphia.)

preferred for biopsying. Some endoscopists use simple round cups or bayonet-type biopsy forceps.

Patient Preparation

Fecal examinations for parasites and ova (e.g., whipworms, *Giardia*), cultures for pathogens (e.g., *Salmonella*, *Campylobacter*), fecal cytologies (e.g., for *Clostridium* spores), and assays (e.g., for *Clostridium perfringens* enterotoxin) should be done before administering enemas or lavage solutions.

The patient should be fasted for 24 to 36 hours. Colons need to be as thoroughly cleaned as possible. Lavage solutions are best for removing food and feces from the alimentary canal. These solutions are isosmotic (same osmotic pressure) and produce an osmotic diarrhea that washes particulate matter out of the colon. One example of a lavage solution is GoLYTELY, which is administered through a gastric or nasoesophageal tube if the patient does not consume the solution orally. GoLYTELY is a concentrated solution of polyethylene glycol and electrolytes that results in virtually no net absorption or excretions of ions or water. GoLYTELY can usually clean a bowel within 4 hours, although some patients may require more than one dosing. Large volumes can be given without causing significant changes in water or electrolyte balance. In addition to lavage solutions, an osmotic cathartic such as magnesium citrate may be used. This combination results in the best colonic preparation and minimizes artifacts induced by enema tubes.

Problems associated with lavage solutions include (1) they are more expensive than enemas, (2) large volumes are needed for some patients, and (3) orogastric intubation administration can be difficult in aggressive animals.

Colonic lavages such as a warm water enema are helpful but may need to be repeated multiple times. Improper technique can easily result in an inadequately prepared patient with possible mucosal artifacts. For this reason, it is best to fast a patient for 36 hours rather than 24 hours. When performing an enema with a well-lubricated enema tube, the tube should not be forced if resistance is encountered because traumatic mucosal hemorrhages will likely occur. If the colon has been lavaged properly, clear water should be evacuated after the last enema. Enemas are helpful for cleaning the descending colon but are inadequate for cleaning the ascending and transverse colon and the ileocolic valve.

Colonoscopy Technique

1. After the patient has been fasted properly (ideally 36 hours) and the colon adequately cleaned, the patient can be anesthetized and intubated and placed in LLR.
2. The flexible endoscope tip is inserted into the rectum, followed by insufflation.
3. As the tip of the scope is advanced central to the lumen, the mucosa and lumen are examined. The endoscope is advanced to its most orad (toward the mouth) limit and then slowly withdrawn so that the mucosa can be thoroughly examined.
4. The splenic flexure is the most orad part of the descending colon and is the area where the descending colon turns and becomes the transverse colon.
5. To enter the transverse colon, the distal tip of the endoscope must be diverted in the direction of the lumen, and then the tip must be carefully advanced using a blind "slide-by" technique. With this technique the distal tip usually pushes lightly against the colonic wall, and visualization is lost for 1 to 2 cm because the lens is too close to the mucosa.
6. In cats the transverse and ascending sections of the colon usually merge. It is difficult to examine the mucosa of this section because the tight bend makes it impossible for the distal tip to stay in the center of the lumen.
7. The blind slide-by technique is used from the descending colon up to the ascending colon, which leads to the cecum and ileocolic valve.
8. When the ileocolic valve is approached, careful observation is necessary, or the valve may be bypassed and the distal tip may enter the cecum.
9. If the area is adequately clean, the ileocolic valve and the cecocolic valve can both be seen (Figure 7-145). In some cases the ileocolic valve appears as another opening adjacent to the cecolic valve. However, this area tends to be less well prepared because mucus and

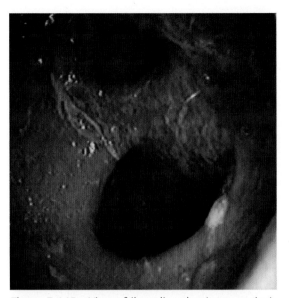

Figure 7-145 View of ileocolic valve (top opening), but dilated; bottom opening is cecocolic valve. (Courtesy MJR-VHUP, Philadelphia.)

debris entering from the ileum may cover and hide the ileocolic valve.

10. As the distal tip reaches the ileocolic valve, minor tip adjustments may be necessary to maintain the ileocolic orifice in the center of the field of view.

11. Minimal forward pressure can be applied to advance the tip directly through the open ileocolic orifice to access the ileum; however, if the ileocolic orifice is closed or slightly open, variable resistance may be encountered.

12. If the cecum is entered and was thought to be the colon, the lumen will make additional bends that cannot be negotiated with the distal tip. No force should be applied to push the distal tip past one of these bends, or the cecum may be perforated.

13. If the working length of the scope has been exhausted in the process of entering the cecum, the endoscope should be retracted slightly and air aspirated to partially collapse the lumen. This should shorten the distance to the cecocolic or ilecolic valve.

14. If rectal lesions are present, a retroflexed view is necessary. This can usually be

performed in dogs that are medium to large breeds. However, a rigid proctoscope is often the better scope for examining rectal lesions.

Biopsy Sampling

Biopsy samples from the ileum, cecum, ascending colon, transverse colon, and descending colon should all be obtained if possible, regardless of how normal the tissues appear. These mucosal biopsy samples are for histopathologic evaluation. However, *Salmonella* organisms sometimes can be cultured from tissue samples if none can be grown from feces.

Attempting to put more distance between the distal tip of the endoscope and the ileocolic valve allows a panoramic view of structures rather than a close-up view. Having the distal tip of the endoscope withdrawn into the descending colon and then reinserted into the ascending colon allows visualization of the ileocolic valve. With this technique, flexible biopsy forceps can be passed through the valve and blind ileal samples obtained.

It is often helpful if the colonic lumen is partially collapsed before the mucosa is grasped with biopsy forceps. This allows the forceps to take a larger, deeper sample that should include the submucosa. It is safe to reinflate the colon after biopsy samples are obtained with flexible forceps. The risk of perforation with flexible biopsy instruments is much less than with rigid instruments.

CANINE AND FELINE CASTRATION

Castration may also be referred to as a "neuter," "alter," or *orchiectomy*.

Routine Feline Castration

Definition: Feline castration refers to the surgical removal of the testicles in the cat.

Indications: The primary indication to perform a castration is for sterilization of the male cat. Other indications include the following:

- Prevention of roaming
- Prevention of aggressive behavior or fighting

- Prevention of urine spraying or marking
- Correction of congenital abnormalities
- Treatment of scrotal neoplasia
- Treatment of scrotal abscess, infection, or trauma
- Treatment of endocrine abnormalities
- Treatment of disease elsewhere in the body related to hormones (e.g., prostatic disease, perineal hernias)

Instrumentation

No special instrumentation is required to perform a feline castration. The surgeon may prefer to use metal clips rather than using the spermatic cord to tie a knot, or may prefer using suture for ligation.

Patient Positioning

The feline patient may be positioned for castration in lateral or in dorsal recumbency with the legs tied cranially. The positioning of the patient is the surgeon's preference.

Patient Draping

A single fenestrated drape should be sufficient for orchiectomy (Figure 7-146).

Feline Castration Procedure

An examination of the testicles should be conducted before inducing anesthesia to ensure that both testicles have descended into the scrotum.

The male cat should be positioned according to the surgeon's instructions (lateral or dorsal recumbency). The testicles should be prepared for surgery by gently plucking the hair from the scrotum. The scrotum should then be prepped and draped with proper aseptic technique. One testicle is held in place while the surgeon makes an incision over the testicle (Figure 7-147). The parietal vaginal tunic is then incised, and the testicle can then be extruded from the scrotum with gentle force (Figures 7-148 and 7-149).

The spermatic cord can be ligated and transected using a couple different techniques. Metal clips can be used for ligation of the spermatic

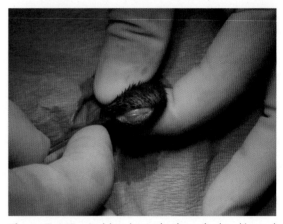

Figure 7-147   Incision is made through the skin and parietal vaginal tunic of the feline scrotum for orchiectomy.

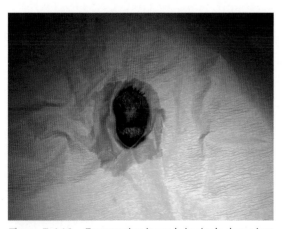

Figure 7-146   Fenestration is made in single drape just large enough to reveal both testicles for feline castration.

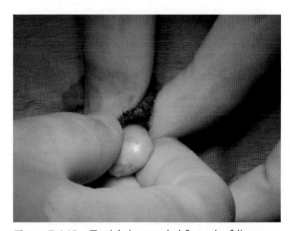

Figure 7-148   Testicle is extruded from the feline scrotum with gentle force.

cord. Once the clips are in place, the testicle can be transected. Another option for ligation of the spermatic cord is using hemostats and suture. Three hemostats are placed on the spermatic cord, and the testicle is then transected. A ligature is placed around the cord just below the forceps.

Another type of procedure uses the reproductive anatomy to tie knots. In one such procedure the ductus deferens and the spermatic vessels are separated and used to tie square knots. Another such procedure uses an overhand technique (Figures 7-150 to 7-152). This is done by placing a hemostat on top of the spermatic cord and wrapping the cord over and around the hemostat. The cord is then grabbed by the hemostats and clamped near the testicle. The testicle is transected and the cord pulled through to make a knot on itself.

All these procedures are acceptable methods for feline castration; the choice is left to the surgeon's discretion. The scrotum itself is left unsutured.

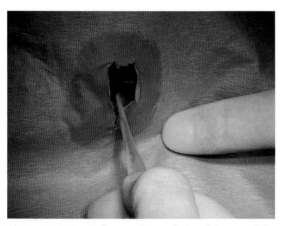

Figure 7-149   Full extrusion of the feline testicle, allowing visualization of the spermatic cord.

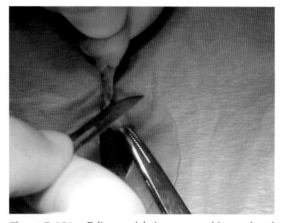

Figure 7-151   Feline testicle is transected in overhand technique.

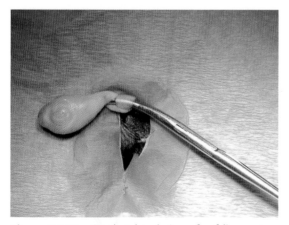

Figure 7-150   Overhand technique for feline castration. Hemostat is placed on top of the spermatic cord, and the cord is wrapped over and around the hemostat. The cord is grabbed with the hemostat and clamped near the testicle.

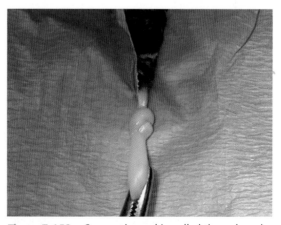

Figure 7-152   Spermatic cord is pulled through and a knot is made with the cord in overhand technique for feline castration.

Postoperative Considerations and Instructions

Scrotal bleeding can be a common complication associated with feline castration. A cold compress can be placed on the scrotum for several minutes to aid in hemostasis. If hemorrhage continues, another surgery may be required to ligate a bleeding vessel. General discharge instructions are listed in Chapter 11. Box 7-18 shows an example of a surgery report for a feline castration.

Routine Canine Castration

Definition: Canine castration refers to the surgical removal of the testicles in the dog.

Indications: The primary indication for performing a canine castration is for sterilization of the dog. Other indications include the following:

- Prevention of roaming
- Prevention of aggressive behavior or fighting
- Prevention of urine marking
- Correction of congenital abnormalities
- Treatment of scrotal or testicular neoplasia
- Treatment of scrotal abscess, infection, or trauma
- Treatment of disease elsewhere in the body related to hormones (e.g., prostatic disease, perineal hernias, perianal tumors)

BOX 7-18   Surgery Report: Feline Castration

Animal Hospital Name

Owner: John Doe

Address: 555 Sterling Lane

Jupiter, NY 55555

Phone number: 555-5555

Animal Name: Kitty

Animal #: 65556501

Species: Feline

Breed: DSH

DOB: 05/05/03

Date of Surgery: 01/03/2004

Primary Surgeon: Dr. Vet

Assistant: Nurse Scrub

Diagnosis or Preoperative Signs: Intact male

Surgical Procedure: Feline castration

Description of Surgical Procedure

Surgical Approach: A 1-cm incision was made through the skin on the left and right caudal scrotum to exteriorize each testicle.

Surgical Pathology: None.

Surgical Procedure: Applying pressure cranially, the right testicle was exteriorized. An incision was made over the testicle, and the spermatic fascia and parietal vaginal tunic were incised. The ligament of the tail of the epididymis was separated from the tunic using a hemostat. The ductus deferens and the vascular cord were then tied to each other and transected distal to the knot. The same procedure was repeated on the left side.

Closure: The scrotal incisions were left open to heal by second intention.

DSH, Domestic shorthair.

Instrumentation

A general-use soft tissue surgical instrument pack should be sufficient for canine castration.

Patient Positioning

The canine patient should be placed in dorsal recumbency for castration.

Patient Draping

A single fenestrated drape is appropriate for orchiectomy. The surgeon may elect to use a four-corner draping method.

Canine Castration Procedure

The scrotum should be examined and palpated for the presence of both testicles before inducing anesthesia. If both testicles are present, a routine castration can be performed. If only one testicle is present, the dog is considered "cryptorchid" and may require an inguinal or abdominal surgery to retrieve the other testicle.

For a routine castration the surgical site should be clipped from the tip of the prepuce to just above the scrotum. The clipped region should extend laterally into the inguinal section on both sides. The scrotum should not be clipped. The skin of the scrotum is delicate and sensitive and may be susceptible to clipper burns or tears. Irritation of the scrotum can cause the animal to lick or bite at the affected region postoperatively. The surgical site should be aseptically prepared and a single fenestrated drape placed over the surgical region (the testicles and scrotum will be draped out of the surgical field).

The surgeon may decide to do an "open castration" or "closed castration." In the closed procedure the tunics are not incised, and the entire spermatic cord encased in its parietal vaginal tunic is ligated and transected. In the open procedure the tunics are incised, and the contents of the cord are ligated and transected separately.

Open Castration

The surgeon selects the first testicle and applies pressure cranially to advance the testicle into the prescrotal region. The skin and subcutaneous tissues and spermatic fascia are incised (Figure 7-153). The surgeon then incises the parietal vaginal tunic (Figure 7-154), and the testicle is gently extruded (Figure 7-155). A hemostat should be

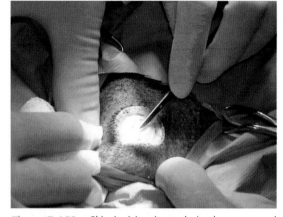

Figure 7-153 Skin incision is made in the prescrotal region for canine castration.

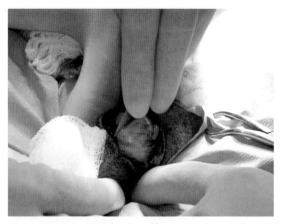

Figure 7-154 Incision into the parietal vaginal tunic of the canine scrotum for orchiectomy.

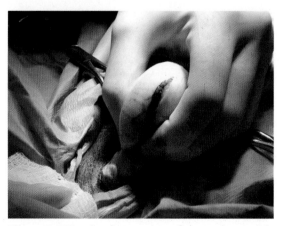

Figure 7-155 Gentle extrusion of the canine testicle for orchiectomy.

placed across the tunic at the attachment of the epididymis. The ligament of the tail of the epididymis is separated from the tunic. Three clamps can be placed across the spermatic cord (Figure 7-156). The vascular cord and the ductus deferens are recognized and can be individually ligated using an absorbable suture. The surgeon may decide to ligate the vascular cord and ductus deferens together. A circumferential ligature is then placed around both the ductus deferens and the vascular cord. A hemostat is placed on the cord close to the testicle. The cord is then transected between the hemostat and ligatures (Figure 7-157). The cord is examined for bleeding and returned within the tunic. The second testicle can be removed in the same manner.

Closed Castration

Closed castration is performed similar to open castration except for the incision of the parietal vaginal tunics. Once the skin, subcutaneous tissue, and spermatic fascia are incised, the spermatic cord is exteriorized. Ligatures are placed around the entire spermatic cord and tunics, and the cord is then transected.

Postoperative Considerations and Instructions

Common complications associated with canine castration include hemorrhage and scrotal hematoma. A scrotal hematoma may be the result of a hemorrhaging vessel (or vessels). Care should be taken during the surgery to provide appropriate hemostasis to avoid such complications. Cold compresses can be placed to aid in hemostasis postoperatively if hemorrhage has occurred. A complete scrotal ablation (removal of scrotum) may be necessary if hemostasis was unsuccessful. Other complications may include self-inflicted trauma to the incision and infection or dehiscence of the incision site.

On discharge of the patient, postoperative instructions for the client should include the same general discharge instructions listed in Chapter 11. Box 7-19 shows an example of a surgery report for a canine castration.

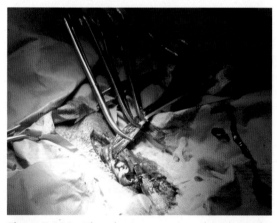

Figure 7-156   Three hemostats are used to clamp the spermatic cord in canine castration.

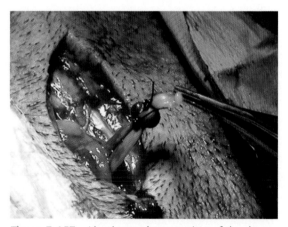

Figure 7-157   Ligation and transection of the ductus deferens and vascular cord in canine castration. The cord is checked for hemorrhage before closing.

BOX 7-19   Surgery Report: Canine Castration

Animal Hospital Name

Owner: John Doe

Address: 555 Sterling Lane

          Jupiter, NY 55555

Phone number: 555-5555

Animal Name: Mikey

Animal #: 65656501

Species: Canine

Breed: Labrador

DOB: 05/05/04

Date of Surgery: 01/03/2005

Primary Surgeon: Dr. Vet

Assistant: Nurse Scrub

Diagnosis or Preoperative Signs: Intact male

Surgical Procedure: Open castration

Description of Surgical Procedure

Surgical Approach: A 3-cm ventral midline incision was made in the prescrotal region while advancing one testicle cranially into the incision line. The incision was extended through the subcutaneous tissues.

Surgical Procedure: The right testicle was pushed up through the incision. The vaginal tunic was then incised and the testicle pushed through. The ligament of the tail of the epididymis was bluntly dissected. The ductus deferens and the vascular cord were individually ligated with 2-0 PDS, then both were ligated together with a circumferential ligature. The testicle was then transected distal to the ligatures. The same procedure was performed on the left testicle.

Closure:

Subcutaneous tissue: 2-0 PDS in simple continuous suture pattern.

Subcuticular tissue: 3-0 Monocryl in simple continuous suture pattern.

Skin: 3-0 nylon in simple interrupted suture pattern.

KEY POINTS

1. To be a competent surgical assistant, the veterinary technician must have proficient knowledge of the surgical procedure, surgical instruments, and aseptic and sterile technique.
2. The intraoperative duties of the surgical assistant include retraction of tissue, bone reduction, wound sponging, suction of the surgical site, and providing hemostasis. Responsibilities also include anticipation of the surgeon's needs and sponge counts before surgery and before closure of the cavity.
3. The use of Balfour retractors during abdominal surgical procedures allows for enhanced exposure to the abdominal cavity.
4. Laparotomy ("lap") sponges should be used to isolate organs during hollow-organ surgery. The use of laparotomy sponges helps reduce contaminants that may enter the abdominal cavity.
5. Stay sutures should be placed during hollow-organ surgeries (e.g., cystotomy, gastrotomy) to

allow for manipulation of the organ as well as to prevent leakage of contaminants within the abdominal cavity.

6. Preoperative blood tests should be performed for any animal undergoing anesthesia and surgery. An animal more than 5 years old should have a more extensive blood analysis (CBC and chemistry) than a patient under age 5 (CBC).

7. Animals should be spayed before their first ovarian cycle to decrease the incidence of mammary tumors.

8. Patients undergoing abdominal procedures should be clipped from the xiphoid process to the pubis. This allows the surgeon to extend the incision as needed.

9. The most common complication reported after an ovariohysterectomy is hemorrhage.

10. Appropriate analgesics should be administered for every surgical patient postoperatively.

11. Abdominal lavage with warm sterile saline before closure of the abdomen helps to dilute any pollutants and to warm the patient.

12. A barium contrast study should never be performed if perforations of the gastrointestinal tract are suspected.

13. During an enterotomy procedure, Doyen clamps or the fingers of an assistant should be used to avoid leakage of intestinal chyme within the abdomen.

14. Abdominal incisions should be monitored daily for swelling, discharge, or malodor. Many postoperative complications are related to the incision site.

15. The patient's bladder should be expressed before entering the OR.

16. The bladder of a traumatic injury patient should not be expressed before entering the OR.

17. Surgical patients may need to be sent home with Elizabethan collars in the event the pet attempts to mutilate the incision site.

18. Patients with gastric dilatation and volvulus (GDV) are considered true surgical emergencies. The immediate treatment for a GDV patient includes decompression of the stomach, correction of fluid and electrolyte imbalances, treatment for shock, and surgery to derotate the stomach and gastropexy.

19. An orogastric tube should never be forced down the esophagus during placement. Gentle placement is necessary to avoid damage to the esophagus.

20. A roll of hospital tape can be placed between the upper and lower jaws of the patient receiving an orogastric tube. The tube can be placed through the hole in the roll of tape. This will keep the jaws of the animal from biting down on the tube or the assistant's hand during placement.

21. The stomach of a dog with a GDV generally rotates in a clockwise direction.

22. Orthopedics involves injuries or diseases of the skeletal system.

23. Orthopedic injuries are usually not considered life threatening unless they involve the skull or spine or unless a long-bone fracture has resulted in great loss of blood.

24. Fracture assessment should include a history, thorough physical examination, and radiographs.

25. When taking radiographs of a long-bone fracture, the joint below and above the fracture site should be included within the film.

26. Open fractures are classified according to mechanism of puncture and the severity of the soft tissue damage.

27. Surgical options for fracture repair include internal fixation and external fixation. Internal fixation includes plates, screws, nails, pins, and wire. External fixation includes casts, rigid splints, and custom-made devices.

28. Casts and splints must be kept dry and clean and should be observed for slippage, self-mutilation, and toe swelling.

29. Hindlimb and forelimb amputations are considered major surgeries and should only be performed with a thorough knowledge of the patient's physical status.

30. Local nerve blocks contribute significantly to postoperative pain control in amputation patients.

31. Cranial cruciate ligament (CCL) ruptures are also referred to as anterior cruciate ligament (ACL) injury or "football player's knee" in humans.

32. The major diagnostic tests for CCL injury include the cranial drawer test and the tibial compression test. Palpation of the affected leg often reveals muscle atrophy, pain, joint effusion, and asymmetry.

33. Biopsy techniques for diagnostic purposes include fine-needle aspiration, impression smears, needle punch, punch, bone, incisional, and excisional biopsy.

34. Lateral ear canal resection involves lateralization and exposure of the horizontal ear canal for drainage purposes, generally in patients with chronic ear infections. Medical management is usually required even after resection.

35. Entropion refers to "rolling in" of the eyelid. Surgery is usually done to alleviate ocular irritation.

36. A meibomian (sebaceous) adenoma is the most common eyelid neoplasm in the dog.

37. Squamous cell carcinoma is the most common feline eyelid tumor and is often found in cats with white or pink eyelids.

38. A wedge resection procedure is the most common procedure performed for eyelid neoplasia.

39. Minimally invasive surgeries include laser surgery, laparoscopy, and endoscopy.

40. The technician's most important role in laser surgery is laser safety. Most practices using laser surgery will appoint a laser safety officer, most likely the technician.

41. Many hazards are associated with laser surgery, including eye, skin, fire, and smoke plume hazards. All safety steps should be taken to avoid potential hazards.

42. Advantages to laser surgery over traditional surgery include more rapid healing time of tissue, less risk of postoperative infection, reduced postoperative pain and swelling, and decreased surgery time.

43. Laparoscopic procedures are performed to examine and biopsy the internal organs or tumors of the abdominal cavity. Laparoscopy can also be used to perform specific surgical procedures, such as a spay and gastropexy.

44. Some advantages to laparoscopic procedures include improved patient recovery, smaller surgical sites, lower postoperative infection rate, and decreased postoperative pain.

45. Patients undergoing laparoscopy should be fasted for 12 hours and have the bladder expressed before entering the OR.

46. When performing endoscopy, handling an insertion tube should always be done carefully. Sharp bends, tight coiling, and striking of the tube against hard surfaces should be avoided.

47. Maintaining endoscopes involves proper cleaning and disinfection, leak testing and inspection, microbial monitoring, and storage.

48. In dogs and cats, gastric and duodenal disorders are more common than esophageal disorders. Because clinical signs of these diseases can overlap, endoscopic examination of the esophagus should extend to the stomach and duodenum for a thorough upper gastrointestinal examination.

49. Patient preparation for colonoscopies is crucial because the whole colon needs to be visualized, and it is more difficult to clean the ileocolic valve area than the descending colon. Also, large debris cannot be aspirated as well with flexible scopes as with rigid scopes.

50. Narcotics (fentanyl, morphine, hydromorphone) should not be used for gastroduodenoscopies because they may cause spasms, and entering the duodenum will be more difficult because of an increase in pyloric tone.

51. Indications for performing a feline or canine castration include eliminating reproductive function, preventing roaming, preventing urine spraying, treating scrotal neoplasia, and treating endocrine abnormalities.

52. Before placing a dog or cat under anesthesia for castration, the testicles are examined to be sure both have descended into the scrotum. If not, an inguinal or abdominal procedure may be necessary for retrieval of the testicle.

53. For cats undergoing castration, the hair of the scrotum should be gently plucked before entering the OR.

54. Scrotal bleeding is the most common complication associated with canine and feline castration.

REVIEW QUESTIONS

1. Which of the following are considered abdominal surgical procedures?
   a. Ovariohysterectomy.
   b. Routine, closed castration.
   c. Incisional gastropexy.
   d. All of the above.
   e. Both a and c.

2. What is the primary indication for an ovariohys-terectomy?
   a. To prevent mammary carcinoma.
   b. To prevent pyometra.
   c. Dystocia.
   d. Reproductive sterilization.
   e. Uterine torsion.
3. Why is it beneficial to spay a dog before her first heat cycle?
   a. To decrease the chance of unwanted litters.
   b. To decrease the chance of the development of mammary gland tumors.
   c. Both a and b.
   d. None of the above.
4. Which of the following breeds of dogs have an increased risk of dystocia?
   a. Golden retrievers.
   b. Pugs.
   c. Bulldogs.
   d. Both b and c.
   e. All of the above.
5. During which of the following surgeries is the uterus removed?
   a. Routine ovariohysterectomy.
   b. Cesarean section without an ovariohys-terectomy.
   c. En bloc resection.
   d. All of the above.
   e. Both a and c.
6. Which of the following is an indication for abdominal exploratory surgery?
   a. Routine ovariohysterectomy.
   b. Splenic tumor.
   c. Ruptured bladder.
   d. All of the above.
   e. Both b and c.
7. Which of the following retractors is routinely used in abdominal exploratory surgeries?
   a. Gelpi.
   b. Senn.
   c. Weitlaner.
   d. Balfour.
   e. None of the above.
8. Which of the following surgeries involves making an incision into the stomach?
   a. Abdominal exploratory.
   b. Gastrotomy.
   c. Enterotomy.

d. Splenectomy.
   e. Laparotomy.
9. Which of the following intestinal surgeries involves removing a piece of the intestine and suturing the ends of the remaining intestines back together?
   a. Enterotomy.
   b. Resection and anastomosis.
   c. Both a and b.
   d. None of the above.
10. *True or False:* Sterile saline can be injected into the surgical site to check for any leakage after the anastomosis site has been closed.
11. Which of the following should be performed before closing the abdomen if peritonitis is suspected?
   a. Bacterial culture swab.
   b. Gastropexy.
   c. Urinalysis.
   d. All of the above.
   e. None of the above.
12. Which of the following refers to surgically attaching the stomach to the body wall?
   a. Gastric dilatation and volvulus (GDV).
   b. Gastropexy.
   c. Splenectomy.
   d. Enterotomy.
   e. Celiotomy.
13. *True or False:* A patient that needs to have an abdominal exploratory for internal hemorrhage resulting from having been hit by a car (HBC) should have its bladder expressed before being moved into the surgery room.
14. Which of the following terms refers to a joint?
   a. Malunion.
   b. Comminuted.
   c. Articular.
   d. Interfragmentary.
   e. None of the above.
15. Which of the following are devices used in *internal* fixation of fractured bones?
   a. Intramedullary (IM) pins.
   b. Ring fixation.
   c. Bone plates.
   d. Both a and c.
   e. All of the above.
16. Which of the following devices are used in *external* fixation of fractured bones?

a. IM pins.

b. Ring fixation.

c. Bone plates.

d. Both a and c.

e. All of the above.

17. Which of the following are possible complications associated with internal fixation of fracture repair?

a. Non-union.

b. Malunion.

c. Delayed union.

d. Aseptic loosening.

e. All of the above.

18. *True* or *False:* Splints are only appropriate for fractures that are distal to the elbow and stifle.

19. Which of the following diagnostic tests may aid in diagnosing a torn cranial cruciate ligament?

a. Cranial drawer test.

b. Palpating the hock joint.

c. Tibial compression test.

d. Both a and c.

e. All of the above.

20. Which of the following diagnostic tests used to evaluate masses does not usually require sedation or anesthesia, is easy to perform, has minimal morbidity associated with it, but has a low diagnostic yield?

a. Needle punch biopsy.

b. Fine-needle aspiration.

c. Excisional biopsy.

d. Both a and c.

e. All of the above.

21. *True* or *False:* Proper fixation of tissue samples requires a ratio of 1 part tissue to 10 parts of 10% neutral buffered formalin.

22. When is a lateral ear canal resection indicated?

a. Chronic otitis externa.

b. Neoplasia of the ear canal.

c. Deafness.

d. Both a and b.

e. All of the above.

23. *True* or *False:* Baby shampoo diluted 1:3 with water is both effective and safe in cleansing the periocular area before ophthalmic surgery.

24. Which of the following breeds are predisposed to protrusion of the gland of the third eyelid, also known as "cherry eye"?

a. Cocker spaniel.

b. Boston terrier.

c. Great Dane.

d. All of the above.

e. None of the above.

25. Which of the following are considered minimally invasive procedures?

a. Laser surgery.

b. Laparoscopy.

c. Endoscopy.

d. All of the above.

e. None of the above.

26. Which of the following is an advantage of using a laser unit over a scalpel handle in surgery?

a. More rapid healing.

b. Simultaneous cauterization of blood vessels when making the incision.

c. Reduced postoperative pain.

d. Both a and c.

e. All of the above.

27. What are some of the workplace hazards associated with laser surgery?

a. Eye and skin damage.

b. Smoke plume hazard.

c. Fire hazard.

d. All of the above.

e. None of the above.

28. What advantage does laparoscopy have over traditional laparotomy?

a. None; the procedures are essentially the same.

b. Smaller surgical incisions.

c. Lower postoperative morbidity.

d. Both b and c.

29. *True* or *False:* A flexible endoscope with a diameter of 8 to 11 mm and a working length of 100 cm is usually adequate for most feline and canine upper gastrointestinal examinations and colonoscopies.

30. *True* or *False:* When the endoscope is not being used, it should be set on the examination table.

31. Which of the following clinical signs refer to possible esophageal disease?

a. Regurgitation.

b. Dysphagia.

c. Odynophagia.

d. All of the above.

e. None of the above.

32. If cytologic samples are collected with a cytology brush during endoscopic procedures, what can be done to prevent contamination and loss of specimen material when the brush is withdrawn through the accessory channel of the endoscope?
    a. Autoclave the endoscope before use.
    b. Use a sheathed cytology brush.
    c. Both a and b.
    d. None of the above.

33. Which of the following can be diagnosed by gastroscopy?
    a. *Helicobacter* infection.
    b. Foreign bodies in the stomach.
    c. Gastric ulceration.
    d. All of the above.
    e. None of the above.

34. How long should a patient be fasted before gastroscopy?
    a. 12- to 18-hour food fast, 4-hour water fast.
    b. 6- to 8-hour food fast, 4-hour water fast.
    c. 24- to 36-hour food fast, 8-hour water fast.
    d. 10-hour food fast; water fast unnecessary.
    e. None of the above.

35. *True* or *False:* Duodenoscopy aids in the diagnosis and treatment of small intestine disease.

36. *True* or *False:* Lymphoma is the most common intestinal neoplasia.

37. Colonoscopy refers to the endoscopic technique of examining the:
    a. Rectum.
    b. Large intestine.
    c. Cecum.
    d. All of the above.
    e. None of the above.

38. Which of the following applies to the patient about to undergo colonoscopy?
    a. It needs to be fasted 24 to 36 hours.
    b. It will receive an enema.
    c. Both a and b.
    d. None of the above.

39. In addition to rendering a male cat unable to reproduce, which of the following is another indication for castrating a male cat?
    a. Prevent aggressive behavior.
    b. Prevent urine spraying.
    c. Prevent roaming.

d. All of the above.
e. None of the above.

40. *True* or *False:* The primary difference between an open and closed castration technique is that the open technique involves incising the parietal vaginal tunic and the closed technique does not incise the tunic.

ANSWERS

1.	e	21.	True
2.	d	22.	d
3.	c	23.	True
4.	d	24.	d
5.	e	25.	d
6.	e	26.	e
7.	d	27.	d
8.	b	28.	d
9.	b	29.	True
10.	True	30.	False
11.	a	31.	d
12.	b	32.	b
13.	False	33.	d
14.	c	34.	a
15.	d	35.	True
16.	b	36.	True
17.	e	37.	d
18.	True	38.	c
19.	d	39.	d
20.	b	40.	True

BIBLIOGRAPHY

American National Standards Institute: *Safe use of lasers* (ANSI Z136.1-1993), New York, 1993.

Bessler M et al: Is immune function better preserved after laparoscopic versus open colon resection? *Surg Endosc* 8:881, 1994.

Bjorab MJ, Ellison GW, Slocum B: *Current techniques in small animal surgery,* Philadelphia, 1998, Williams & Wilkins.

Blood DC, Studdert VP: *Saunders comprehensive veterinary dictionary,* ed 2, London, 1999, Saunders.

Brockman DJ, Washabau RJ, Drobatz KJ: Canine gastric dilatation/volvulus syndrome in a veterinary critical care unit: 295 cases (1986-1992), *J Am Vet Med Assoc* 207:460, 1995.

Burrows CF, Bright RM, Spencer CP: Influence of dietary composition on gastric emptying and motility in dogs: potential involvement in acute gastric dilatation, *Am J Vet Res* 46:2609, 1985.

Darvelid AW, Linde-Forsberg C: Dystocia in the bitch, *J Small Anim Pract* 35:402, 1994.

Doverspike M et al: Contralateral cranial cruciate ligament rupture: incidence in 114 dogs, *J Am Anim Hosp Assoc* 29:275, 1993.

Flanders JA, Harvey HJ: Results of tube gastrostomy as treatment for gastric torsion in the dog, *J Am Vet Med Assoc* 185:74, 1984.

Fossum TW et al: *Small animal surgery,* ed 2, St Louis, 2002, Mosby.

Gaudet DA: Retrospective study of 128 cases of canine dystocia, *J Small Anim Pract* 21:813, 1985.

Gelatt KN: *Essentials of veterinary ophthalmology,* Philadelphia, 2000, Lippincott Williams & Wilkins.

Glickman LT et al: Analysis of risk factors for gastric dilatation and dilatation volvulus in dogs: a practitioner/owner case-control study, *J Am Anim Hosp Assoc* 33:197, 1997.

Glickman LT et al: Multiple risk factors for the gastric dilatation-volvulus syndrome in dogs, *J Am Vet Med Assoc* 216:40, 2000.

Gross ME et al: Effects of abdominal insufflation with nitrous oxide on cardiorespiratory measurements in spontaneously breathing isoflurane-anesthetized dogs, *Am J Vet Res* 54:1352, 1993.

Gualtieri M: Esophagoscopy, *Vet Clin North Am Small Anim Pract* 31:605, 2001.

Harvey CE: The ear and nose. In Harvey CE et al, editors: *Small animal surgery,* Philadelphia, 1990, Lippincott.

Hitz CB: An overview of laser technology. In *Understanding laser technology: an intuitive introduction to basic and advanced laser concepts,* ed 2, Tulsa, Okla, 1991, Pennwell.

Holt TL, Mann FA: Soft tissue applications of lasers, *Vet Clin North Am* 32:569, 2002.

Jacques SL: Laser-tissue interactions: photochemical, photothermal, and photomechanical, *Surg Clin North Am* 72:531, 1992.

Johanningmeier JP: TPLO repair method for CCL tears, *Vet Tech,* October 2003, p 682.

Johnson JA, Austin C, Bruer GJ: Incidence of appendicular musculoskeletal disorders in veterinary teaching hospitals from 1980-1989, *Vet Comp Orthop Trauma* 7:56, 1994.

Johnson JM, Johnson AL: Cranial cruciate ligament rupture: pathogenesis, diagnosis and postoperative rehabilitation, *Vet Clin North Am* 23:717, 1993.

Katzir A: Medical lasers. In *Lasers and optical fibers in medicine,* San Diego, 1993, Academic Press.

Katzir A: Single optical fibers. In *Lasers and optical fibers in medicine,* San Diego, 1993, Academic Press.

Lettow E: Laparoscopic examinations in liver diseases in dogs, *Vet Med Rev* 2:159, 1972.

Live MS et al: Circumcostal gastropexy for preventing recurrence of gastric dilatation-volvulus in the dog: an evaluation of 30 cases, *J Am Vet Med Assoc* 187:245, 1985.

Lucroy MD, Bartels KE: Using biomedical lasers in veterinary practice, *Vet Med* 95:4, 2000.

Lumenis LX-20SP NovaPulse Laser System operator's manual, 2002.

Macoy DM et al: A gastropexy technique for permanent fixation of the pyloric antrum, *J Am Anim Hosp Assoc* 18:763, 1982.

Magne ML, Tams TR: Laparoscopy: instrumentation and technique. In Tams TR, editor: *Small animal endoscopy,* ed 2, St Louis, 1999, Mosby.

Marsolais GS, Dvorak G, Conzemius MG: Effects of postoperative rehabilitation on limb function after cranial cruciate ligament repair in dogs, *J Am Vet Med Assoc* 220:1325, 2002.

Matthiesen DT: Partial gastrectomy as treatment for gastric volvulus, *Vet Surg* 14:185, 1985.

Mehler SJ, Bennett A: Surgical oncology of exotic animals, *Vet Clin Exotic Anim Pract* 2005 (in press).

Monnet E, Twedt DC: Laparoscopy, *Vet Clin North Am* 33:1147, 2003.

Moore KW, Read RA: Rupture of the cranial cruciate ligament in dogs, *Compend Contin Educ Pract Vet* 18:223, 1996.

Morrison WB: *Cancer in dogs and cats,* Baltimore, 1998, Williams & Wilkins.

Muir WW: Gastric dilatation-volvulus in the dog, with emphasis on cardiac arrhythmias, *J Am Vet Med Assoc* 180:739, 1982.

Nasisse MP, Moore CP, Constantinescu GM: Surgery of the adnexa, *Vet Clin North Am* 27(5), 1997.

Nelson R, Couto C: *Small animal internal medicine,* ed 2, St Louis, 1998, Mosby.

Osborne CA et al: Analysis of 77,000 canine uroliths, *Vet Clin North Am Small Anim Pract* 29:1, 1999.

Pearce J, Thomsen R: Rate process analysis of thermal damage. In Welch AJ, van Gamert MJC, editors: *Optical-thermal response of laser irradiated tissue,* New York, 1995, Plenum.

Pearson H: The complications of ovariohysterectomy in the bitch, *J Small Anim Pract* 14:257, 1973.

Phillips BS: Bladder tumors in dogs and cats, *Compend Contin Educ Pract Vet* 21:540, 1999.

Richter KP: Laparoscopy in dogs and cats, *Vet Clin North Am* 31:707, 2001.

Robben JR, Stokhof AA, van Sluisjs FJ: Arrhythmias after surgery of gastric dilatation volvulus in dogs, *Tijdschr Diergenneeskd* 118(suppl):67S, 1993.

Roberts SM, Severin GA, Lavach JD: Prevalence and treatment of palpebral neoplasms in the dog: 200 cases (1975-1983), *J Am Vet Med Assoc* 189:1355, 1986.

Rothuizen J: Laparoscopy in small animal medicine, *Vet Q* 3:225, 1985.

Sammarco JL et al: Postoperative analgesia for stifle surgery: a comparison of intraarticular bupivacaine, morphine or saline, *Vet Surg* 25:59, 1996.

Schneider R et al: Factors influencing canine mammary cancer development and post surgical survival, *J Natl Cancer Inst* 43:1249, 1969.

Schumway R, Broussard J: Maintenance of gastrointestinal endoscopes, *Clin Tech Small Anim Pract* 18:254, 2003.

Slatter D: *Fundamentals of veterinary ophthalmology,* ed 3, Philadelphia, 2001, Saunders.

Slatter D: *Textbook of small animal surgery,* ed 3, Philadelphia, 2003, Saunders.

Smeak DD: The Chinese finger trap suture technique for fastening tubes and catheters, *J Am Anim Hosp Assoc* 26:215, 1990.

Smith GK, Torg JS: Fibula head transposition for repair of cruciate-deficient stifle in the dog, *J Am Vet Med Assoc* 187:375, 1985.

Stasi K, Melendez L: Care and cleaning of the endoscope, *Vet Clin North Am Small Anim Pract* 31:589, 2001.

Sullins KE: Diode laser and endoscopic laser surgery *Vet Clin North Am* 32:639, 2002.

Tams T: *Handbook of small animal gastroenterology,* ed 2, Philadelphia, 2003, Saunders.

Tams T: *Small animal endoscopy,* ed 2, St Louis, 1999, Mosby.

Theran P: Early-age neutering of dogs and cats, *J Am Vet Med Assoc* 202:914, 1993.

Troncy E et al: Results of preemptive epidural administration of morphine with or without bupivacaine in dogs and cats undergoing surgery: 265 cases (1997-1999), *J Am Vet Med Assoc* 221:666, 2002.

Welch AJ, van Gemert MJC: Introduction to medical applications. In *Optical-thermal response of laser irradiated tissue,* New York, 1993, Plenum.

Welch AJ et al: Definitions and overview of tissue optics. In Welch AJ, van Gamert MJC, editors: *Optical-thermal response of laser irradiated tissue,* New York, 1995, Plenum.

Whittick WG: *Canine orthopedics,* ed 2, Philadelphia, 1990, Lea & Febiger.

Willard MD: *Small animal clinical diagnosis by laboratory methods,* Philadelphia, 2004, Saunders.

Withrow SJ, MacEwen EG: *Small animal clinical oncology,* ed 3, Philadelphia, 2001, Saunders.

Withrow SJ, Postorino NC, Straw RC: Tumors of the gastrointestinal system. In *Clinical veterinary oncology,* Philadelphia, 1989, Lippincott.

Witney WO et al: Belt-loop gastropexy: technique and surgical results in 20 dogs, *J Am Anim Hosp Assoc* 25:75, 1989.

Young WP: Feline onychectomy and elective procedures, *Vet Clin North Am* 32:601, 2002.

Zepp CP: Surgical technique to establish drainage of the external ear canal and correction of hematoma of the dog and cat, *J Am Vet Med Assoc* 115:91, 1949.

PART III

Postoperative Considerations

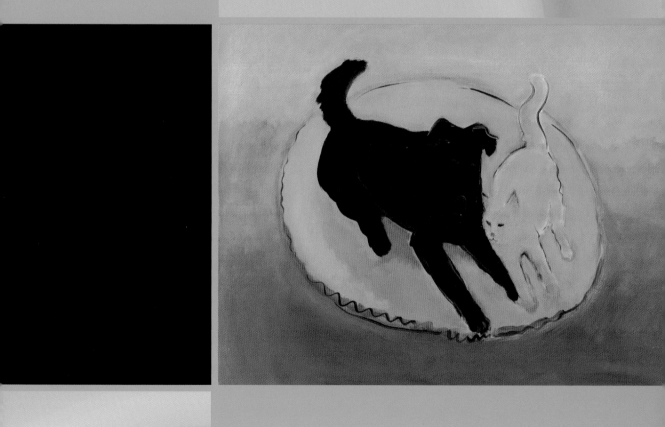

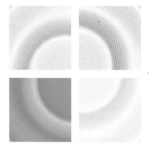

CHAPTER 8

The Postoperative Patient

Gail Hartman, Nancy Shaffran

LEARNING OBJECTIVES

After studying this chapter, the reader should be able to do the following:

- Monitor the patient during the anesthesia recovery period.
  - Identify the proper time to extubate the patient.
  - Safely extubate the patient.
  - Recognize and administer prescribed treatments for postanesthesia complications, such as hypothermia, emergence delirium, and prolonged recovery.
- Recognize and administer prescribed treatments for postsurgical complications, such as hemorrhage, seroma, dehiscence, self-trauma, and infection.
- Thoroughly and properly cleanse wounds, understanding the principles of lavage and debridement.

- Maintain and monitor bandages, casts, splints, and slings.
- Maintain and monitor surgical drains.
- Maintain and monitor indwelling venous and urinary catheters.
- Understand the basic forms of physical therapy.
- Provide nutritional support for postoperative patients through the techniques of force-feeding and tube feeding.
- Provide effective postoperative analgesia.
- Understand the importance of preemptive, presurgical analgesia on the success of postoperative analgesia.
- Safely combine different classes of analgesics to provide effective postoperative pain management.

The work of the veterinary surgical assistant is still far from complete even when the last suture is placed and the surgeon leaves the surgical table. The patient still needs to recover from the anesthesia. The surgical wounds need to heal. The surgical procedure has yet to be proved successful. The patient and the owner need help and guidance during the recuperation period. Careful patient monitoring and owner mentoring are important responsibilities of the veterinary technician.

Compassion, caring, and concern are the hallmarks of an excellent technician. All hospitalized patients need an advocate. The observant nurse

who advocates for the patient's needs and points out changes in the patient's physical status to the attending veterinarian is an invaluable asset to both the patient and the veterinarian.

RECOVERY FROM ANESTHESIA AND EXTUBATION

Shepherding the patient from the surgical plane of anesthesia back to consciousness is the first step in the recovery process. The recovery period starts with the cessation of anesthesia and continues until the patient's vital signs and level of consciousness have returned to normal.

First, the patient must be safely extubated. The steps in the process of extubation are as follows:

1. Turn off the anesthetic vaporizer and leave the patient on oxygen for 5 minutes, if possible. Flush anesthetic gas out of the anesthesia machine by quickly disconnecting the patient from the machine. Open the pop-off valve all the way, place the thumb or heel of the hand over the patient attachment site, and press the oxygen flush button. The oxygen rushes through the machine and out the exhaust, carrying off the anesthetic gas. Reconnect the patient to the anesthesia machine.
2. Untie the endotracheal (ET) tube attachment from the patient's head or muzzle.
3. Find an empty syringe with the plunger depressed completely. Attach a syringe to the cuff if using a silicon tube with a spring valve in the pilot tube (non–red rubber tube). Do not deflate the ET tube cuff yet.
4. Check the patient's reflexes. Not every patient will stay under for the full 5 minutes. The anesthetist must know whether or not the patient is close to jumping off the table.
5. Untie the patient from the table, and detach all monitoring devices and fluid administration lines. Remove the V-trough or sandbags and place the patient in lateral recumbency. When rotating the patient into lateral recumbency, guard the tube and do not let it rotate in the patient's trachea. It is important to prevent twisting injury to the trachea. Small patients are especially prone to this injury.
6. The immediate postoperative temperature is taken at this point. Anesthetic monitoring of the vital signs continues every 5 minutes until the patient is sufficiently recovered to be returned to the cage.
7. Once the 5 minutes of oxygen administration are completed, disconnect the patient from the anesthesia machine while the oxygen is flowing. This will ensure that the patient always has a source of oxygen in case of an emergency. Place your hand over the end of

the Y-piece and squeeze the reservoir bag. This will empty the circuit of most of the gas through the exhaust system.

8. *Now* shut off the oxygen at the flowmeter.
9. Recheck the reflexes and determine the patient's stage of anesthesia. If the patient is still "asleep," stimulate the patient by rubbing its thorax, stroking the neck, and gently pulling the tongue or ears.
10. Once the patient swallows two or three times, deflate the cuff and gently pull the ET tube down and out of the mouth. (See exception for brachycephalic breeds noted below.) The ET tube cuff should never be deflated before the patient regains the ability to swallow. A patient that cannot swallow is vulnerable to aspiration of material that has pooled in the pharynx. A properly inflated ET tube cuff prevents such aspiration.
11. Check the end of the ET tube for blood, regurgitated stomach contents, and food. If the animal has regurgitated material in the mouth, hang the head down off the surgical table to allow the material to drip out of the mouth. Quickly determine if the patient needs to be reintubated or have the pharynx suctioned. Carefully rinsing the mouth gently with water may suffice, provided this does not cause the patient to gag and choke from the rinsing process.
12. Take the patient to the recovery cage.
13. Continue to monitor the patient every 5 to 10 minutes to ensure the recovery is a safe and smooth event until complete. At this point, give postoperative pain medications as instructed. Generally, if the patient's temperature is below 98° F postoperatively, opioid drugs will not be given. Hypothermia concerns are discussed later.

Brachycephalic breeds of dogs, such as English bulldogs, pugs, and Pekingese, are prone to developing complications while recovering from anesthesia. These short-headed dogs frequently have stenotic nares and elongated soft palates and are predisposed to laryngeal obstruction during sedation. An elongated soft palate can occlude the larynx and prevent the passage of air through the mouth. The stenotic nares do not allow sufficient air to pass through the nasal passages (Figure 8-1). When managing a brachycephalic dog under anesthesia, the best course of action is to delay extubation as long as possible. Many anesthetists will extubate brachycephalic dogs only after they can lift their heads by themselves. Allow these patients to recover as fully as possible before pulling the ET tube. Once the ET tube is out, closely monitor the patient for any signs of dyspnea and cyanosis (blue mucous membranes).

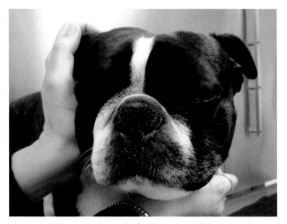

Figure 8-1   Brachycephalic breeds of dogs and cats frequently have nasal openings that are extremely small. Breathing through the nose is difficult. This condition is known as stenotic nares.

POSTOPERATIVE MONITORING

Close monitoring and documentation of vital sign values is usually discontinued after the patient is extubated and placed in the recovery cage. The patient is not completely recovered until all physiologic parameters, including neurologic responses, are normal. The recovery period lasts for hours. Potential complications include airway obstruction, hypotension, thermoregulatory problems (primarily hypothermia), and cardiac arrhythmia. Although patient monitoring may not need to be as frequent, regular monitoring should continue.

The recovery area should be a separate and quiet area in the animal hospital dedicated to anesthetic recovery. The recovery area should be constantly staffed with one or more technicians. The area should be fully stocked with drugs and equipment necessary to handle any emergency. In small hospitals with limited personnel, the recovering patients should be placed in a staffed area where the patient will be observed frequently.

At-risk patients (ASA status III, IV, or V; see Chapter 5) should be monitored closely while recovering. A charting system should be used to help the recovery technicians identify trends and initiate appropriate treatments. The vital signs may be plotted on a graph similar to the anesthesia form, or the vital sign readings may be written in a chart (Figure 8-2).

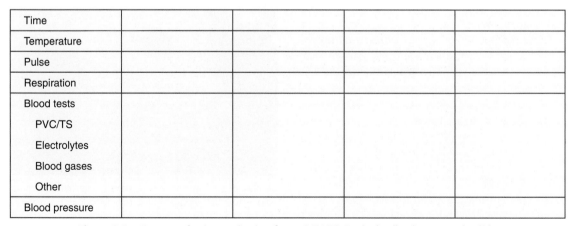

Time				
Temperature				
Pulse				
Respiration				
Blood tests				
PVC/TS				
Electrolytes				
Blood gases				
Other				
Blood pressure				

Figure 8-2   Postanesthesia monitoring form. *PCV/TS,* Packed cell volume, total solids.

COMPLICATIONS RELATED TO ANESTHESIA

Hypothermia

Most patients lose body heat while they are anesthetized. Mild hypothermia, or body temperature no lower than 36° C (about 97° F), is expected and is usually well tolerated by the patient. A body temperature below 34° C (about 93° F) is worrisome and can affect the patient's recovery adversely. As the body temperature decreases, the amount of anesthetic required decreases. The metabolism of the body cells functions best at normal body temperature. As the body temperature drops, normal metabolism slows down, adversely affecting the functioning of all organs of the body. The brain and heart are particularly sensitive to hypothermia.

When body heat loss exceeds heat production, hypothermia results. Causes of hypothermia are related to the effects of anesthesia and the consequences of surgery. Preanesthetic and analgesic drugs can alter the thermoregulatory center in the brain, thus interfering with the maintenance of a constant, optimum body temperature. As the body cools, the anesthetized animal cannot compensate by shivering or seeking a warmer environment. Muscular activity involved with shivering increases body heat. The anesthetized patient is lying still, so body heat production from muscular activity is absent.

All animals undergoing a surgical procedure are at risk of developing hypothermia. Neonates, very lean animals, and geriatric animals are at greatest risk for hypothermia. Numerous procedures are performed on the surgical patient that augment the loss of body heat and include the following:

1. The surgical site is shaved.
2. The surgical site is cleaned with surgical scrub and water followed by alcohol. The evaporation of these cleansing agents quickly cools the skin.
3. The patient may be maintained on gas anesthesia carried by cold oxygen. The source of the oxygen is a compressed oxygen tank. Any gas stored under pressure is cold. The cold gases entering the lungs cool the body.
4. Room-temperature fluids administered intravenously will lower body temperature.
5. A body cavity may be opened, exposing the internal organs to room-temperature air.

Various means to prevent hypothermia during surgery are discussed in Chapter 5. Treatment of hypothermia is discussed below. Many of the treatment measures are similar to the measures used to prevent hypothermia. The hypothermic patient needs to be monitored closely and frequently. Placing pads or blankets with circulating warm water or air under, over, and around the patient is a first step (Figure 8-3). Snuggle Safe discs, sacks of rice or lentils heated in a microwave oven, and warm water bottles or bags can supplement other measures. The patient, including its head, can be placed under a "tent" made by blankets and warming objects. The air under the blankets is warmer than the room air; breathing in the warmed air helps to warm the body. Fluids administered subcutaneously or intravenously should be warmed to approximately 98° to 99° F. The fluid temperature can be tested on the person's wrist, as in testing for the proper temperature of baby formula before feeding. Warming devices for intravenous (IV) fluids are also available.

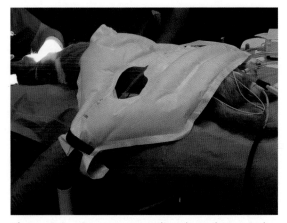

Figure 8-3 Gaymar convection-air patient-warming system blanket is placed over cat recovering from anesthesia. The warm air diffuses around the patient, providing a warm microenvironment.

Water-filled balloons or latex gloves can be used instead of bottles. Expired fluid bags can be heated in a microwave oven and are effective in warming the patient. These are softer than bottles and mold to the contours of the patient's body. Towels or blankets can be warmed in the dryer and then wrapped around the patient with an outer blanket to help trap the heat.

Uncooked rice or lentils can substitute for the water in bottles, balloons, or gloves. The rice-filled containers are placed in a microwave oven for several minutes. The time required depends on the power level used, the oven's wattage, and the size of the bottle or bag. The technician must experiment beforehand to determine the proper heating time needed. These containers tend to remain warmer for a longer time than water bottles. Be careful not to leave plastic containers in the microwave too long; overheating could melt the plastic.

As the warm water bottle cools and its temperature falls below the temperature of the hypothermic patient, the bottle that was warming the patient will now be cooling the patient. Rewarm the water bottles frequently. Also, leaking of the warm water on to the patient is a concern. A wet patient is at risk of becoming a colder patient.

Electric heating pads should not be used. These pads can become too hot for the recumbent patient. Severe thermal burns of the skin may occur. These burns usually do not become evident until several days later. Large areas of skin that were in contact with the electric heating pad may be affected. Significant skin sloughing can be a serious complication.

Emergence Delirium

Occasionally when recovering from general anesthesia, the animal will exhibit signs of excitement, possibly with exaggerated and uncontrollable movements. The patient may thrash around in the cage, cry out, or "paddle" all four legs. This phenomenon is called *emergence delirium* (Figure 8-4).

Emergence delirium occurs for several reasons. During the recovery process the animal will travel back through the stages of anesthesia. Stage II is the "excitement" stage of anesthesia. In some cases the patient passes slowly through stage II and spends several minutes exhibiting signs of excitement. Analgesic and anesthetic side effects contribute to the development of emergence delirium. Opioids are given for their analgesic effects, but these drugs can sensitize the patient to loud auditory stimuli and bright visual stimuli. When stimulated, these patients may be aroused and may exhibit erratic behavior. Dissociative anesthetic agents are known to cause hallucinations in humans, so animals also may undergo hallucinations when given these agents.

If the patient thrashes violently in the cage, problems may arise. The surgical site may undergo severe trauma and possibly dehiscence. The animal may smash its head against the hard side of the cage, causing bruising, scraped skin, and even fractured teeth. Toes can become wedged into the bars of the cage. The patient that is wildly thrashing in the cage may also become hyperthermic, so a body temperature reading should be taken as soon as possible. Howling and screeching may become loud and may disturb other patients, hospital personnel, and clients.

The animal undergoing emergence delirium needs to be approached carefully. This animal is capable of hurting itself as well as the staff. Nevertheless, this patient needs to be calmed down; in some cases, "tincture of time" and holding the animal are sufficient. Some animals benefit from administration of a tranquilizer. Notify the

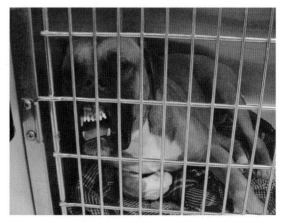

Figure 8-4   Dog exhibiting emergence delirium. Between thrashing in the cage, the dog pressed its nose against the cage door.

veterinarian in charge of the case for a consultation if the animal has injured or may injure itself or if the delirium is lasting several minutes.

Prolonged Recovery

Some animals may take an unexpectedly long time to recover from the anesthesia. Most animals are able to maintain sternal recumbency and lift their head within several minutes after extubation. The patient that is unable to raise its head or be aroused while recovering in its cage is a concern for the recovery room nurse. There are many reasons why a patient may have a prolonged recovery from anesthesia.

Anesthesia-Related Causes
Excessive Depth of Anesthesia
   If the patient was maintained for a long time under anesthesia (>1 hour) and the depth of anesthesia was maintained at a deep level (stage III, plane 3), the patient will have a high concentration of the anesthetic in the body tissues. Gas anesthetics must pass out of the body tissues into the bloodstream and be eliminated by the lungs. A small percentage of the gas anesthetic is metabolized by the liver.
Breed Predisposition
   "Sight hounds" are sensitive to barbiturate anesthetics. In most dogs, barbiturates are redistributed from the vessel-rich tissues of the brain and muscles to the fat stores. Once in the fat stores, the barbiturate slowly reenters the bloodstream and is eventually metabolized in the liver. Sight hounds do not have much fat on their bodies. Therefore, when the muscles become saturated, the barbiturate has no place for storage and is recirculated back to the brain, thus prolonging anesthetic recovery.

Patient-Related Causes
Hypotension, Poor Perfusion, or Shock
   The patient that is in shock or has hypotension is not effectively perfusing the organs and tissues. The anesthetic is therefore not being delivered to the organs that will eliminate it.
Liver or Kidney Disease
   Many anesthetics are metabolized and eliminated through the liver or kidneys. Patients with compromised liver or kidney function will eliminate these anesthetic agents more slowly than patients with healthy organs. Preanesthetic blood tests will help to identify such patients. The dose of anesthetic should then be reduced for these patients, or that anesthetic should not be used.
Intracranial Disease
   Patients with an altered level of consciousness caused by central nervous system (CNS) disease are especially sensitive to the side effects of certain anesthetics. Some anesthetics increase intracranial pressure. Patients with a history of head trauma or seizures may not be able to tolerate anesthetic agents that lower the seizure threshold. In these patients a different anesthetic protocol should be used.
Hypoglycemia
   The neonatal patient is extremely susceptible to developing hypoglycemia. These patients should not be fasted, or only fasted for a few hours before anesthesia. Hypoglycemia will adversely affect the patient's recovery from anesthesia and predispose the patient to seizures.
Hypothermia
   The cells of the body function best at normal body temperature. The cellular enzymes involved in metabolizing anesthetic drugs are less active when the body temperature falls. Bradycardia and subsequent perfusion abnormalities are other consequences associated with hypothermia. If perfusion and circulation are adversely affected, the anesthetic cannot be redistributed to the organs that will eliminate it.

Therapeutic Measures
The patient recovering slowly from anesthesia needs to be assessed by the veterinarian, who may order laboratory tests. Additional nursing care measures may be instituted as well. Close monitoring is important because this is a fragile patient that could develop a life-threatening complication. Several methods can be used to hasten the patient's recovery from anesthesia.
Physical Stimulation
   Physical stimulation by rubbing, massaging, and turning is a simple way to increase the patient's level of consciousness.

Ventilation

The patient that is still intubated can be manually ventilated with pure oxygen. Gas anesthetic agents are mainly eliminated through the lungs. Ventilating the patient with pure oxygen and increasing the frequency of respirations increase the rate at which the gas anesthetic leaves the body.

Fluid Therapy

A bolus of IV fluids can help increase the blood pressure of the hypotensive patient and improve perfusion of internal organs such as the lungs, liver, and kidneys. Warmed fluids can help raise the core body temperature.

Reversal Agents

Some injectable anesthetic agents have reversal agents. Consult with the veterinarian before administering a reversal agent. Giving an opioid antagonist, such as naloxone, will reverse all the effects of the opioid, including its analgesic effects. The loss of analgesic effects could be detrimental to the patient. Doxapram is a respiratory stimulant that helps to arouse the deeply anesthetized patient; it is not a specific reversal agent.

Warming Measures

The hypothermic patient will recover slowly from anesthesia and will benefit from warming measures (see earlier discussion).

Dextrose

Hypoglycemia may be documented through a blood test or may be suspected based on the patient's symptoms and risk factors. Clinically, patients with hypoglycemia may appear disoriented, may gaze blankly off into space, may be slow to respond to noxious stimuli, or may have a prolonged recovery from anesthesia.

Dextrose solution administered intravenously is the preferred treatment. For IV administration of sterile 50% dextrose, dilute 1:1 with sterile water. Administer slowly to patients with marked hypoglycemia at a rate of 1 to 4 ml/kg of body weight over 15 minutes, to effect. The desired effect includes increased awareness and consciousness almost immediately. A constant-rate infusion (CRI) of 2.5% to 5% dextrose solution may be required to maintain blood glucose levels high enough to eliminate signs of hypoglycemia (see Appendix A for instructions).

Beware of administering dextrose orally. Oral administration may lead to aspiration if the gag reflex is diminished or absent. Do not give dextrose by intramuscular (IM) or subcutaneous (SC, SQ) injection. The dextrose solution is hypertonic and will draw fluid into the tissues, and the dextrose will not be efficiently absorbed into the bloodstream.

COMPLICATIONS RELATED TO SURGERY

Hemorrhage

The surgical incision should be routinely inspected during postoperative monitoring. Attend to any bleeding at the surgical site (Figure 8-5). If direct pressure applied to the site for 5 to 10 minutes does not stop the bleeding, apply a bandage if possible, and notify the surgeon. Excessive bleeding at the surgical site that does not stop may indicate that bleeding is also occurring internally.

Internal bleeding can manifest with the following clinical signs: pale mucous membranes, rapid respiratory rate, abdominal bloating, swelling at or around the surgical site, and hypotension, ultimately culminating in hypovolemic shock. An abdominocentesis (abdominal tap, "belly tap") can be performed using a 22-gauge needle and syringe. Collecting frank blood from the

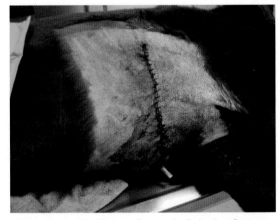

Figure 8-5   Bleeding at the surgical site is often seen when drains are placed. It is important to clean the blood from the surgical site or cover the site with a bandage temporarily. Dogs and cats will be driven to lick at the surgical site covered with blood.

abdominocentesis is a positive diagnosis for internal bleeding into the peritoneal cavity. A thoracocentesis ("chest tap") is performed if internal bleeding is suspected after thoracic surgery.

Excessive postsurgical bleeding occurs for several reasons. The patient may have a coagulation disorder. A surgical ligature around a major vessel may have dislodged. Smaller arteries that were not bleeding intraoperatively because of hypotension may begin to bleed as the patient regains normal blood pressure and the effects of anesthesia wear off.

Coagulation disorders may predispose the patient to hemorrhage. Certain breeds, such as Doberman pinschers, may have a genetic disorder called von Willebrand's disease, which manifests as a blood-clotting problem. Animals with chronic liver disease may have coagulation problems caused by a clotting-factor deficiency. Preanesthetic assessment of animals with chronic liver disease usually includes a coagulation profile. Certain toxins, such as rodenticides, can cause coagulation disorders. Platelet disorders caused by immune-mediated disease (e.g., immune-mediated thrombocytopenia) or infectious disease (e.g., Rocky Mountain spotted fever) will predispose the patient to hemorrhage.

In some cases the surgeon may decide to reanesthetize the patient and "go back in." The patient may need to be surgically explored to find the bleeding vessel or vessels. This patient is at high risk. Fluid therapy should be maintained, and colloid fluids may replace the crystalloid fluids. It is important to be prepared for emergent situations and to work efficiently. An additional venous access site may be needed for administering a blood transfusion or blood component therapy. In general, a "blood transfusion" refers to administering whole blood (fresh or stored) from one patient to another. Depending on how recently the whole blood was collected from the donor and when it is administered to the recipient, it may contain red blood cells (RBCs), white blood cells (WBCs), platelets, plasma proteins, and functional coagulation factors. Blood component therapy involves separating out the parts of whole blood and administering only those parts the patient needs (e.g., plasma, packed RBCs) and that will extend the usefulness of the blood collected from the donor.

The blood pooling in the abdomen or thorax can be aseptically collected, filtered, and readministered to the patient. This procedure is called an *autotransfusion*. If an exogenous source of blood is needed, ideally crossmatched units of blood will be administered. Whole blood will increase the colloid pressure and oxygen delivery to the tissues. Administering blood rich in clotting factors will improve coagulation. Some practices have blood products such as fresh plasma, fresh frozen plasma, and platelet-rich plasma available for administration.

Another manifestation of excessive bleeding is the formation of a hematoma at the surgical site, such as in the scrotal sac after a castration procedure (Figure 8-6). The surgical site may be traumatized if the patient has a difficult recovery (e.g., emergence delirium). Clots covering the cut ends of small subcutaneous blood vessels can dislodge, and blood pools under the skin at the suture site. Initially, a soft, fluctuant swelling is observed. Aspirating the lump with a 22-gauge needle and syringe shows the lump to be filled with blood. The presence of the hematoma will impede the healing process.

The surgeon may order warm, moist compresses applied to the area multiple times daily. The surgeon may choose to suction the blood with a needle and syringe, followed by application of a pressure bandage. Alternatively, a Penrose drain can be surgically placed for continuous drainage.

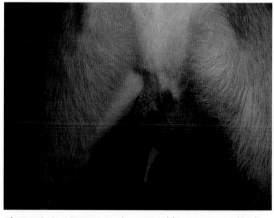

Figure 8-6   Postoperative scrotal hematoma: Bleeding into the scrotal sac has occurred. This picture was taken 18 hours after the castration surgery.

Seroma

A seroma is a collection of tissue fluid in a pocket under the skin that forms at areas of excessive movement. A patient that is overactive postoperatively may develop a seroma at the surgical site, with the skin-layer suture line rubbing against the muscle-layer suture line. The irritation from the scraping of rough sutures causes inflammation. When tissues are inflamed, serum leaks from the capillaries. The serum collects in the potential space between the skin and muscle layers (Figure 8-7). This seroma interferes with the normal healing process. If the serum leaks through the skin suture line, bacteria from the skin may contaminate the serum in the pocket, and an abscess may form.

Seromas appear as a lump at the surgical site. An abscess, hematoma, or hernia can resemble a seroma. Aseptically aspirating the mass with a 22-gauge needle and syringe will allow a differential diagnosis. A straw-colored or light red fluid will be seen if the mass is a seroma. Hematomas are filled with blood. Purulent fluid will fill the syringe when the swelling is caused by an abscess. The syringe will appear empty or will have a small drop of liquefied fat if the lump results from herniation of omentum.

Seromas are treated in a similar manner as hematomas. Small seromas can be managed by warm, moist compresses applied multiple times during the day. The pocket can be drained using a syringe and needle, followed by a pressure bandage. Large seromas will need to be drained surgically (Figure 8-8). Surgical drainage also allows the surgeon to explore the surgical site to ensure that all the muscle-layer sutures are intact.

Dehiscence

Postoperative dehiscence is the premature loss of sutures that allows the surgical site to open. Dehiscence exposes underlying tissues to contamination. Any or all layers of the surgical closure may undergo dehiscence. If a thoracic surgical site dehisces, pneumothorax can follow. Dehiscence can have serious and even fatal consequences.

The animal can cause dehiscence by excessively licking at the surgical site. Infection of the site can also weaken the tissues, and the suture can tear through the skin and muscles. Blunt trauma to the surgical site can cause sutures to rip through healthy tissue. Active playing with other dogs or falls while climbing steps postsurgically can create blunt trauma extensive enough to lead to dehiscence.

Self-Trauma

Self-trauma may be a problem in the postoperative patient. Excessive licking, scratching, or

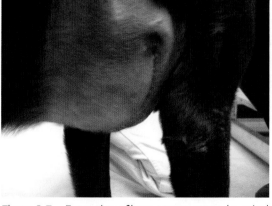

Figure 8-7   Formation of large seroma around surgical site caused by dog scratching at site over 24-hour period.

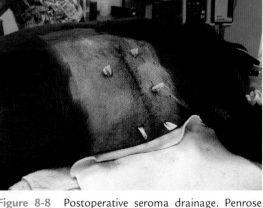

Figure 8-8   Postoperative seroma drainage. Penrose drains were placed on each side of the surgical incision to allow drainage of the seroma fluid.

rubbing of the surgical site will slow the healing process and can lead to dehiscence.

Animals instinctually lick their wounds. Sutures are at risk of being removed by the animal before healing is complete. When licking occurs, bacteria from the mouth can be deposited deep into the surgical incision. The surgical site becomes contaminated, and the animal runs the risk of infection.

Preventive Measures

Prevention of self-trauma is essential. The strategy for keeping the postoperative patient free of self-trauma requires two tactics: (1) preventing the animal from reaching the surgical site and (2) preventing the animal from *wanting* to reach the surgical site.

Block Access to Surgical Site

- *Elizabethan collar.* The flat, plastic "E-collar" is placed around the neck. It is attached to the animal's collar, or a gauze strip is threaded through the collar stays. The plastic shield blocks the patient from licking surgical sites caudal to the neck (Figure 8-9). The animal can still scratch or rub the site. It is important to make sure that the patient can eat and drink with the E-collar. The pet will be awkward and have no peripheral vision while wearing the collar. Do not let the pet loose outside while wearing an E-collar. Expect the pet to knock things over and collide with door frames.

- *Bite Not collar.* While fitted with this brand-name device, the patient is unable to bend its neck to reach any part of its body and lick. As with an E-collar, the pet wearing the Bite Not collar can still scratch or rub at the site.

- *Bandaging the area.* A bandage may be enough to block the patient from licking the area. Surgical sites are not always in areas that can be easily bandaged. A pet may find a way to remove the bandage or may even eat the bandage. Thus it is essential that the bandage be monitored closely for signs of slipping or wetness, and for tooth marks (Figure 8-10).

- *Basket muzzle.* A dog can be fitted with a basket muzzle, which prevents the patient from chewing at the site. The dog may rub the site with the muzzle and may also be able to lick. However, this type of muzzle may act as an effective psychological barrier.

- *Hobbles.* Taping the hind legs together can prevent the patient from scratching at the surgical site (see Figure 8-10).

Block Desire to Reach Surgical Site

- *Foul-tasting product applied around the site.* Bitter-apple liquid and Yuk ointment are examples

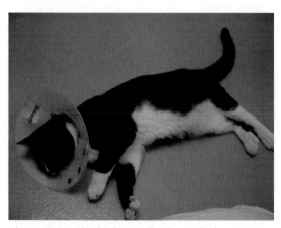

Figure 8-9 Elizabethan collar is applied to prevent licking and chewing on a drain.

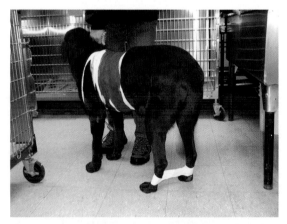

Figure 8-10 This pet had a bandage applied that encircled the chest. The bandage covered Penrose drains that had been placed to drain a seroma. The bandage also helped to keep the dog clean during the first 12 hours postoperatively. The hind legs are taped together ("hobbled") to prevent scratching at the chest area with the rear paws.

of bitter-tasting applications that can be placed on the skin around the surgical site. The foul taste may deter the patient from licking the area.

- *Sedation.* "Chemical restraint" can be very effective. Chronic tranquilization during the recuperative period may be necessary to prevent licking as well as overactivity.

- *Stainless steel suture or staples.* The surgeon may anticipate a problem with licking and elect to place staples in the skin rather than close with sutures. Stainless steel sutures prick the tongue when licked. Staples can withstand more licking than sutures or tissue adhesive ("skin glue").

Infection

When the surgical site becomes infected, healing is delayed. The patient is in pain and may have a fever. The surgical site is swollen, red, and draining, and the sutures are at risk of falling out.

Surgical debridement and resuturing may be necessary. Some animals may have an allergic reaction to the absorbable sutures that has the appearance of an infected wound. The surgeon will cut away the dead tissue and suture healthy tissue together using less reactive suture material. The patient will most likely receive systemic antibiotic therapy. Warm, moist compresses and cleaning the site with dilute antiseptic solution also may be prescribed.

POSTOPERATIVE NURSING CARE

Successful wound healing depends on minimal microbial contamination of the wound. Invasion by microbes into the wound is unavoidable, but large numbers of opportunistic microbes must not be allowed to overwhelm the patient's immune system. Bacterial numbers within a wound can be minimized through attentive wound care. In addition, preventing the animal's access to the wound diminishes ongoing trauma and contamination to the wound through contact with bacteria-laden saliva.

Wound Cleansing

Surgical site preparation, sterile gloving, sterile draping, use of sterile instruments, and adherence to aseptic technique all minimize initial contamination of the surgical wound. Circumstances such as immunosuppressed patient status, self-mutilation, or unavoidable intraoperative contamination can render the surgical wound contaminated. Cleansing of contaminated wounds will facilitate healing. Whether caused by surgery or trauma, contaminated wounds are cleansed of debris and protected from microorganisms through numerous means, including debridement, lavage, dressings, and antimicrobial agents.

Debridement

Debridement (also débridement) is the removal of adhered debris and dead tissue from the wound. *Surgical debridement* is the cutting away of dead tissue from the living tissue until fresh bleeding edges are exposed. After the area is debrided, the fresh skin edges are sutured together. Usually, surgical debridement is performed under anesthesia. General anesthesia is used if the animal is stable and the involved area is large. Local anesthesia is often administered with debilitated animals and smaller wounds (see anesthesia texts for specific techniques).

During the early phase of wound healing, debridement may need to occur. The primary layer of bandage material can provide a means of debridement. Dry mesh gauze directly applied to an open wound with embedded foreign material or necrotic tissue is called a *dry-to-dry bandage*. Removal of the dry-to-dry bandage can be painful.

Mechanical debridement can also be accomplished on a daily basis through the use of wet-to-dry bandaging techniques. The *wet-to-dry bandage* is used with open wounds that have embedded foreign material, devitalized tissue, and viscous exudates. A primary layer of sterile, saline-soaked gauze sponges is applied directly to the wound. A secondary layer of dry gauze sponges and rolled-cotton batting is layered onto the primary layer and then secured to the animal with rolled gauze and tape. The dressing is changed two or three times daily. When the primary layer is removed, the foreign matter and necrotic debris is dried to the gauze and thus pulled off the wound. As with dry-to-dry bandaging, the patient may need to be sedated for bandage changes because this procedure tends to be painful.

Wet-to-dry and wet-to-wet bandages have the disadvantage of possible bacterial growth in the bandage. A moist environment at the wound surface dilutes the viscous exudates, which allows the secondary layer to absorb the fluid more readily.

Enzymatic preparations of trypsin or chymotrypsin can be applied to wounds to digest and remove necrotic tissue. This technique is indicated when (1) further surgical debridement may damage important nerves and blood vessels, (2) deeper fistulas exist, or (3) the patient is a poor anesthetic risk.

Lavage

Lavage is the procedure of forceful rinsing of a wound (Figure 8-11). Anesthesia may be necessary if the patient is in pain and struggles. Thorough lavage will flush out foreign debris, purulent fluid, and microorganisms from a wound. The goal of a successful lavage is to reduce the number of microorganisms in the wound to a level that the immune system can handle.

Solutions used to lavage external wounds include tap water, sterile saline, lactated Ringer's,

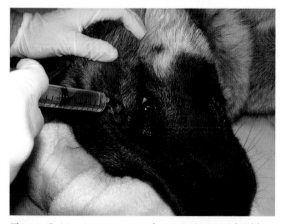

Figure 8-11   Lavage procedure. Syringe with dilute chlorhexidine solution (1:40 dilution) is flushed around the wound to rinse debris and blood from the area.

diluted chlorhexidine, and diluted povidone-iodine. Although tap water is not sterile, it is still a safe and effective lavaging agent for external wounds that do not penetrate a body cavity (thorax or abdomen) or joint. Two percent chlorhexidine solution is diluted 1:40 with water to make a 0.05% concentrated solution for lavage. Povidone-iodine (10% stock solution) is diluted 1:10. These diluted solutions should be prepared fresh daily; their potency diminishes with time.

Wound Dressings

Wound dressings are categorized as two types: semi-occlusive and occlusive. Wound dressings are the contact, or primary, layer of a bandage. *Semi-occlusive* dressings include the wet-to-dry dressings used to debride wounds mechanically. Cotton and polyester gauze pads, petroleum jelly–coated gauze pads, antibiotic ointment–coated polyethylene glycol sponges, and polyurethane foam sponges are examples of nonadherent, semi-occlusive dressings. Semi-occlusive dressings allow excess fluid to be absorbed by the secondary layer.

Occlusive wound dressings are impermeable to air and produce a moist environment that facilitates wound healing. These dressings are used in the later stages of wound healing when the bandage needs less frequent changing. Examples of occlusive dressings are natural cellulose and gelatin, as well as polyethylene polymers attached to a synthetic film. These occlusive wound dressings do not adhere to the wound.

Antimicrobial Agents

Antimicrobial agents may be applied topically to superficial wounds. However, the use of antimicrobial agents is not a substitute for appropriate and careful debridement and lavage. Dispensing these antimicrobial agents from large multidosing tubs may create problems unless aseptic technique is used when retrieving the contents from the container. Large multi-use tubs of antimicrobial agents may be a source of patient-to-patient contamination. Topical treatment is discontinued once granulation tissue appears in the wound.

Bandages, Splints, Casts, and Slings

Bandages, splints, casts, and slings are frequently applied after surgical procedures or trauma to a limb. The purposes of these applications are to protect wounds, speed the healing process, and immobilize the extremities. Immobilization helps the patient by decreasing pain and facilitates healing by securing bone fragments and soft tissue pieces close together to allow healing.

Bandages have three basic layers: primary (contact) layer, secondary (padded) layer, and tertiary (outer) layer. The *primary layer* is in contact with the wound. This contact layer may adhere to the open wound or may be nonadherent. Adherent materials such as cotton gauze are usually applied early in the healing process and allow debridement when the bandage is changed. Nonadherent dressings are used later in the healing process or to cover wounds closed by sutures.

The *secondary layer* secures the contact layer to the wound and provides an absorptive layer for blood, serum, and purulent fluid. This padded layer also provides support to the extremity. It applies pressure to the wound, thus compressing any dead space and preventing hemorrhage. Rolled cotton, synthetic polyester batting, multilayer absorbent pads, or cast padding may be used. Rolled gauze is used to hold the layer in place, with pressure applied to compress the padding underneath. It is important not to use too much pressure and occlude the blood supply to the extremity. Mastering the technique of applying the proper pressure and placing a comfortable, supporting bandage on a patient requires practice. Thus an experienced technician or veterinarian should supervise the first few bandage wrappings attempted by personnel.

When a bandage, cast, or sling is applied immediately after trauma to an extremity, swelling of the limb is expected. When the limb is confined by such a stabilizing measure, swelling may result in cessation of blood flow to the extremity. Toes can be left exposed at the distal end of the bandage or cast to monitor the amount of swelling under the bandage. The nails of the two middle toes should be only a few millimeters apart. If the nails are farther apart, the toes are swollen. If the toes look swollen, the bandage should be removed immediately.

The tertiary layer of the bandage is made of porous adhesive tape or elasticized tape (e.g., Vetrap, Elastikon). This layer provides protection to the secondary layer. If this outer layer becomes wet, either from moisture on the outside (e.g., soiled by rainwater) or seepage from the inside, the entire bandage must be changed immediately.

It is important to keep these bandages intact, secure (no slipping down the leg), and dry. The animal may try to remove the wrappings by gnawing, violently shaking the extremity, or prying off the bandage. After several days, stretching of the outer layer and compression of the inner padding will loosen the bandage, which may slip or shift position. Also, the skin adjacent to the edges of the bandage, sling, splint, or cast may become abraded. Wetness, staining, and odor may also be noted. If any of these problems occurs, the bandage, cast, or splint should be changed.

Drains

A drain is a surgically placed implant that is temporarily affixed in the wound. The drain provides a channel through which unwanted fluid or gas may leave the wound. When surgery or other trauma to the skin disrupts the hypodermis, the skin may no longer adhere to the underlying fascia. This creates a potential space that the body will try to fill with tissue fluid. Healing will occur most rapidly if the fluid is evacuated. Drawing the fluid out through a needle is only effective temporarily. Continuous drainage needs to be provided.

The two basic categories of drains are passive and active. *Passive drains* use gravity and overflow gradients to evacuate the fluid or gas. *Active drains* create negative-pressure gradients to the area and suck the fluid and gas from the wound.

Passive drains are typically made of soft, pliable latex tubing. Red rubber tubes and silicon tubes are stiff, less compliant, and potentially more irritating. "Teat cannulas," originally made to drain purulent fluid from infected mammary glands in cows, are also used to drain

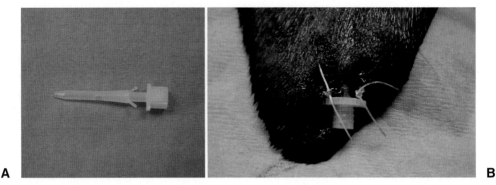

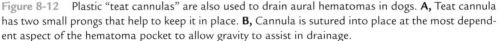

A   **B**

Figure 8-12   Plastic "teat cannulas" are also used to drain aural hematomas in dogs. **A,** Teat cannula has two small prongs that help to keep it in place. **B,** Cannula is sutured into place at the most dependent aspect of the hematoma pocket to allow gravity to assist in drainage.

aural hematomas in dogs. Teat cannulas are made of polyethylene plastic and are quite hard (Figure 8-12).

The passive drain exits the skin at the most ventral (gravity-dependent) spot possible. The drain does not exit from the primary surgical incision. A small stab incision is made through the skin adjacent to the surgical incision. The drain is secured to the skin by one or two sutures. The opposite end of the drain may remain buried below the skin or may exit at the opposite end of the wound. Whether the end of the drain is buried or exits to the surface, a suture secures the end of the drain (Figure 8-13).

The active drain is usually made out of Silastic, red rubber, polyethylene, or polypropylene plastic. The drain is fenestrated (has holes) in multiple places. The fenestrated section of the drain is placed in the area that requires draining. Many commercial suction devices are available. Attaching a syringe to the tube can make a simple, homemade suction device. The plunger of the syringe is pulled back and secured by a pin placed through a predrilled hole in the plunger's shaft to hold the plunger in place.

All drains must be kept clean. Dried fluid will accumulate around the drain where it exits the skin. Place a warm, moist cloth over the drain to loosen the dried material. The cloth is soaked in a bowl of water or dilute solution of an antiseptic such as chlorhexidine (1:40 dilution). This procedure

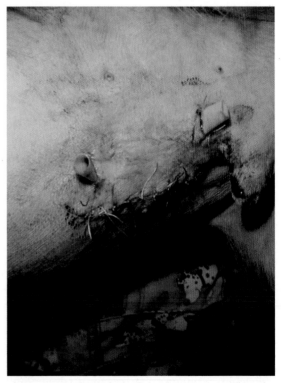

Figure 8-13   Each end of the drain is sutured to the skin to keep it in place.

may need to be repeated several times daily. The skin surrounding the drain may become raw and irritated from contact with the serous or purulent fluid. Petrolatum-based ointments applied to the skin can facilitate cleaning and protect the skin from further damage.

The veterinary surgeon will determine the best time to remove the drain. Usually, the drain is removed 3 to 5 days after surgery. Any dried fluid is cleaned out, and all sutures securing the drain are cut. The drain is firmly grasped and pulled out with one swift motion. If the proximal end of the drain is not buried, one end is freed and pulled as much as possible from the incision and cut. The opposite end is then freed and the remainder of the drain removed.

If the patient has removed the drain prematurely, ask the owner to bring the drain in for inspection. It is import to determine that the pet has removed the entire drain. A piece of drain left under the skin will fester. The immune system will treat the piece of drain as a foreign invader, surrounding it with fluid and inflammatory cells. This drain piece will need to be surgically removed.

Intravenous Catheter Maintenance

Intravenous catheters are placed and maintained for extended periods in some surgical patients. Common veins used for *peripheral* catheter placement include the left and right cephalic, left and right lateral saphenous (dogs), and left and right medial saphenous (cats). The left and right jugular veins are generally used for *central* catheters. Central catheters ("central lines") allow the technician to measure central venous pressures and collect blood samples for frequent blood glucose checks without a separate venipuncture for each sample collected.

All IV catheters provide direct access to the patient's vascular system, and therefore all catheters should be placed using aseptic technique. (See Chapter 1 for more information on IV catheterization techniques.) All connections among the catheter, connector sets, and IV lines need to be left untaped but securely connected to each other. Access to these connections must be available at all times without untaping the connections. The patient will often attempt to pull or chew out the catheter. Sufficient taping and restraint devices (e.g., E-collar) can prevent many

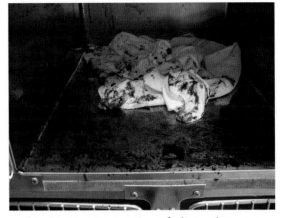

Figure 8-14   Consequence of a lost catheter cap.

problems. Figure 8-14 shows a cage that was occupied by a cat that pulled off the catheter cap (catheter remained intact).

Most types of IV catheters require replacement every 3 days (72 hours) with a new catheter placed in a different vein. The old catheter is removed only after the new catheter is secured in place. If no continuous infusion is being administered through the catheter, the catheter is flushed with 1 to 5 ml of heparinized saline every 6 to 8 hours. This procedure helps to ensure that the catheter remains patent the entire 72 hours. Bandages securing catheters in place should be changed if they become soiled with vomitus or other contaminants.

Each time the catheter is flushed, the leg and all connections should be checked. If the tape is soiled, it should be retaped. If swelling is noted in the paw, the tape may be wrapped too tightly, and it should be replaced. If swelling is noted proximal to the catheter, the catheter may be perivascular (not in the vein). If the catheter bandage is soaked, the entire catheter should be replaced at a different site. The old catheter site is covered for a few minutes with a piece of gauze. A spot of antibiotic ointment can be applied to the gauze, which is secured by adhesive tape.

When administering medication through the catheter, check for patency using a heparinized saline flush. After administering the medication, the catheter is flushed again with heparinized saline.

Blood samples are often collected through the IV catheter, but the clinician must keep in mind that residues from medications administered through the catheter could interfere with test results.

Urinary Catheter Maintenance

Patients recovering from back surgery, urinary tract surgery, and orthopedic procedures may have a urinary catheter in place. The urinary catheter helps to ensure urethral patency, allows for quantification of urine production, and helps to keep the patient clean.

The catheter is placed aseptically. The distal end is secured to the patient with tape and sutures. An empty, sterile IV fluid bag and administration set are connected to the distal end of the catheter. The bag is suspended below the level of the bladder for urine flow by gravity.

It is important to check the patency of the urine collection system regularly. The tubing may become kinked. As the patient turns in the cage, the collection tubing may become twisted and cause the tube's lumen to collapse. The collection tube can be pinched in the cage door as it is closed. Blood clots can be passed and form obstructions in the tubing. The catheter and tubing should be checked for leaks. Often the patient will attempt to pull out the catheter, and tooth marks may be detected. Leaking systems are replaced, and the patient is fitted with an Elizabethan collar to prevent further problems.

Physical Therapy

Physical therapy techniques can benefit most patients. Immobility resulting from sickness, trauma, or surgical procedures can complicate recuperation. Physical therapy techniques enhance patient comfort, prevent complications from disuse, and hasten healing. The success of many orthopedic procedures rests on the rehabilitation of the patient. Veterinarians, veterinary technicians, and owners can perform many physical rehabilitation techniques to improve surgical outcomes and ensure client satisfaction. Some states have limited the practice of physical therapy on animals to licensed physical therapists.

Therefore, many veterinarians prefer to use the term "physical rehabilitation" when referring to the following techniques.

Massage, application of heat or cold, bandaging, range of motion (ROM) exercises, and physical exercise are all therapeutic techniques that may be prescribed. Under the supervision of the attending veterinarian, the veterinary technician or owner may perform the techniques with the patient. Detailed descriptions of these techniques are found in other texts and articles; this section briefly describes the various types of physical therapy that may be used postoperatively.

In the first 72 hours after surgery, opioid analgesics, anti-inflammatory drugs, passive ROM exercises, and cryotherapy are used to decrease pain, prevent edema formation, and gradually improve range of motion. Pain management is discussed later. *Cryotherapy* is the application of cold, such as ice packs wrapped in a towel, to the affected limb. The packs can be affixed to the limb using elastic wraps. The cold packs are applied for up to 30 minutes two to four times a day. The cold causes vasoconstriction, which decreases blood flow and limits edema formation. The cold temperature of the tissue also reduces nerve conduction, producing analgesia.

Passive ROM exercises are exercises that support a joint while moving it to the extent of its limitations (Figure 8-15). The best time to perform passive ROM exercises is shortly after administration

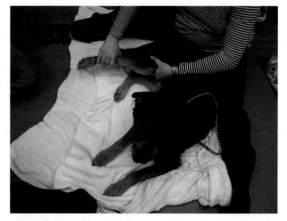

Figure 8-15   Physical therapist demonstrating passive range of motion movements.

of analgesic drugs. This procedure should be performed slowly with the muscles relaxed. While supporting the limb, slowly and gently flex and extend each joint one at a time, taking care to keep all the joints in the working extremity in their normal anatomic alignment throughout the exercise. Flex and extend each joint only to the extent that the joint just begins to resist the degree of flexion or extension applied to it. Passive ROM helps to prevent contracture, improve blood and lymph flow, maintain normal range of joint movement, and stimulate sensory awareness. Ten to 15 repetitions should be performed two or three times daily. Treat every joint of the affected limb, starting with the joint distal to the injury or surgical site.

Between 3 and 5 days after surgery, other physical therapy procedures may be added. Cryotherapy is replaced with *thermotherapy*. Warm, moist heat is applied to the injured area. The heat will cause vasodilation, increase local circulation, and provide mild pain relief. Thermotherapy should be applied for 10 to 20 minutes before passive ROM, massage, or exercise. *Massage therapy* relaxes muscles, breaks down adhesions, improves blood and lymph flow, and relieves pain. The massage session starts with *gently* running the hands over the surface of the animal's skin (effleurage, frottage). The stroking movements should start distally and move proximally. The second massage method kneads the muscles in small circles using the pads of the fingers (not the fingertips) or the heel of the hand with a gradual increase in pressure (petrissage, pétrissage). The massage session lasts about 20 minutes and is done every 24 to 48 hours (Figure 8-16).

Exercise that elevates the heart rate and increases muscle tone can be initiated about 2 weeks after surgery. Initial exercise is assisted by slings and harnesses. Swimming is also a good initial exercise; the buoyancy of the water helps to support the patient. This low-impact exercise is replaced in a few weeks with unassisted exercise, such as leash walks. As the patient's stamina increases, the length of time spent exercising also increases.

Although physical therapy has many benefits, contraindications do exist. Massage should not be performed over open wounds, infected areas, or malignant tumors. Animals with thromboembolic disease and those receiving anticoagulants should not be massaged. Cryotherapy is avoided in patients with ischemic injury, diabetes mellitus, vasculitis, or indolent pressure sores. ROM procedures should not be performed on nonstabilized legs after a severe orthopedic injury (e.g., fracture, ligament rupture). Bandaging to prevent or reduce edema needs to be performed carefully to prevent vascular compromise of the limb. Exercise regimens and active ROM procedures must start slowly and increase gradually in length and frequency.

Nutritional Support

All animals recuperating from surgery and serious illness need to maintain a good plane of nutrition. Wound healing will not proceed smoothly if nutrients are not available. Voluntary food intake may not fulfill the caloric requirements for prompt healing. Additional intake may be accomplished through force-feeding, pharmacologic appetite stimulants, and tube feedings.

Force-feeding is best accomplished with pureed or liquid diets. The food may be smeared on the animal's lips to initiate licking and cleaning. A lump of food may be applied to the roof of the mouth. A liquid diet may be squirted through a syringe into the cheek pouch. Force-feeding is

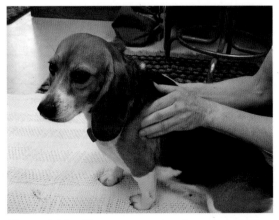

Figure 8-16   Massage can relax the pet as well as increase blood and lymph flow, relieve pain, and break down adhesions.

a labor-intensive and time-consuming process and frequently falls short of the required caloric goal. The animal often fights the feedings and may become stressed. Aspiration of the food in the mouth during the struggling is a major concern. If the patient does not start to eat sufficiently on its own within 1 or 2 days, a different approach should be considered.

Several pharmacologic agents are thought to increase the appetite of dogs and cats. The benzodiazepine tranquilizer *diazepam* has been shown to stimulate the appetite of cats. An IV injection will generally induce the cat immediately to eat food within reach. *Cyproheptadine* is a serotonin antagonist that stimulates the appetite of both dogs and cats. Corticosteroids and progestational steroids (e.g., megestrol) work well in humans but are seldom used in dogs and cats because of potential adverse side effects, such as diabetes mellitus, immunosuppression, and delayed healing.

Acupuncture also may stimulate a surgical patient's appetite postoperatively, in addition to providing some pain relief. A veterinary acupuncturist should be consulted for these cases.

The amount of food that the patient will need per day is calculated in the following way:

$$\text{Daily energy requirement} = 70(\text{Body weight in kg})^{0.75}$$

$$\text{Food quantity} = \frac{\text{Daily energy requirement}}{\text{Caloric density of food}}$$

Tube feeding may be necessary to meet nutritional needs. Neonatal animals adapt well to repeated orogastric tubing. Juvenile and adult animals deal better with the placement of a semipermanent, indwelling feeding tube. The feeding tube may be placed through the nose, pharynx, or esophagus. A tube placed through the abdominal wall into the stomach is known as a *gastric tube* and is the easiest of all feeding tubes to maintain.

Using an indwelling feeding tube is convenient and less time-consuming than force-feeding, but these indwelling tubes can develop problems. The tube that passes down the esophagus may irritate the stomach wall and initiate vomiting. The tube can come out the mouth, and the patient may chew through it. An improperly positioned

pharyngostomy tube may interfere with the epiglottis, preventing complete closure of the larynx. A nasogastric tube must be very small in diameter and therefore can easily become obstructed. The nasogastric tube can cause nosebleeds, sneezing, and inflammation of the nasal passage with mucous discharge. Premature removal of the tube by the patient is a complication inherent in all types of feeding tubes.

The pureed or liquid diet may be homemade or commercially purchased. When the tube feedings are initiated, the amounts should be small (2-10 ml depending on animal's size) and administered frequently (about every 2 hours). Use of a gastric tube should be postponed for 24 hours after it is placed to allow a seal to form internally between the visceral and the parietal peritoneum. Vomiting occurs most frequently in the first or second day. Once the feedings are tolerated, larger amounts and less frequent feedings can be done. The food is slowly injected through the tube to allow the stomach to accommodate gradually to the presence of the food. After injecting the food, water is slowly injected to rinse the inside of the tube. The tube is closed using an adapter plug or syringe. The end of the feeding tube is secured with tape to the bandage covering the tube's exit from the skin. The exception is the nasogastric tube, which is secured to the bridge of the nose and forehead by sutures.

POSTOPERATIVE ANALGESIA

The ease and success of managing postoperative pain are directly related to preoperative analgesia. That is, the more successful the attempts to preempt surgical pain, the easier it is to control postoperative pain with minimal additional analgesics. Assuming adequate preemptive analgesia, the overall goal of postoperative pain management should be to maintain the analgesic plane achieved throughout surgery.

The patient should recover quietly and calmly without displays of overt signs of pain (e.g., vocalization, excessive movement, abnormal body posturing). At no time should the patient be required to return to a painful state and "request" additional analgesics during the immediate postoperative period. Some patients will experience pain that persists or develops despite adequate doses of analgesics and must be treated with additional analgesia or analgesic techniques. This type of pain is termed *breakthrough pain* because it has "broken through" the usual analgesic barriers.

Postoperative pain management also includes medications dispensed for home use. This is a service and level of care that veterinary medicine has not sufficiently advocated, until recently. Now, with veterinarians' increased awareness of the options available for take-home pain medication and the benefits to the patient, effective pain management can continue throughout the at-home recovery period.

Common Analgesic Classes

The two classes of analgesia most often used postoperatively are opioids and nonsteroidal anti-inflammatory drugs (NSAIDs). These two classes of agents can be used individually, but the drugs may be most efficacious when used in combination with each other. Postsurgical pain should be managed aggressively for 24 hours up to a full week or more, depending on severity of pain. In general, experts agree that most patients with soft tissue elective surgery should receive opioids for 24 hours and NSAIDs for 3 to 4 days postoperatively. Patients that have emergency or nonroutine soft tissue surgeries (e.g., thoracotomy, gastric dilatation-volvulus repair) may be managed initially with opioids alone until their cardiovascular health is restored. A major concern is the effect of opioids on gastrointestinal (GI) motility. Although morphine may slow GI motility, the benefit of opioids outweighs the risk of altered GI function, because stress and pain are likely to play a larger role in decreasing GI motility than short-term postoperative opioid administration. Patients with severe GI disease may benefit from the addition of a constant-rate infusion (CRI) of lidocaine for systemic analgesia, provided the patient does not have cardiovascular disease (see Chapter 5 and Appendix A).

Patients may also benefit from postoperative local anesthetics, such as bupivacaine, which can be instilled through indwelling chest tubes or by soaker catheter.

Patients undergoing orthopedic procedures will benefit from 24 to 72 hours of postoperative opioids and NSAIDs for at least 1 week. The exact type of opioid is matched to the expected level of pain (see Chapter 1). Appendix A provides specific protocols for postoperative pain management, including take-home medications.

"Wind-Up"

Patients who do not respond satisfactorily to maximum dose and frequency of opioids and require additional analgesia may have experienced the phenomenon known as "wind-up." In this condition the spinal cord has become hypersensitized to incoming pain signals as a result of constant bombardment. Once hypersensitization occurs, traditional analgesia may no longer be adequate. There are several effective techniques for managing wind-up, including CRI of morphine, ketamine, or lidocaine. Ketamine blocks sensitization of neurons in the spinal cord, essentially "unwinding" it, and may allow the patient to become responsive to usual dosing regimens, as described earlier.

"Take-Home" Analgesia

Nonsteroidal Anti-Inflammatory Drugs
The availability of veterinary NSAIDs has greatly improved outpatient pain management. These relatively inexpensive analgesics provide long-lasting perioperative and chronic pain relief in convenient oral formulations. Once-daily administration tends to improve owner compliance. NSAIDs will provide adequate pain relief to many patients during the at-home recovery period, especially if therapy was instituted preoperatively. Some patients require additional take-home medications, most often opioids.

Opioids
Several oral opioids are available for take-home use; however, because of the potential for human abuse of these controlled drugs, care must be taken in prescribing this type of drug. Sustained-release

morphine is available and can be used in dogs, but morphine is difficult to obtain in sufficiently small doses to administer safely to cats. Based on research at the University of Florida, *buprenorphine* can be safely and efficaciously administered to cats by the transbuccal (sublingual) route. Small, single-dose aliquots can be prepared for administration by owners at home. The opioid *fentanyl* is available in a transdermal patch (Duragesic, Janssen Pharmaceuticals), which can be applied in the hospital to provide up to 3 days of postoperative analgesia for hospitalized as well as discharged patients.

Butorphanol tablets are not recommended for take-home analgesia because of butorphanol's extremely short duration of action.

The synthetic opioid *tramadol* is available in tablet form. Tramadol is gaining popularity for long-term use in dogs and cats as an effective non-scheduled take-home analgesic. Tramadol can be used as an adjunct to NSAIDs for the treatment of moderate to severe pain. Optimum dosages and dose schedules are being determined. Oral dosages of 4 mg/kg two or three times daily in the dog and 2 mg/kg twice daily in the cat are currently being used with apparent success.

KEY POINTS

1. When monitoring recovery of a patient intubated with an endotracheal (ET) tube, the technician must be prepared for the animal to awaken quickly. The ET tube is untied from the head or muzzle. All limbs should be untied and the patient placed in lateral recumbency. A syringe is at hand if needed to deflate the ET tube cuff. The technician should *never* leave the patient unattended on the table, and it is best to have a hand on the patient at all times.

2. The ET tube cuff should not be deflated until the patient has regained the ability to swallow.

3. The patient that is a moderate to high anesthetic risk (ASA status III, IV, or V) should be closely monitored (every 5 minutes) until fully recovered.

4. Extubation of brachycephalic breeds should be delayed until the patient can raise its head without assistance.

5. When the body temperature is below 97° F, immediate and active measures should be taken to warm the patient. Additional postoperative opioid analgesics should not be given until the patient's temperature is above 98° F.

6. When treating an animal for hypothermia, do not assume the measures are successful. Monitor the patient's body temperature, and confirm that the body temperature is rising.

7. A patient thrashing in a cage during recovery must be protected from injury, but the staff should ensure the animal does not cause injury to others.

8. The technician who thinks a patient is not recovering as expected should notify the attending veterinarian. The cause of the delayed recovery needs to be identified and corrected.

9. Attention to the surgical wound is an important part of the recovery process. Any change in the wound's condition should be reported immediately to the surgeon.

10. Debridement and lavage are important steps in the wound-cleansing process.

11. Bandages, casts, splints, and slings must be monitored closely for displacement, patient mutilation, wetness, and odor.

12. Drains must be kept clean so that drainage can continue as long as needed and the skin around the exit wound for the drain does not become irritated by the draining fluid.

13. Indwelling IV and urinary catheters need regular inspections to ensure that they are functional and have not been disturbed by the patient.

14. Physical therapy techniques used during the recuperative period can greatly improve patient outcome and enhance client satisfaction.

15. A patient that will not eat will not heal quickly and is predisposed to developing complications.

16. Providing adequate preoperative analgesia ("preemptive analgesia") makes it easier to achieve successful postoperative pain management.

17. Postoperative pain management should continue at home. Oral analgesics and transdermal analgesic patches can provide continued pain relief after the patient leaves the veterinary hospital.

18. The best pain relief is achieved by combining different classes of analgesics that block or prevent pain by different mechanisms of action. Postoperatively, these typically include oral opioids and NSAIDs.

REVIEW QUESTIONS

1. When does the postoperative recovery period begin for the surgical patient?
   a. As soon as the surgeon begins closing the incision.
   b. On discontinuation of anesthesia.
   c. On regaining full mental capacity.
   d. On return of normal vital signs (temperature, pulse, respiration) and consciousness.
   e. None of the above.

2. At what point should the endotracheal tube's cuff be deflated in preparation for extubation?
   a. As soon as the gas anesthetic is discontinued.
   b. As soon as the ties keeping the tube in place are untied.
   c. When the patient regains the ability to swallow (except for brachycephalic breeds).
   d. On discontinuation of oxygen.
   e. Before moving the patient off the surgery table.

3. *True* or *False:* Brachycephalic breeds should have the endotracheal tube removed at the first sign of return of the ability to swallow.

4. *True* or *False:* Brachycephalic breeds should be extubated only after they can lift their heads by themselves.

5. *True* or *False:* Once the patient is extubated, the anesthetist can relax because all risks associated with anesthesia immediately cease on extubation.

6. *True* or *False:* All animals that undergo an anesthetic/surgical procedure are at risk for hypothermia.

7. What phrase is used to describe the excitement and exaggerated and uncontrollable movements some patients exhibit during the recovery phase of anesthesia?
   a. Drug-induced dysphoria.
   b. Endorphin euphoria.
   c. Emergence delirium.
   d. Reverse induction.
   e. None of the above.

8. Which of the following can contribute to a prolonged recovery from anesthesia?
   a. Hypoglycemia.
   b. Liver disease.
   c. Kidney disease.
   d. All of the above.
   e. Both b and c.

9. Which of the following can hasten a patient's recovery from anesthesia?
   a. Physical stimulation.
   b. Oxygen supplementation with or without manual ventilation.
   c. Warming measures.
   d. Reversal agents.
   e. All of the above.

10. Which of the following postoperative complications involves premature suture loss and surgical site opening?
    a. Dehiscence.
    b. Hemorrhage.
    c. Seroma.
    d. Hematoma.
    e. Both c and d.

11. Debridement is:
    a. The process of removing dead tissue and debris from a wound.
    b. The name given to a divorce caused by a household of too many dogs.
    c. A way to check for a fluid wave in the abdomen of animals with suspected ascites or hemoabdomen.
    d. Necessary in all cases of neoplastic surgery.
    e. None of the above.

12. Topical antimicrobial medications are usually:
    a. Not used on wounds.
    b. Discontinued once granulation tissue appears in the wound.
    c. Only used once granulation tissue appears in a wound.
    d. Only applied to anesthetized patients with wounds.
    e. None of the above.

13. Which of the following statements is *true*?
    a. Bandages, splints, and casts are used to immobilize bones and joints.
    b. Immobilization helps decrease pain associated with fractures.
    c. Immobilization facilitates healing by securing bone fragments close together.
    d. All of the above.
    e. None of the above.

14. With a bandaged limb, leaving the toes exposed:
    a. Is useful to monitor the amount of swelling that may occur under the bandage.
    b. Is an example of a poorly placed bandage.
    c. Allows the animal's caregiver to compare the toes on the bandaged limb to the toes on the other limb.
    d. Both a and c.
    e. None of the above.
15. Which of the following statements regarding drains is *true*?
    a. Drain are usually removed 3 to 5 days after surgery.
    b. Petrolatum-based ointments applied to the skin around the drain's exit site helps prevent exudates from accumulating and clogging the drain's exit site.
    c. All types of drains have hollow lumens to allow for the fluid to drain out of the wound through this lumen.
    d. All of the above.
    e. Both a and b.
16. Which of the following statements regarding urinary catheters is *true*?
    a. Catheters help to ensure urethral patency.
    b. Catheters allow measurement of urine production, which reflects the condition of the kidneys.
    c. Urinary catheters help to keep the patient clean and dry.
    d. Both a and c.
    e. All of the above.
17. *True* or *False:* Physical therapy should be performed shortly after analgesics have been administered to the surgical patient.
18. *True* or *False:* Cold generally is applied to recent wounds and heat to wounds at least 3 to 5 days old.
19. Massage provides which of the following benefits to the surgery patient?
    a. Muscle relaxation.
    b. Improved blood and lymph flow.
    c. Pain relief.
    d. Both a and b.
    e. All of the above.
20. The terms *effleurage* and *petrissage* refer to which physical therapy modality?
    a. Cryotherapy.
    b. Passive range of motion exercises.
    c. Massage.
    d. All of the above.
    e. None of the above.
21. Which of the following may be useful in stimulating a patient's appetite?
    a. Diazepam.
    b. Steroids (megestrol).
    c. Acupuncture.
    d. Serotonin antagonist (cyproheptadine).
    e. All of the above.
22. *True* or *False:* Feeding tubes can be placed semipermanently through the nose, pharynx, esophagus, or stomach.
23. How can a veterinary surgical technician determine if a patient's pain was successfully managed through surgery and into the postoperative phase?
    a. Recovery from anesthesia is smooth.
    b. The patient is calm and quiet postoperatively.
    c. Signs of overt pain (e.g., vocalization, excessive movement) are absent.
    d. All of the above.
    e. Both a and c.
24. Which of the following statements regarding postoperative analgesia is *true*?
    a. Patients undergoing soft tissue elective surgery should receive opioids for 24 hours and NSAIDs for 3 to 4 days postoperatively.
    b. Patients undergoing emergency or nonroutine soft tissue surgery should never receive opioids.
    c. Patients undergoing surgery of the gastrointestinal tract should never receive NSAIDs.
    d. Patients undergoing orthopedic surgery should receive opioids and NSAIDs only for the first 24 to 72 hours postoperatively.
    e. None of the above statements is true.
25. *True* or *False:* NSAIDs are the only class of analgesics that are safe to be sent home with the owner for at-home pain management following surgery.

ANSWERS

1. b
2. c
3. False

4. True
5. False
6. True
7. c
8. d
9. e
10. a
11. a
12. b
13. d
14. d
15. e
16. e
17. True
18. True
19. e
20. c
21. e
22. True
23. d
24. a
25. False

BIBLIOGRAPHY

Clark B, McLaughlin RM: Physical rehabilitation in small-animal orthopedic patients, *Vet Med* 96:3, 2001.

Davidson EB: Managing bite wounds in dogs and cats. Part II, *Compend Contin Educ Pract Vet* 20:9, 1998.

Fowler D, Williams JM: *Manual of canine and feline wound management and reconstruction,* Shurdington, 1999, British Small Animal Veterinary Association.

Manning AM, Rush J, Rudnick D: Physical therapy for critically ill veterinary patients. Part II. The musculoskelatal system, *Compend Contin Educ Pract Vet* 19:7, 1997.

Simpson AM, Radlinsky M, Beale BS: Bandaging in dogs and cats: basic principles, *Compend Contin Educ Pract Vet* 23:1, 2001.

Slatter D: *Textbook of small animal surgery,* ed 3, Philadelphia, 2003, Saunders.

Taylor R, McGehee R: *Manual of small animal postoperative care,* Baltimore, 1995, Williams & Wilkins.

CHAPTER 9

The Surgery Room

Paige A. Jones

LEARNING OBJECTIVES

After studying this chapter, the reader should be able to do the following:

- Explain the ideal layout of a surgery room and adjacent areas.
- Differentiate between nonmovable (permanent) and movable equipment in a surgery room.
- Explain the cleaning of the equipment located in the surgery room.
- Describe the ideal cleaning procedure for a surgery room.
- Identify the different types of disinfectants and the microorganisms they target.
- Identify the supplies that should be stocked in a surgery room.
- Explain supply rotation in the surgery room.

LAYOUT OF THE SURGERY SUITE

The American Animal Hospital Association (AAHA) recommends three distinct and separate areas for a surgical facility: the preparation area, the scrub area, and the surgery room. Although AAHA certification is not a legal requirement for veterinary facilities, a surgical facility should create the best environment for the patient. In addition, some state licensing boards have specific requirements regarding surgical facilities that a veterinary hospital must meet to pass inspection and to receive authorization to offer surgery.

Preparation Area

Ideally, the preparation area should be adjacent to the surgery room. The "prep" room can be used for patient preparation and the storage of surgical supplies. AAHA also recommends placement of storage and cabinets in the prep area, not the surgery room. The surgeon can use the preparation area to scrub and gown for surgery if a separate scrub area is not available. It is ideal to have a separate anesthesia machine for the prep room so that cross-contamination does not occur by moving the machine from one room to another. The prep area is used for clipping the patient. Procedures classified as "dirty" should be done in the prep area. Surgeries such as abscessed wound care, debridement of old wounds, and impacted anal sacs are often defined as "dirty surgeries."

Scrub Area

The scrub area may be a small area with the scrub sink, autoclave, and room to gown and glove (Figure 9-1). This is a transitional area where the veterinarian and technician can prepare to move into the surgery room. Adding the autoclave to the space makes it a dual-purpose area that works well for personnel, because the counter area would not be in use for pack preparation while the surgeon is gowning and gloving for surgery.

Surgery Room

Ideally, the surgery room is a separate room that should be used only for surgery. The AAHA recommends that the surgery room be easily cleanable and be closed off as needed. Closing the door minimizes traffic, maximizes cleanliness, and helps to ensure the surgery room is used only for aseptic procedures. The room should be a "dedicated" room reserved for clean surgical procedures. It should be used only for surgery, not for other types of procedures that may introduce bacteria into the room. The surgery room should be large enough that personnel can easily move around the surgery table and not contaminate the surgical field or the surgeon. If present, cabinets should be off the floor and constructed of nonporous material. Keeping cabinets off the floor allows for adequate cleaning underneath and prevents dust and debris from collecting around the base of the cabinets. The cabinets that hold sterile supplies should have doors that can be closed to protect the packs and other supplies from dust, debris, and other contaminants (Figure 9-2).

The surgery room should also be free of clutter and items that may collect dust or harbor bacteria. It should have a door that can be closed, and this

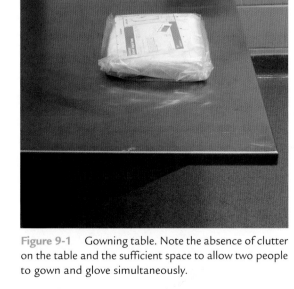

Figure 9-1   Gowning table. Note the absence of clutter on the table and the sufficient space to allow two people to gown and glove simultaneously.

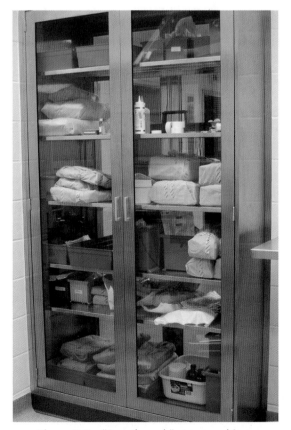

Figure 9-2   "Pass-through" storage cabinet.

door should be opened only when necessary to limit the amount of traffic and air flow in and out of the room. "Tacky mats" have a strong adhesive coating for dirt removal and historically have been used to decrease the amount of debris entering the surgery room. However, the Centers for Disease Control and Prevention (CDC) found that tacky mats in operating rooms do little to minimize the overall degree of floor contamination. If possible, the air pressure should be greater in the surgery room to reduce the influx of bacteria from the rest of the veterinary facility.

EQUIPMENT CLEANING

Different types of equipment are located in a surgery room. Some equipment is nonmovable (i.e., permanently affixed), and some is movable. Cleaning of these pieces of equipment varies depending on their use and design.

Nonmovable (Permanent) Equipment

Permanent items are pieces of equipment that are attached to the floor, wall, or ceiling in the surgery room. These pieces are usually not moved from the room because of their weight or the physical difficulty of moving them. These items should be wiped down daily before surgery with a damp cloth to remove any dust that may have accumulated. Nonmovable pieces of equipment include the following:

- Surgery lights (Figure 9-3)
- Surgery table (Figure 9-4)
- Radiographic view box

Movable Equipment

Movable pieces of equipment can be transported to other areas of the hospital. Ideally, movable items should not leave the surgery room, but in many veterinary facilities, they serve dual purposes and are moved to other areas of the hospital. If these items must be moved, it is essential to clean and disinfect them thoroughly before returning them to the surgery room. Movable equipment

items include the following:

- Anesthesia machine (Figure 9-5)
- Monitoring equipment
  —Electrocardiogram (ECG) machine (Figure 9-6)
  —Blood pressure (BP) cuffs and monitors
  —Airway tubes and monitors
- Heating pads
- Intravenous (IV) drip stand (or IV pole)
- Instrument table (Figure 9-7)
- Suction unit
- Cautery unit
- Kick bucket (Figure 9-8)

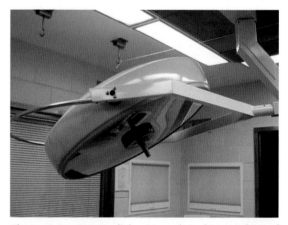

Figure 9-3   Surgery light. Note that shiny surface of the lamp is dust free.

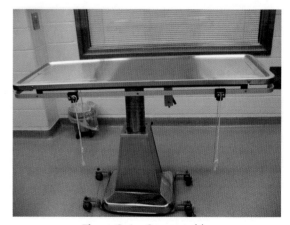

Figure 9-4   Surgery table.

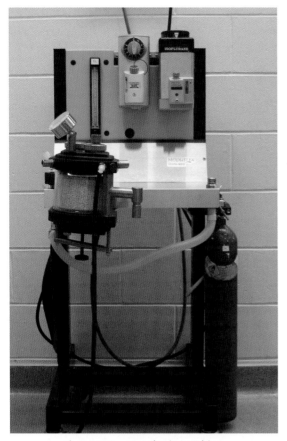

Figure 9-5   Anesthesia machine.

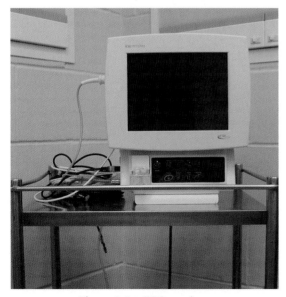

Figure 9-6   ECG monitor.

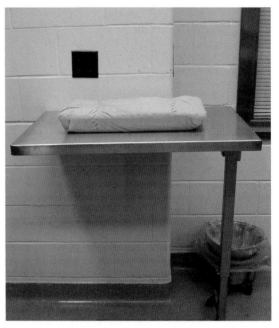

Figure 9-7   Mayo stand, or instrument table.

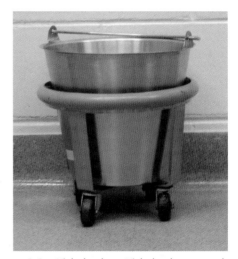

Figure 9-8   Kick bucket. Kick buckets are cleaned after every surgery and prepared with a new plastic liner before every surgery.

General Cleaning Instructions

All equipment should be wiped daily before surgery using the appropriate cleaning or disinfecting solution. It is important to follow the manufacturer's instructions because improper cleaning or use of inappropriate solutions may damage the equipment. The CDC states that the manufacturers of medical equipment should provide care and maintenance instructions that are specific to the equipment. This information should include the equipment's compatibility with chemical germicides, whether it can be immersed for cleaning, and how it should be decontaminated. The CDC also states that in the absence of any instructions from the manufacturer, items that are considered noncritical (stethoscopes, BP cuffs, knobs of equipment) can be cleaned and then disinfected with alcohol.

CLEANING OF SURGERY ROOM

Ideally, the equipment used to clean the surgery room should be used *only* in the surgery room to prevent cross-contamination from other areas of the veterinary facility. Various agencies or organizations that evaluate human medical facilities provide recommendations that the veterinary facility can use when setting up a protocol for the cleaning and maintenance of the surgery room.

The Association of periOperative Room Nurses (AORN) publishes recommended practices for environmental cleaning in the surgical setting. Although these recommendations may be difficult to meet in all veterinary practices, it is important to the veterinary patient's health that guidelines for cleanliness and disinfection of the surgical area include as many recommended practices as possible.

The CDC has no recommendation for disinfecting the surgery room after each surgery in the absence of visible soiling and contamination. However, wet vacuuming the surgery room floor is recommended at the end of the day. The CDC also states that the actual physical removal of microorganisms and soil by scrubbing is more important than the antimicrobial effect of the cleaning agent used.

AORN recommends cleaning a 3- to 4-foot perimeter around the surgical field when it is visibly soiled, with the cleaning area extended as necessary. Also, the entire floor should be cleaned each day. The following AORN recommendations,

including a *rationale* (purpose) to clarify some practices, may be useful as a protocol for the cleaning of a surgery area in a veterinary facility:

1. Cleaning is performed on a regular basis to reduce the amount of dust, organic material, and microbial presence in the surgery room.
2. The operating room (OR) should be cleaned before and after each surgical procedure.
3. All horizontal surfaces in the OR should be damp-dusted before the first surgery of the day. In "damp dusting" a lint-free cloth dampened with water is used to wipe down the horizontal surfaces.
   Rationale: Proper cleaning of horizontal surfaces helps reduce airborne contaminants that may travel on dust and lint.
4. OR equipment and furniture that are visibly soiled should be cleaned at the end of each procedure.
   Rationale: Items used for surgery are considered contaminated through contact with the patient's blood, tissue, and body fluids and should be cleaned before admittance of the next patient to the surgery room.
5. Surgery rooms should be "terminally cleaned" daily. *Terminal cleaning* is cleaning that is performed at the completion of the daily surgery schedules. It includes all the equipment in the surgery and prep areas and all the permanent and movable equipment.
6. Surgery rooms should be cleaned daily whether they are used or not.
   Rationale: A clean surgical environment reduces the number of microbial flora present.
7. Mechanical friction (a scrubbing motion) should be used to clean all surfaces, including (but not limited to) the following:
   - Surgical lights
   - Any fixed equipment
   - All furniture and equipment, including wheels, casters, step stools, foot pedals, telephones, and light switches
   - Handles of cabinets
   - Ventilation faceplates
   - Horizontal surfaces (doorway ledges)

- Areas adjacent to surgery room
- Scrub sinks
8. Refillable soap dispensers are not recommended because they can harbor bacterial growth.
9. Surgery rooms should be wet-vacuumed at the end of the day.
   Rationale: Terminal cleaning in the surgery room reduces the number of microorganisms, dust, and organic debris from the environment.
10. Cleaning equipment (mops, wet vacuums) should be disassembled, cleaned, and dried before storage.
    Rationale: This practice prevents growth of microorganisms during storage and subsequent contamination of the surgery room.

DISINFECTANTS

Definitions

The following basic definitions are needed to understand how the different disinfectants work and interact with bacteria, viruses, spores, and even each other:

- **Anionic detergent:** Soap that has free, negatively charged ions that precipitate when combined with calcium and magnesium in hard water.
- **Antiseptic:** Chemical that inhibits or prevents the growth of microbes on living tissue; compare with *disinfectant.*
- **Bactericide:** Agent that destroys (kills) bacteria.
- **Bacteriostat:** Agent that inhibits the growth of bacteria.
- **Biocide:** Agent that kills living organisms.
- **Cationic detergent:** Contains positively charged ions that remain suspended in solution (e.g., quaternary ammonium).
- **Detergent:** Chemical that contains free ions and leaves a film on surfaces.
- **Disinfectant:** Chemical used to inhibit or prevent the growth of microbes on inanimate objects; compare with *antiseptic.*

- **Fungicide:** Agent that kills fungi.
- **Sanitize:** To reduce the number of microbes to a safe level.
- **Sporicide:** Agent that kills spores.
- **Sterilize:** To eliminate all microbes by death or inactivation.
- **Virucide:** Agent that kills viruses.

The ideal disinfectant should have the following characteristics:

- Broad spectrum
- Nonirritating
- Nontoxic
- Noncorrosive
- Inexpensive

Effectiveness

The effectiveness of any disinfectant depends on the following factors:

1. *Type of microorganism.* Some microorganisms are more resistant to certain types of disinfectants.
2. *Degree of contamination.* This may affect the length of time and the amount of chemical disinfectant necessary to disinfect effectively.
3. *Amount of protein in area.* Proteins may absorb or inactivate the disinfectant.
4. *Organic matter.* Hair, feces, litter, and other organic matter will decrease the effectiveness or render the disinfectant ineffective. Therefore, all organic matter should be removed from the area, and the area should be sanitized before applying the disinfectant.
5. *Additional sanitizing compounds.* Other compounds used to sanitize the area may inactivate or react with the disinfectant. Therefore, thorough rinsing and drying after sanitizing should be attempted before applying a disinfectant.
6. *Concentration and quantity of chemical.* Improper dilution or inadequate amount of the correct dilution may result in ineffective disinfection.
7. *Contact time and temperature.* Incorrect contact time or the temperature of the surface may result in ineffective disinfection.

Types of Disinfectants

Many types of disinfectants are available for use in a veterinary facility. Each facility should research the product information and decide the best policy for the facility. Most disinfectants require some form of dilution. The manufacturer's recommendations should be followed so that each disinfectant is used at its maximum effectiveness against bacteria, viruses, and other infective agents.

An example of a *chlorine-based* disinfectant is bleach (Figure 9-9). It can be used for cleaning as well as disinfecting. Bleach does corrode metals and causes fabrics to deteriorate. It can be irritating to eyes, mucous membranes, and skin. Bleach can be deactivated by fecal matter. Decreased temperature and the pH of the water in which the bleach is diluted may alter its efficacy.

Phenol-based disinfectants include common household disinfectants (e.g., Lysol, Pine-Sol). Phenols are able to work in the presence of organic material. These disinfectants are relatively safe but can cause skin irritation. They are infrequently used in veterinary medicine.

An example of *quaternary amine–based* disinfectant is Roccal-D Plus (Figure 9-10). These disinfectants bind to and are inactivated by organic material, so the area must be cleaned before disinfection. They also react with soaps, so the area must be well rinsed. Hard water may also deactivate quaternary amine disinfectants.

Iodine disinfectants such as povidone-iodine are not generally used as disinfectants, but in veterinary medicine they are frequently used as antiseptics (Figure 9-11). The iodines can stain fabric and floors and can irritate tissue. They are also corrosive. Iodines are inactivated by organic material.

Chlorhexidine disinfectants are widely used in veterinary medicine as disinfectants for examination tables and for the disinfection of instruments for minor procedures (Figure 9-12). Chlorhexidine maintains its effectiveness in the presence of organic material but is not as effective against some bacteria and viruses as other disinfectants. It also has residual activity, which can be important. One drawback is that chlorhexidine must have sufficient contact time to be effective.

Table 9-1 compares types of various disinfectants.

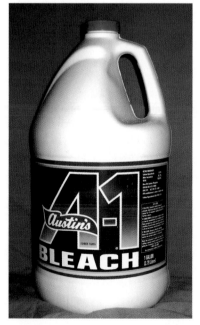

Figure 9-9   Chlorine-based disinfectant.

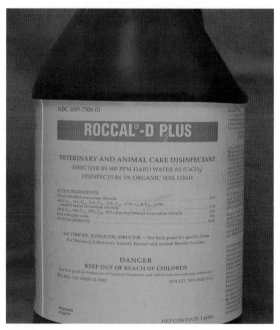

Figure 9-10   Quaternary amine–based disinfectant.

ROTATING AND RESTOCKING SUPPLIES

Supplies in the surgery room should be limited to an amount that would be used over a short time. Necessary supplies in the surgery room vary greatly between veterinary facilities depending on the number and types of surgeries performed and what is needed for each surgery. Supplies should not be excessive because increased inventory can tie up the facility's money unnecessarily. The veterinary technician plays a vital role in communicating with the veterinarians on staff about their needs for the surgery area. The veterinary technician is often the person who restocks and organizes the room. It is important to keep open lines of communication and to monitor closely the supplies used in the room. Supplies can be broken down into two categories: disposable and reusable.

Disposable Supplies

Disposable supplies consist of the supplies purchased for single-time use, such as scalpel blades, suture, and surgical gloves. These items are purchased as sterile items and usually include a date specifying when they should be "used by" or when they are considered "outdated." These items need to be checked and rotated each time the surgery area is stocked. Items with expiration dates that are shortest (or closest) should be rotated so that they are used before items with longer (further) dates. If too much stock of one item is kept in the area, the potential for outdating increases. For this reason, keep only a minimum of what is needed in a day. This keeps the stock rotated, and the potential for outdated items decreases.

Reusable Supplies

Reusable supplies are the items that the veterinary facility uses and resterilizes between patients. These items consist of surgery packs, clean and laundered reusable cloth drapes, hand towels, and separate instruments. These items are often cleaned after surgery, repackaged, sterilized, and

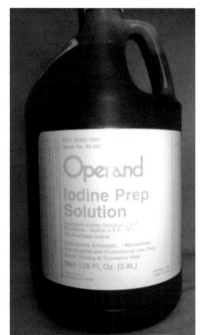

Figure 9-11   Povidone-iodine disinfectant.

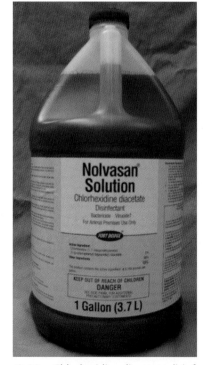

Figure 9-12   Chlorhexidine diacetate disinfectant.

TABLE 9-1   Comparison of Different Types of Disinfectants

DISINFECTANT	EFFECTIVENESS	ADVANTAGES	DISADVANTAGES
Chlorine based	Viruses: enveloped, nonenveloped Fungi Bacteria Algae *Not effective against:* Spores	Wide germicidal activity Relatively nontoxic Effective at low concentrations Low cost	Corrodes metal Deteriorates fabric Irritates mucous membrane, eyes, and skin Inactivated by organic material Area must be cleaned before use.
Phenol based	Bacteria Viruses: enveloped *Not effective against:* Viruses: nonenveloped Spores	Maintains effectiveness with organic matter Wide germicidal activity Relatively noncorrosive Limited toxicity Low to moderate cost	Poor or limited residual activity Not sporicidal
Quaternary amine based	Bacteria: gram positive, gram negative Viruses: enveloped *Not effective against:* Viruses: nonenveloped Spores Fungi	Low toxicity Wide germicidal activity Noncorrosive Good for use on cleaned surfaces Low cost	Binds to organic material and soaps Deactivated by hard water Areas must be cleaned and rinsed free of soap.
Iodine (iodophor)	Bacteria Spores (some) Viruses Fungus	Wide germicidal activity Relatively nontoxic Better as sporicidal than chlorine Low cost	Inactivated by organic material Must be applied multiple times Stains fabric Poor residual activity Corrosive
Chlorhexidine	Bacteria Viruses: enveloped Fungus (some) Spores	Nonirritating to tissue Maintains effectiveness with organic matter Wide germicidal activity, but ineffective against some important species Nontoxic Effective at low concentrations Low cost	Less effective than other agents Must be in contact for 5 minutes Hard or alkaline water causes precipitation of active ingredients.
Alcohols	Bacteria: gram positive, gram negative Viruses: enveloped *Not effective against:* Viruses: nonenveloped Spores	Wide germicidal activity Noncorrosive Excellent instrument, disinfecting at 70%-95% concentration	Requires time to work Does not penetrate organic material Irritates tissue Denatures protein, which may promote bacterial growth in open wounds Too expensive for general use

placed back in the storage cabinets of the surgery room. For reusable supplies, as with disposable items, place the oldest packs so that they are used first and the stock is continually rotated. If the veterinary facility has more than one spay pack, it is important to rotate the packs so that they do not fall out of the rotation.

Current thinking in human medicine is that packs do not automatically become outdated after a certain number of days. An event must occur to cause the item to become nonsterile. An "event" is something that occurs to cause a breach of the item's sterility. Examples of events are opening of the pack, the pack coming in contact with moisture, and the pack being dropped on the floor. Many veterinary facilities still operate on the assumption that an item is outdated after a certain arbitrary period, such as 30 days. For items sterilized in a veterinary facility, is it necessary to keep everything wrapped and sterilized, just in case it might be needed? It would be a better practice for the facility to sterilize only the items that will be needed in the next few days or weeks. Although the veterinary profession is not always predictable and emergencies do occur, all the spay packs do not need to be sterile unless multiple spays are scheduled for the next day. This practice would save on storage of sterile items in the surgery room and facilitate a more organized rotation of supplies.

SUMMARY

The veterinary profession has few legal guidelines in surgery room cleanliness and supply rotation compared with the human medical profession, but this does not mean these areas can be ignored. For the well-being of the patients and the financial well-being of the veterinary facility, it is important that veterinary technicians take a proactive role in establishing protocols for cleanliness, stock rotation, and sterilization of surgical items. A breakdown in any of these areas can be costly for the veterinary facility. By being organized, efficient, and detail oriented, the veterinary technician can serve the best interests of the patient, the client, and the veterinary facility.

KEY POINTS

1. The surgery suite ideally should consist of a preparation area, a scrub area, and a surgery area.
2. The preparation area should be next to the surgery room and used for patient preparation and the storage of supplies.
3. Surgical procedures classified as "dirty" should be done in the prep area, not in the surgery room.
4. The scrub area can also be used as the sterilization area and the place for gowning and gloving.
5. Ideally, the surgery room should be a separate room. (Some state licensing boards require the surgery room be a separate room.)
6. There should be minimal cabinets in the surgery room, and if possible the cabinets should be mounted on the wall.
7. Permanent (nonmovable) equipment consists of surgery lights, surgery table, and radiographic view box.
8. Movable equipment consists of anesthesia machine, monitoring equipment (ECG, blood pressure, airway), heating pads, intravenous (IV) drip stand, instrument table or Mayo stands, suction unit, cautery unit, and kick bucket.
9. All equipment should be damp-wiped daily before surgery.
10. Always follow the manufacturer's instructions for cleaning of equipment.
11. Surgery rooms should be spot-cleaned between each procedure.
12. Surgery rooms should be terminally cleaned at the end of each day.
13. Mechanical friction should be applied when cleaning.
14. Disinfectants should be used according to the manufacturer's instructions.
15. There is no "ideal disinfectant," but there are many good disinfectants that meet most of the criteria of an ideal disinfectant.
16. The effectiveness of a disinfectant depends on many factors (e.g., microorganisms, contamination, organic matter).
17. The stock of disposable surgical supplies should be limited so that expiration does not occur.
18. Reusable supplies are items that are cleaned and resterilized.

19. All surgical supplies should be rotated so that the items are used in a rotating order (oldest first).
20. In event-related contamination, an event must occur to cause an item to become nonsterile (contaminated).

REVIEW QUESTIONS

1. Where should anal sac surgeries and abscessed wounds be lanced and flushed?
   a. In the surgery room.
   b. In the preparation room.
   c. In the scrub room.
   d. In the examination room.
2. What items should be located in the scrub area/room?
   a. Hair clippers.
   b. Scrub sink.
   c. Autoclave.
   d. Table/counter to hold open gown packs.
   e. Answers b, c, and d.
3. *True* or *False:* All surgeries should be performed in the surgery room, whether the surgery is considered "clean" or "dirty."
4. *True* or *False:* The surgery room needs to have easy access, so doors should not be placed between surgery rooms and scrub or prep areas.
5. *True* or *False:* The air pressure in the surgery room should be greater than that in the rest of the hospital to reduce the influx of bacteria into the surgery room.
6. *True* or *False:* Movable equipment (i.e., equipment that is not permanently affixed) in the surgery room should not leave the surgery room.
7. When movable equipment is removed from the surgery room:
   a. It should not be brought back into the surgery room.
   b. It should be thoroughly cleaned and disinfected before being returned to the surgery room.
   c. It is considered contaminated and must be sterilized before being returned to the surgery room.
   d. It can be returned directly to the surgery room when it is no longer needed outside the surgery room.

8. In the absence of cleaning instructions from the manufacturer, stethoscopes and blood pressure cuffs and other noncritical items can be cleaned in what manner for use in the surgery room?
   a. Autoclaved.
   b. Immersed in high-level disinfectants.
   c. Cleaned and then disinfected with alcohol.
   d. Put through a cycle on a washing machine or dishwasher.
   e. None of the above.
9. How often should the surgery room floor be cleaned?
   a. Only as needed.
   b. Daily.
   c. Morning and evening.
   d. Weekly.
   e. It does not matter.
10. *True* or *False:* Surgery rooms should be cleaned daily whether they are used or not.
11. Why are refillable soap dispensers not recommended for use in the surgery prep or scrub area?
    a. They always run out just when they are needed.
    b. They take too long to refill should they run out of soap during the hand prep process.
    c. They can harbor bacterial growth.
    d. All of the above.
    e. None of the above.
12. What is the difference between antiseptics and disinfectants?
    a. Antiseptics are intended for use on living tissues, and disinfectants are intended for inanimate objects.
    b. Antiseptics are intended for use on inanimate objects, and disinfectants are intended for living tissues.
    c. There is no difference, and they are used interchangeably.
    d. Antiseptics are used daily, and disinfectants are only used weekly.
    e. Disinfectants are sporicidal, bactericidal, and virucidal, whereas antiseptics are only bactericidal and virucidal.
13. Regarding disinfectants, what does "contact time" refer to?
    a. The time required for the disinfectant to be in contact with the microorganisms to achieve

its intended effect (i.e., significantly reduce the number of microorganisms).

b. The time of day when the manufacturer can be contacted for assistance.

c. The time required for a microorganism to develop resistance to the disinfectant.

d. The latent phase of microorganisms, giving the disinfectant a "window of opportunity" to kill the microorganisms.

14. Which of the following affect a disinfectant's effectiveness?

a. Amount of protein present in the area.

b. Type of microorganisms present.

c. Concentration of the disinfectant.

d. Both b and c.

e. All of the above.

ANSWERS

1. b
2. e
3. False
4. False
5. True
6. True
7. b
8. c
9. b
10. True
11. c
12. a
13. a
14. e

BIBLIOGRAPHY

Catanzaro T: *Veterinary practice building design starter kit,* ed 2, Denver, 1990, American Animal Hospital Association.

Copich W: Avoiding the common errors made in the designing of animal hospitals, *Vet Clin North Am* 2(3):537, 1972.

Centers for Disease Control and Prevention (CDC), Healthcare Infection Control Practices Advisory Committee (HICPAC): *Draft guidelines for environmental infection control in healthcare facilities,* Atlanta, 2001, CDC.

Crawford L et al: A comparison of commonly used surface disinfectants, *Infect Control Today,* 2000. http://www.infectioncontroltoday.com/articles/0b1feat2.html.

Kennedy J, Bek J, Griffin D: *Selection and use of disinfectants,* Lincoln, 2000, Institute of Agriculture and Natural Resources, University of Nebraska. http://ianrpubs.unl.edu/animaldisease/g1410.htm.

Recommended practices for environmental cleaning in the surgical practice setting, *AORN J* 67(2):448, 1998.

Recommended practices for environmental cleaning in the surgical practice setting, *AORN J* 76(6), 2002.

Sacred cow survey, *OR Manager* 14(9):1, 1998.

CHAPTER 10

Instrument Cleaning and Sterilization

Pat Weinman, Paige A. Jones

LEARNING OBJECTIVES

After studying this chapter, the reader should be able to do the following:

- Describe the steps to prepare instruments for use in surgery.
- Describe the cleaning methods used for preparing instruments for sterilization.
- Identify which method is best for sterilizing instruments.

- Demonstrate how to wrap a pack for sterilization.
- Describe the types of expiration dating.
- Explain the different types of sterilization indicators.

BASIC CLEANING PROCEDURES

Cleaning, decontaminating (or sanitizing), and sterilizing are the three cornerstones to providing sterile instruments in the surgery room. Each of these processes contributes to the overall destruction of microorganisms that could cause serious postoperative complications, including the death of the patient.

Basic cleaning procedures for instruments include presoaking, decontaminating, and ultrasonic cleaning. In the cleaning and sterilization of instruments, it is imperative to begin the process of presoaking immediately after a surgery.

Presoaking of Instruments

Presoaking involves placing the soiled instruments in distilled water or water mixed with a detergent solution that is specifically approved for use with surgical instruments (e.g., Haemo-Sol; Figure 10-1), without using mechanical agitation. The purpose of presoaking is to prevent blood and other surgical debris from drying on the instruments or to soften dried blood and debris on the instruments.

Presoaking or precleaning can make the cleaning process more efficient. *Precleaning* involves rinsing the instruments in distilled water to rid them of tissue and blood. If this is not done, processing the instruments may take longer. Allowing tissue and blood to dry on the instruments makes cleaning much more difficult, especially in hinged areas and box locks. Debris can build up and harden in crevices, making decontamination more difficult as well.

Decontamination of Instruments

The decontamination process is the manual cleaning of an instrument in a detergent solution

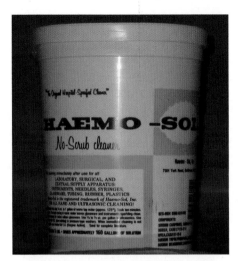

Figure 10-1 Example of product approved for use as a cleaning solution for surgical instruments.

to assist in the breakdown of biologic debris. Because this may be the only cleaning before sterilization, the instrument must be cleaned thoroughly. When cleaning instruments by hand, take care not to damage the more delicate items, and pay special attention to cleaning areas that have box locks or joints. Instruments should be decontaminated using the following procedural steps:

1. Prepare a basin with warm water and a detergent approved for use on surgical instruments.
2. Open all box locks and unlock ratchets as each instrument is gently placed in the basin.
3. Wash all surfaces of each instrument with a soft bristle brush. Pay special attention to box locks, joints, and serrations because biologic debris will build up in these areas. Use a brushing motion, directed away from you, to scrub the instruments. This will prevent biologic debris from splashing back toward you.
   - Never use a wire brush on instruments because it will damage the instrument's surface and cause crevices that can harbor pathogens (microorganisms).
   - Instruments have a protective coating of chromium oxide to extend their usefulness as properly functioning devices. If the

coating is removed, the instrument will be compromised, and then its surface can harbor pathogens that adversely affect the patient's health.

4. Rinse each instrument thoroughly with distilled water. This will prevent the buildup of "scale" on the instruments. If tap water is used, scale will eventually build up on instruments, and they will not work properly.
5. With locks and ratchets opened, place the instruments flat on an absorbent surface to drain and dry.
6. Cover the draining instruments with another layer of lint-free absorbent material.
7. When the instruments are clean and dry, check each for its general condition and its ability to function properly. Box locks should open and close smoothly; ratchets should engage and disengage easily; scissors should cut easily and smoothly; and the jaws and teeth should mesh as designed. One way to check the integrity of ratchets is to close them and firmly tap the ringed end of the instrument against a firm, smooth surface. If the ratchets pop open when tested, they cannot be trusted to hold the target tissue in surgery and should not be included in the surgery pack.

Instruments with broken or missing parts, malfunctioning parts, pitted or discolored parts, or rusted surfaces should be set aside for repair or replacement. When purchasing new instruments, it is best to buy high-quality instruments that will withstand repeated and excessive use.

Ultrasonic Cleaning of Instruments

After the decontamination process has been completed, the next step is ultrasonic cleaning with a solution of distilled water and chemicals (enzymes) (Figure 10-2). Several brands of enzymatic solutions are available, and the solution chosen should contain a *surfactant,* a product that reduces surface tension. The brand used at Purdue's Veterinary Teaching Hospital is MetriClean2 (Figure 10-3). *Enzymes* are organic substances that cause a particular chemical reaction. Enzymes assist in the

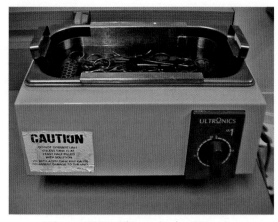

Figure 10-2   Ultrasonic cleaning unit.

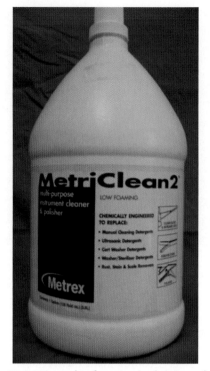

Figure 10-3   Example of enzymatic cleaning solution used in ultrasonic cleaning unit.

breakdown of soils and are generally formulated with a surfactant to improve their penetration into dried soil. Enzymes work most effectively when kept in water at a temperature recommended by the manufacturer. If the temperature is too high or too low, the enzymes may be inactivated. Enzymes can clean without mechanical action and are therefore used to clean instruments with lumens, such as endoscopes.

The benefit of ultrasonic cleaning is best demonstrated with hinged instruments or those with inaccessible areas (e.g., box lock), including hinged retractors and bone-cutting instruments. These devices should be in the open position for cleaning. An ultrasonic cleaner uses sound waves higher than those heard by the human ear, which create tiny bubbles. These bubbles form and collapse thousands of times each second, producing a scrubbing effect, known as *cavitation,* on the surface of items immersed in the liquid. Particles that have been agitated from instruments are suspended in solution and are subjected to negative pressure or suction. As a result, proteins are coagulated, the cell walls are disrupted, and microorganisms are destroyed.

The typical processing time of instruments in the ultrasonic machine is 3 to 6 minutes. Based on the manufacturer's recommendation, the temperature of the solution should be maintained in the range of 110° to 130° F. The temperature at which the chemical has greatest effect varies with the enzyme used. The instrument may be damaged if the enzyme is maintained at too high a temperature. Additionally, if the solution is not maintained at the correct temperature, soil may be "heat set" on the instrument, making it more difficult to clean.

After the ultrasonic cleaning is complete, rinse the instruments with distilled water to remove mineral deposits left behind. It is appropriate at this point to apply a lubricant to prolong the life of the instruments and help prevent rust and corrosion. Many different types of instrument lubricants are available. Some are used as a bath for soaking the instruments; other lubricants are sprayed on opened instruments spread out on a lint-free towel, then left to air-dry. Regardless of the type used, it is important to use only fresh, clean lubricant and to follow the manufacturer's directions. Lubricants can penetrate into difficult-to-reach areas such as box locks and leave a lubricating, microscopic film on the instrument.

Most lubricants are steam permeable and do not interfere with the sterilization process.

The instruments are now ready for wrapping.

PACK WRAPPING

Recipes

Typically, each instrument pack has a "recipe" detailing pertinent information that is maintained in a procedures manual. The recipe should include the names of all the instruments contained in each pack and the quantity of each type of instrument required to complete the pack. Additionally, the recipe should include the types and quantity of supplies that are necessary for pack completion, such as the number of gauze squares to include. It should contain a photo or illustration of each instrument and should specify whether linen or paper material should be used to wrap the pack. The procedures manual should also include the manufacturer's guidelines for any instrument in the pack that requires special handling and maintenance, any warranty that may be appropriate for items in the pack, and the manufacturer's telephone number.

Wrapping Material

Wraps used for sterilizing instruments are usually made of cotton or linen textiles and paper. These materials are able to sustain the heat and moisture of steam sterilization. For technicians working in a small animal facility that relies on steam sterilization for in-house procedures, the choice is usually linen or paper. The ideal wrap should have the following qualities:

- *Selective permeability.* Steam or gas must be able to penetrate the wrapping for sterilization to occur and must be easily "exhausted" from the pack once the sterilization process is completed. Microbes and dust particles must not be able to penetrate from the outer surface of the wrap to the inner surface.
- *Resistance.* The material should be resistant to damage when handled. Rips, punctures, or worn areas should be readily visible, which helps ensure contaminated packs will not be used.
- *Flexibility.* The material should be able to conform to the shape of the pack.
- *Memory.* After the pack has been opened, the wrapping material should return to the original flat position. This will help prevent accidental contamination of the pack contents.

Textile wraps traditionally are cotton textiles with a thread count of 140 to 288 threads per square inch. Textile wraps must be laundered, dried, and inspected for any damage before reuse as an instrument pack wrap. The advantage of using textile wraps is that they are more resistant to rips and punctures than paper and generally have a higher degree of flexibility and memory. When purchasing textile wrappers, cotton is the best option. Synthetic wrap may contribute to static electricity in the operating room. Gray, light tones of green, and medium tones of blue are often preferred because they result in less eyestrain over time than white. Select fabric by thread count, not by its weight or texture.

Personnel may be reluctant to discard textile wraps that have become torn or ripped and may attempt to mend them. Continued use of damaged textile wrap is not recommended because each stitch in the wrap creates a passage for microbes. If heat-sealed patches are used, steam cannot penetrate the patches during sterilization as easily as it penetrates the body of the wrap.

There are many types of paper wraps, but crepe paper is preferred over the noncrepe papers. Crepe paper should not be reused because continuous autoclaving can destroy the integrity of the paper fiber.

Sealing of Pack

Steam indicator tape is recommended when securing the wrapping material in place. Pretreated strips on the steam indicator tape change color from a pale yellow to black when the pack has been autoclaved. This indicates that conditions were met for sterilization. The name of the

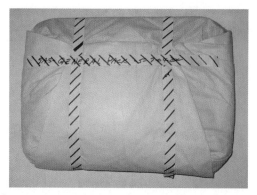

Figure 10-4   Sterilized pack with labeling information. black strips along the indicator tape show this pack has been autoclaved.

pack, the date the pack was sterilized, and the initials of the person who wrapped the pack should be written on the tape (Figure 10-4).

Packs can be wrapped with one wrap (single-wrapped) or with two wraps (double-wrapped). If a pack is double-wrapped, only the outer layer is sealed with steam indicator tape. Generally, when a pack is double-wrapped, the circulating nurse unwraps the outer layer, and the scrubbed-in assistant unwraps the inner layer. If inadvertent contamination occurs when unwrapping the outer layer (circulating nurse accidentally touches outer surface of inner wrap), double-wrapped packs have the advantage of an additional layer of material protecting the instruments. The circulating nurse may then open the interior layer, and as long as contamination does not occur, the surgeon can use the pack. The disadvantage of double wrapping is the additional cost of the material used to wrap the pack.

When securing a wrapped package, personnel may attempt to use ordinary masking tape instead of indicator tape. This is not advisable because the adhesive on masking tape will not adhere adequately during steam sterilization.

The following guidelines should be followed in the preparation of packs:

1. All items to be sterilized must be clean and in good condition.
2. The wrap material used must be durable for the sterilization process.

3. Contents of frequently used packs should be standardized so that the same pack can be used for the same surgical procedure from session to session.
4. Pack size must be compatible for the size of the autoclave chamber.
5. Soft items such as towels and drapes should be folded using the *accordion pleat technique* (Figure 10-5). Items that have been folded in this manner can be lifted by one corner and allowed to fall open. No elaborate unfolding or shaking is necessary, which reduces the potential for air currents that may circulate microbes.
6. All packs should be wrapped using the same method so that they can be unwrapped in the same way. One common method uses *angled wrapping* (Figure 10-6).
7. A sterilization indicator strip should be placed in the middle of the pack to verify conditions were met for sterilization.
8. The outer wrap should be sealed with indicator tape to indicate the pack has been autoclaved and to keep the pack from opening (Figure 10-7).

Each step of this process is critical in providing sterile instruments; that is, each method used in these steps fulfills a particular function that cannot be omitted. Box 10-1 provides directions on how to wrap a surgical gown and towel pack.

Expiration Dating

Much debate surrounds the issue of how long an item can be stored and still can be considered sterile. Shelf-life expiration and event-related expiration are the two types of dating for sterilized items. *Shelf-life expiration* includes a predetermined date that identifies how long an item should be considered sterile. For items wrapped in woven (linen) or nonwoven (crepe paper) materials, a shelf life of 2 weeks is an acceptable time to expiration. Items placed in peel-away pouches have an expiration date of 7 weeks.

In contrast, *event-related expiration* is determined from an environmental perspective. If damaged in any way, the pack would be considered nonsterile.

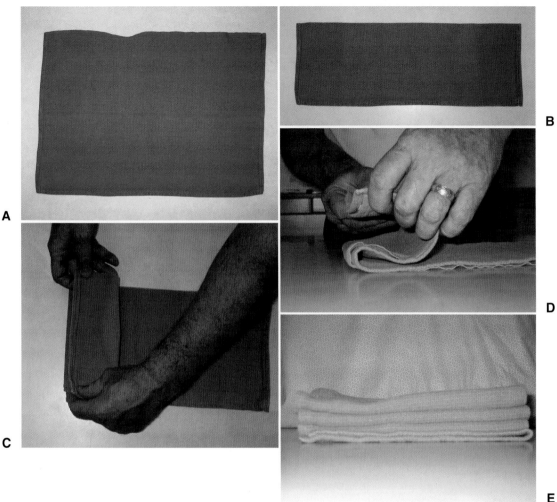

Figure 10-5 Steps in accordion pleat folding of a hand or field towel. **A,** Spread towel flat on table. **B,** Fold towel in half lengthwise. **C,** Make first fold of accordion. **D,** Lateral view of first accordion fold. **E,** Completed accordion folding.

Excessive handling of the pack, causing it to fall onto the floor, or accumulation of dust on the pack would lead personnel to question if the pack is still sterile. Even under these conditions, packs have been found to be sterile after 50 weeks. However, whenever a pack's sterility is in question, it must be assumed that the pack is contaminated. Products that break down or alter over time, such as latex tubing, require expiration dating.

STERILIZATION

The last step in the cleaning process after presoaking/precleaning and decontamination is sterilization. Sterilization is defined as the use of a process to rid an object of all living microbes.

Two types of sterilizers (autoclaves) are typically used in small animal practices: gravity air-displacement autoclaves and high-vacuum sterilizers (also known as *prevacuum sterilizers*). Both types

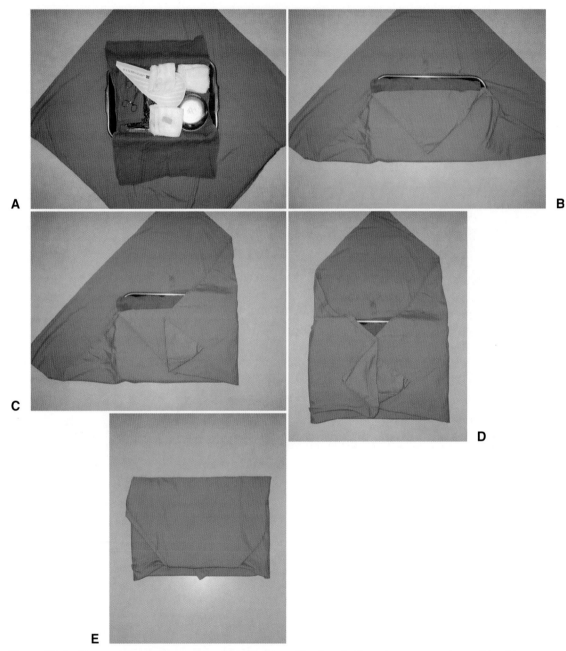

Figure 10-6   Five steps in angle wrapping of a pack for sterilization. **A,** Spread wrap on a clean table with tray centered in middle of wrap. **B,** Bring bottom flap on top of tray, and fold back the corner to create a tab. **C,** Bring first side flap to center, and fold back the corner to create another tab. **D,** Bring second side flap to center, and fold back the corner to create another tab. **E,** Make final fold of pack wrap, and tuck under other flaps, leaving a short tab untucked to allow for easier unwrapping of the pack when opened for surgery.

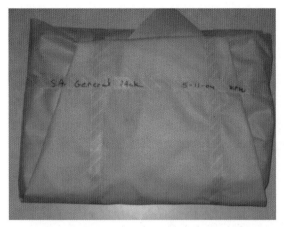

Figure 10-7   Wrapped and taped pack, ready for sterilization. Yellow strips on the indicator tape used to seal this pack have not yet changed to black, indicating this pack has not yet been autoclaved.

use steam under pressure to kill microorganisms. Some autoclaves are capable of performing both methods of sterilization. With both types of sterilizers, proper sterilization depends on the following three factors:

1. Proper operation of the sterilizer
2. Proper preparation of the packs
3. Proper loading of the sterilizer

Gravity Air-Displacement Sterilizer

The gravity air-displacement sterilizer found in most small animal hospitals is typically a table-top-sized autoclave (Figure 10-8). Distilled water is placed in the bottom of the sterilizer and then heated electrically. As the water turns to steam, the steam forces air out of the sterilizer through a port. Once the air is out of the sterilizer, the steam pressure builds up until the operating temperature is reached. Once the cycle has been

---

BOX 10-1   Wrapping Gowns and Hand Towels

Gowns
1. Place a clean gown flat on a surface with the outer surface facing up.
2. Straighten out the sleeves and cuffs.
3. Fold the near edge of the gown to the center.
4. Fold the far edge of the gown toward the center to meet the near edge.
5. Fold the gown in half lengthwise.
6. Fold the gown lengthwise in accordion fashion into thirds.
7. Ensure neck ties are easily accessible on the uppermost surface of the gown.

Hand Towels
1. Place a clean hand towel flat on a clean surface.
2. Use the accordion pleat technique to fold the towel on its long axis.
3. Fold the towel in accordion fashion into thirds or quarters.
4. Fold back a corner tab.

Gowns and Towels Together
1. Flatten out a clean outer wrap on a clean surface (single-layer wrap).
2. Place the folded gown in the center.
3. Place the folded hand towel on top of the gown.
4. Place an indicator strip inside the towel.
5. Wrap in same fashion as an instrument pack.*
6. Seal with tape, label "gown pack," note gown's size and the date, and initialize.

---

*Most instrument packs are wrapped in two layers (double-wrapped). Gown packs typically are wrapped with one layer (single-wrapped).

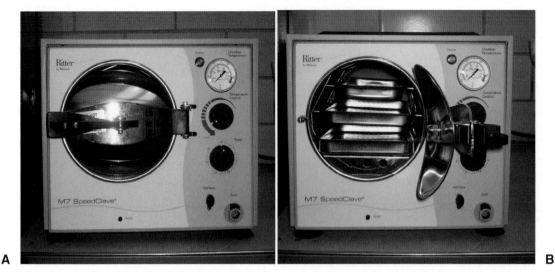

A   **B**

Figure 10-8   **A,** Tabletop gravity air-displacement sterilizer, with door closed. **B,** Same autoclave, with door opened.

completed, the steam is removed and condenses back to water.

Several settings can be used in gravity air-displacement sterilization. The typical temperature is 250° to 270° F, and typical pressure is 15 to 27 pounds per square inch (psi). The cycle will run approximately 15 minutes to achieve the proper temperature and will sterilize between 3 and 15 minutes depending on the item. At the completion of the cycle, the door should be cracked open for approximately 15 minutes to allow any moisture to evaporate and prevent condensation on the pack.

High-Vacuum Sterilizer

Proper operation of a high-vacuum gravity displacement sterilizer includes setting the sterilizer between 250° and 272° F for 4 minutes at 32 psi (Figure 10-9). The sterilizer should run through (1) a conditioning phase for about 17 minutes, (2) a sterilization phase for 4 minutes, (3) a high-vacuum exhaust for about 4 minutes, and (4) a drying cycle for about 20 minutes. The total sterilization process should take about 45 minutes. To ensure proper settings for specific types of packs (e.g., instruments, soft items), consult the manufacturer's operating manual.

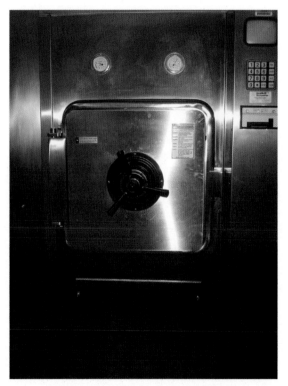

Figure 10-9   High-vacuum sterilizer.

The main difference between gravity air-displacement and high-vacuum sterilizers is that the high-vacuum sterilizer *forces* steam into the sterilizing chamber, which causes steam to penetrate the pack more quickly. Additionally, after the sterilization cycle has been completed, the steam is vacuumed out of the chamber. This pulls the steam out of the pack to prevent condensation in or on the pack. This avoids a wet pack, which could compromise the pack's sterility.

Preparation and Loading

Proper pack preparation should be done in an area reserved for this purpose. For many small animal practices, however, this is not always possible. An acceptable alternative is to combine both the pack preparation area and the area used for preparation of operating room personnel. Traffic to and from this area should be minimized, and routine cleaning procedures should be in place to reduce the microbial load in the area as much as possible.

Proper loading of the sterilizer is a critical step in the sterilization process. The chamber of the sterilizer must not be overloaded. The outer wraps of the packs should not touch the inner surface of the chamber. Steam will not be able to penetrate the packs effectively if they are crammed too tightly into the chamber.

"Flash" Sterilization

Flash sterilization is an abbreviated version of a regular sterilization cycle. Instruments sterilized by this method are not wrapped and are usually sterilized one or two instruments at a time. Special "flash sterilization" autoclaves are available, or the autoclaves just discussed can also be used to "flash-sterilize" individual, unwrapped instruments. The autoclave settings should be 272° F, 32 psi, and timed for 4 minutes. The conditioning phase is approximately 10 minutes, with a 4-minute sterilization phase. This is followed by a gravity exhaust of approximately 1 minute, then a 1-minute dry cycle. The dry cycle is shortened because no linen or paper was present for the steam to penetrate.

Typically, this process is used for individual instruments that have been dropped during surgery. Flash sterilization should not take the place of regular steam sterilization.

Ethylene Oxide (Gas) Sterilization

In the past a popular form of sterilization used ethylene oxide (EtO), a colorless gas at room temperature. EtO is a toxin that can cause skin and mucous membrane irritation, however, and it is therefore considered a health hazard and has fallen out of favor.

EtO penetrates paper and plastic film packaging without melting these materials. EtO destroys metabolic pathways in the cells and is capable of killing all microorganisms. Effective sterilization with EtO depends on the concentration of gas, exposure time, temperature, and relative humidity. Moisture is necessary for the lethal action of EtO, and optimal relative humidity for this type of sterilization is 40%. Exposure time varies from 48 minutes to several hours, but 3 to 4 hours of exposure is typically used when sterilizing at room temperature. After EtO sterilization, materials should be quarantined in a well-ventilated area for a minimum of 24 hours. The aeration time can be reduced to 4 hours with the use of aerators that vent the gas outside the work environment (Figure 10-10).

Plasma Sterilization

The three most common states of matter are solid, liquid, and gas. The fourth, plasma, often occurs in nature, as lightning and the aurora borealis (northern lights), for example. The plasma state of matter is produced through the action of a strong electric or magnetic field.

Low-temperature plasma sterilization with hydrogen peroxide (H_2O_2) gas is produced when the gas is stimulated under a deep vacuum with radiofrequency (RF) or microwave energy. The plasma system uses H_2O_2 to form the reactive components to kill microorganisms. After a liquid solution of H_2O_2 is vaporized in a chamber, RF energy is applied to create an electric field that then creates low-temperature gas plasma (Figure 10-11).

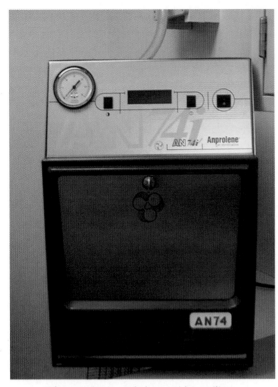

Figure 10-10   Ethylene oxide sterilizer.

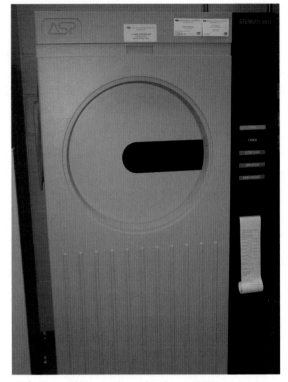

Figure 10-11   Plasma sterilizer.

Within the plasma, H_2O_2 is broken into reactive components, including hydroperoxy-free and hydroxyl-free radicals. These radicals interact with cell membranes, killing the microorganisms in the process. After the components lose their energy, they recombine to form harmless by-products of oxygen and water.

One limitation to gas plasma sterilization is that it cannot penetrate the walls of an instrument with a lumen, and thus the area within the lumen is not sterilized.

Sterilization Indicators

Chemical and biologic indicators help determine if items have been properly sterilized. *Chemical indicators* come in the form of strips or tape. Strips are placed inside the pack next to the instruments, whereas the tape is placed on the outside of the pack. The strips and tape will turn black if the conditions have taken place for sterilization. This does not mean that the instruments are sterile, but only that the conditions were met for sterilization to have occurred.

Biologic indicators, on the other hand, demonstrate that the sterilizer has met all the sterilization parameters. A vial of *Bacillus stearothermophilus* is typically placed in the sterilizer with the first load to be sterilized for the day. At the end of the sterilization cycle, the vial is removed and placed in an incubator for 24 hours and checked for microbial colony growth. The vial should demonstrate that all the microorganisms have been killed, providing reassurance that the sterilizer worked appropriately at that time.

SPECIALTY INSTRUMENT CLEANING

High-Level Disinfection

Cold sterilization is more of a high-level disinfection process than a true sterilization process. Cold sterilization is defined as the practice of immersing

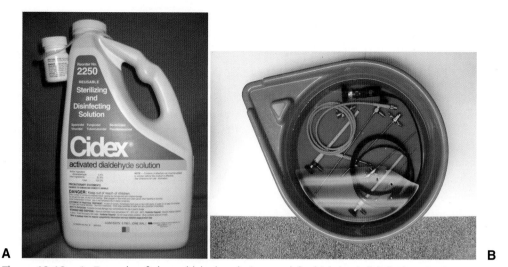

A **B**

Figure 10-12 **A,** Example of glutaraldehyde solution used for high-level disinfection. **B,** Instruments soaking in high-level disinfectant.

items in a disinfectant solution to reduce the level of contamination. Some instruments are cold-sterilized because they will not withstand repeated exposure to high-temperature steam sterilization. *Alcohol,* if used properly, exhibits strong bactericidal properties because of its ability to coagulate protein. Ethanol and isopropanol can be effective in a wide variety or applications. If used properly, alcohol solutions are effective against vegetative bacterial cells, including the bacterium that causes tuberculosis. However, alcohol cannot be relied on to kill bacterial spores or viruses and therefore should be used with caution.

Glutaraldehyde solution is considered a high-level disinfectant but not a sterilizing agent (Figure 10-12). Glutaraldehyde is bactericidal, tuberculocidal, and virucidal with an exposure time as short as 10 minutes. If exposure time is increased to several hours, the action is considered sporicidal. Prolonged exposure may adversely affect items made of rubber and plastic.

Drill Cleaning

Power drills (e.g., 3M's Mini and Max Drivers) are used in orthopedic surgery. Drills are not to be

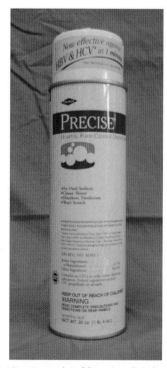

Figure 10-13 Example of foaming disinfectant used to disinfect power drills.

submerged in water or ultrasonically cleaned. They should be disassembled and inspected for any tissue or blood debris. If there is dried debris on the instrument, use a foam disinfectant cleaner (e.g., Precise) on the drill (Figure 10-13). Allow the foam to loosen the debris so that it can be removed with a clean, lint-free towel. The drill should then be wiped with a clean, lint-free cloth moistened with isopropyl alcohol. Generally, power drills are wrapped and autoclaved according to the manufacturer's instructions in preparation for their use in orthopedic surgery. Frequently, this involves doubling the standard sterilization time used for soft tissue instrument packs.

Endoscope Cleaning

Another specialty item that requires special care in its cleaning process is an endoscope. Items such as endoscopes undergo high-level disinfection rather than sterilization. Chapter 7 provides directions for leak-testing, cleaning, and disinfecting endoscopes.

KEY POINTS

1. Appropriate cleaning procedures begin with a thorough presoaking of instruments to rid the items of any blood or tissue.
2. Decontamination of instruments is vital in removing debris from the instrument's box locks and hinges.
3. Lubricants make instruments easier to open and close and help prevent the buildup of protein on the instruments.
4. Ultrasonic cleaning is a critical step in removing microbes from instruments.
5. Enzymes are used to assist in the breakdown of debris to allow more thorough ultrasonic cleaning of instruments.
6. Each instrument pack should contain a "recipe" that includes the types of instruments, quantity of each, type of wrapping material, manufacturers' guidelines, and any warranty.
7. Pack wraps are made of linen or paper and should have selective permeability, flexibility, memory, and resistance to damage.

8. Textile wraps are selected based on thread count (140-288 threads/in^2), not weight or texture.
9. Torn wraps repaired by stitching can allow an avenue for microbes to penetrate the pack, and patches can hamper steam penetration during sterilization; torn wraps should be discarded and replaced.
10. Steam indicator tape is used in securing wraps; a black stripping effect indicates that conditions were met for sterilization.
11. Guidelines for preparing a pack for sterilization address the items' condition, wrap material, standardization of contents, compatibility with autoclave, folding of soft items, use of similar wrapping methods, placement of indicator strips, and sealing of the outer pack.
12. Expiration dating may be used for packs with items that degrade over time (e.g., latex tubing).
13. Sterilization takes place after presoaking, decontaminating, and ultrasonic cleaning. The sterilization process rids the instruments of any living microbes.
14. Sterilization depends on three factors: proper sterilizer operation, proper pack preparation, and proper loading.
15. Gravity air-displacement sterilization is typically done on a tabletop. Steam enters the chamber by gravity and is set at a lower pressure.
16. High-vacuum sterilizers force steam into the sterilizer chamber for quicker penetration.
17. If a separate area is unavailable for proper pack preparation, this can be done in the preparation area for surgical personnel.
18. Flash sterilization is used for items dropped in the surgery suite.
19. Ethylene oxide is an excellent means to sterilize instruments and supplies wrapped in paper and plastic, but health and environmental risk factors have decreased its use over the years.
20. Plasma sterilization offers a safe technique for sterilization, but it is not an effective means of sterilizing items with lumens.
21. Chemical and biologic indicators determine if items have been properly sterilized. Biologic indicators show that the sterilizer has met all the sterilization parameters.
22. Alcohol exhibits strong bactericidal properties but may not kill spores or viruses. Glutaraldehyde

is considered a high-level disinfectant and is bactericidal, tuberculocidal, and virucidal.

23. Orthopedic drills should not be immersed in liquid and should be cleaned with a foaming disinfectant and alcohol before sterilization.

REVIEW QUESTIONS

1. What is the correct order of events used to achieve the level of disinfection required for surgical supplies and instruments?
   a. Decontaminate → sanitize → sterilize.
   b. Clean → sanitize → sterilize.
   c. Sterilize → sanitize → decontaminate.
   d. Sterilize → sanitize → clean.
   e. None of the above.

2. Basic cleaning of surgical instruments involves which order of the following steps?
   a. Presoaking → decontaminating → ultrasonic cleaning.
   b. Ultrasonic cleaning → rinsing → lubricating.
   c. Decontaminating → ultrasonic cleaning → presoaking.
   d. None of the above.

3. What is the purpose of presoaking?
   a. To scrub the instruments with mechanical cleaning.
   b. To prevent blood and other surgical debris from drying on the instruments.
   c. To soften blood and other surgical debris already dried on the instruments.
   d. Both b and c.
   e. All of the above.

4. What process involves manually cleaning surgical instruments in a detergent?
   a. Presoaking.
   b. Decontaminating.
   c. Sterilizing.
   d. All of the above.
   e. None of the above.

5. After ultrasonic cleaning, instruments:
   a. Are ready for sterilizing.
   b. Should be rinsed with distilled water.
   c. Should be individually inspected and towel-dried.
   d. Should be rinsed in tap water and air-dried.

6. *True* or *False:* Steam indicator tape is recommended when securing the wrapping material of an instrument pack.

7. *True* or *False:* Both the inner and the outer wraps of a surgical pack should be closed with steam indicator tape.

8. What are two methods used to identify how long a previously sterilized item is considered sterile?
   a. Expiration dating and event-related expiration of sterility.
   b. Double wrapping or single wrapping.
   c. Autoclaving or ethylene oxide sterilizing.
   d. Paper- or linen-wrapped packs.
   e. High-level disinfecting or gas plasma disinfecting.

9. Which of the following are acceptable ways to sterilize items for use in surgery?
   a. Gravity air-displacement autoclave.
   b. High-vacuum autoclave.
   c. Ethylene oxide unit.
   d. All of the above.
   e. None of the above.

10. What is an example of a chemical sterilization indicator?
    a. Steam indicator tape.
    b. Vial of *Bacillus stearothermophilus*.
    c. Both a and b.
    d. None of the above.

11. *True* or *False:* Power drills used in orthopedic surgery should not be submerged in liquids (high-level disinfectants) or cleaned in ultrasonic units.

12. *True* or *False:* Endoscopes are routinely submerged in high-level disinfectants rather than steam-sterilized.

ANSWERS

1. b
2. a
3. d
4. b
5. b
6. True
7. False
8. a

9. d
10. a
11. True
12. True

BIBLIOGRAPHY

Adler S, Scherrer M, Daschner FD: Cost of low temperature plasma sterilization compared with other sterilization methods, *J Hosp Infect* 40(2):125, 1998.

Blankenau R: Shedding light on flash sterilization, *Mater Manag Health Care* 3(12):32, 1994.

Carlile F: Sterilization or disinfection: that is the question, *Surg Technologist* 27(11):8, 1995.

Detwiler MS: Ultrasonic cleaning in the hospital, *J Healthc Mater Manage* 7(3):46, 1989.

Frey KB: The new alternative: plasma sterilization, *Surg Technologist* 26(9):8, 1994.

Harrison SK et al: Cleaning and decontaminating medical instruments, *J Healthc Mater Manage* 8(1):36, 1990.

Klapes NA et al: Effects of long term storage on sterile status of devices in surgical packs, *Infect Control* 8:289, 1987.

Lind D: Steam sterilization, *J Healthc Mater Manage* 12(11):56, 1994.

Lind N: Cleaning in decontamination, *J Healthc Mater Manage* 12(4):48, 1994.

Mathias JM: Draft guideline on processing practices, *OR Manager* 18(6):7, 2002.

O'Connor LM: Event-related sterility assurance, *Surg Technologist* 26:8, 1994.

Reichert M, Schultz JK: Coping with drills and other powered equipment, *OR Manager* 18(11):21, 2002.

Reichert M, Schultz JK: When and how to use ultrasonic cleaning, *OR Manager* 14(2):20, 1998.

Simmons BL: Fundamentals of cleaning: the effects of water and detergents, *J Sterile Serv Manage* 5(1):16, 1987.

Thro E: Surgical instruments: their care and characteristics, *J OR Res Inst* 3(9):3, 1983.

CHAPTER 11

Client Education for Postoperative Care

Gail Hartman

LEARNING OBJECTIVES

After studying this chapter, the reader should be able to do the following:

- Provide instructions to the owner describing the proper care of a patient after general anesthesia.
- Provide instructions to the client describing proper care of a patient with postoperative drains.
- Describe client education for postoperative care of a patient with a bandage, splint, or cast.
- Provide instructions to the owner describing proper care of a patient after the following

surgical procedures:
  Tooth extraction
  Gastrointestinal surgery
  Feeding tube placement
  Cystotomy
  Declaw
  Orthopedic surgery
  Aural hematoma
  Ear canal resection or ablation
  Cesarean section

DISCHARGE INSTRUCTIONS

When the surgical patient is ready to go home, the owner (client) must be taught how to care for the animal properly. The responsibility for explaining the patient's aftercare to the owner is often assigned to the veterinary technician. This is a logical policy because the technician has been the postoperative caregiver and understands the patient's needs and reactions. Every patient cannot be treated in the same manner. The approach to providing the prescribed treatments is dictated by the patient's reaction and willingness to cooperate. The veterinary technician assigned to care for the patient has determined which restraint

techniques work, what method to use to administer oral medication, and how effective the analgesic drugs have been for the patient. Areas to discuss with the client include timing of drug administration, wound care, and daily walks. For example, antibiotics and analgesics may be administered with a meal. The wound care should be delayed for about an hour after the analgesic is given. This technician knows the patient, can advocate for the patient, and can best educate the owner on how to care for the patient.

Written instructions explaining how to care for the postoperative patient should be sent home with the client. The hospital often has generic instructions that are prepared for all routine postoperative patients. Special instructions will be added for certain nonroutine surgical procedures or medical conditions. However, each patient is an individual, and each client appreciates and deserves an explanation of the specific observations of the pet's reactions and the specific care techniques used. The veterinary technician personally discharging the pet to its owner can provide this communication. It is best to explain the discharge instructions in a quiet area of the clinic. The client's full attention needs to be directed to the technician's instructions, so the animal should not be brought to the client until all the information has been provided. Alternatively, the veterinary technician can write out special instructions and add these to the generic instructions (Figure 11-1).

GENERAL POSTANESTHESIA INSTRUCTIONS

All patients that have been under sedation or general anesthesia should go home with instructions regarding their care for at least the first 24 hours. The instruction sheet should address (1) confinement, (2) feeding, (3) medications, (4) signs of possible adverse reactions, and (5) how to reach the hospital or 24-hour emergency clinic.

The client may need to confine the pet to a recovery crate or room. The pet may still be sedated and unable to walk normally. The pet may need to be accompanied or carried up and down stairs. Other pets in the household may disturb the patient, and it may be preferable to have the patient isolated from other animal housemates for a specified time. Over the long term it may be necessary to keep cats inside and to walk dogs only with a leash.

The owner needs instructions regarding when and how much to feed the animal after returning home. The time to resume the normal feeding schedule should also be addressed. Special diets may be prescribed and may be introduced gradually. Specific instructions regarding the special diet should be written in the space provided on the postoperative form.

Medications may be sent home with the patient. Specific instructions regarding their administration are written on the label of the medication bottle. The instructions are repeated on the discharge instructions with more details, including whether the medication should be administered with food or on an empty stomach. In addition, the necessity of giving one medication at a separate time from other medications can be explained to the owner at discharge. Also, possible side effects of the medication should be addressed.

Animals under anesthesia or sedation may experience undesirable side effects. Gastrointestinal motility may be slowed down (ileus), which may cause inappetence, vomiting, constipation, or bloating. Lethargy, ataxia, or depression may be symptoms of prolonged recovery from anesthesia. These symptoms should be discussed with the client or listed on the instruction sheet. The informed owner will be an observant advocate for the patient.

Finally, instructions should be clearly provided regarding how to reach the hospital or a referral emergency center 24 hours a day.

GENERAL POSTSURGICAL INSTRUCTIONS

In addition to the postoperative instructions already mentioned, the client is instructed on the need to observe the patient's surgical site. The integrity of the surgical site should be monitored at least twice daily. The number of sutures should be counted. The client should observe for swelling, redness, and discharge. If sutures are missing or if excessive swelling, discharge, or redness is noted, the owner should be instructed to call the veterinary hospital. The owner is encouraged to call for advice regarding the management of the patient and any changes involving the surgical site.

Specific instructions on confining the pet should be discussed with the owner. Each situation is unique, and residences vary, for example, in the presence and number of stairs to the outside. Other pets in the household may necessitate new routines regarding feeding, litter boxes, and walks outside. Children may need to be restricted from handling the pet until the patient is fully recovered. During the pet's recuperative phase at home,

DISCHARGE INSTRUCTIONS
Elsewhere Veterinary Clinic
123 Street Road
Somewhere, USA
123-555-1234

Client name:_____ Patient's name: _____

Date admitted: _____ Date discharged: _____

Procedure or diagnosis: _____

Medications:
- ☐ None dispensed
- ☐ Dispensed—directions on medication bottle
- ☐ Start medication _____

Food and water:
- ☐ Only offer ___ cup water and _____ food today
- ☐ Offer normal meal tonight
- ☐ Normal feeding may resume _____

  Special diet _____

Exercise:
- ☐ Restrict running, jumping, playing until _____
- ☐ If cat, confine indoors for _____ days
- ☐ If dog, leash walk only for _____ days

Sutures:
- ☐ Discourage your pet from licking or chewing at incision site.

  If excessive licking or chewing occurs, please call the clinic for a collar to prevent this.

- ☐ Check the incision daily for swelling, redness, or discharge.

  If it appears irritated, swollen, or bleeding please notify us.

- ☐ **Please make an appointment for suture removal in ____ days.**

- ☐ Sutures are absorbable and do not need to be removed.

- ☐ No sutures.

Please notify the clinic if any of the following occur:

- ☐ Loss of appetite for more than ____ days
- ☐ Pain
- ☐ Straining to urinate/defecate
- ☐ Excess drainage from incision
- ☐ Excessive vomiting/diarrhea
- ☐ Depression

*Special instructions: _____
_____
_____
_____
_____

Emergency clinic numbers:_____

Veterinarian's signature: _____

Figure 11-1   Example of general postoperative instructions for clients (owners) after a veterinary patient's discharge.

the family's routines and lifestyle will be disrupted, which can be stressful. If possible, before leaving the hospital, dates are scheduled for rechecks, suture removal, and drain removal.

Postoperative Care of Patients with Drains

Many surgical procedures involve the implanting of drains. These devices are temporarily placed to channel unwanted fluid or gas from a wound or body cavity. Often the patient is sent home with a passive drain. The owner is required to clean the discharge from the drain site and ensure that the drain is not disturbed by the patient. Clear and detailed instructions regarding drain care are important.

The owner needs a demonstration as well as written instructions regarding the care of the surgical site with the drain. Warm soaks to loosen and remove dried serous discharge will be necessary (Figure 11-2). The skin may need to be protected from the development of a moist dermatitis caused by contact with the discharge. A thin film of petroleum jelly can be spread over the area where the discharge tends to dry to the skin. The petrolatum serves as a protective barrier and facilitates skin cleaning.

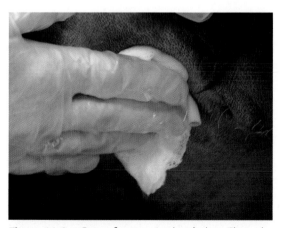

Figure 11-2   Care of postoperative drains. Clean the area where the drain exits the wound with a warm compress of gauze. Apply warm soaks to the area to soften the discharge. Once the discharge is soft and loose, the area is wiped clean.

Inadequate cleaning of discharge can prevent the drain from functioning and block further discharge. Fluid then becomes trapped under the wound or body cavity. This will slow the healing process or compromise a successful outcome in other ways. The veterinary technician must emphasize to the client the importance of proper and thorough cleaning of the drain site.

The client also requires instructions about effective restraint of the pet while the drain is being cleaned. The technician who has been caring for the patient knows the most effective means to restrain the patient safely and effectively. If possible, this technician should be present when the patient is discharged. These "customized" instructions can be written on the discharge information form in the area for special instructions.

If the pet pulls out the drain, the owner should report this to the clinic. The owner should search for any parts or pieces of the drain. These pieces can help the veterinary technician determine if a portion of the drain is still in the patient. If a piece of the drain remains deep in the wound or body cavity, it will need to be surgically retrieved.

Postoperative Care of Patients with a Bandage, Splint, or Cast

When a bandage, splint, or cast has been applied to a limb, the pet should be kept quiet. Cats are confined indoors and restricted from jumping. Dogs may need to be confined in a recovery crate. Play with other dogs and humans in the household must be suspended. Dogs are walked only by leash.

The owner is instructed to examine the pet carefully each day, making the following observations:

1. *Position of bandage.* Check to be sure that the bandage, cast, or splint has not slipped or shifted.
2. *Irritation of adjacent skin.* Check the skin adjacent to the edge of the bandage, cast, or splint by parting the fur and looking for redness or feeling for moisture.
3. *Discoloration of bandage.* The bandage, cast, or splint can become discolored because of

staining from wetness on the outside or discharge soaking through from the inside.

4. *Moisture.* A wet bandage, cast, or splint should be replaced immediately.

5. *Odor.* A foul odor associated with the bandage, cast, or splint may be caused by infectious discharge.

6. *Signs of chewing on bandage.* Torn areas of tape or spots of discoloration or moisture are telltale signs of chewing. The patient chewing at the bandage, splint, or cast may have discomfort or pain. Replacement of the bandage (splint, cast) may be necessary, and an Elizabethan collar may be needed for the animal.

The owner is given instructions regarding how to protect the cast, bandage, or splint from wet grass, snow, puddles, and other sources of moisture. A plastic bag taped to the limb can effectively cover and protect the bandage (cast, splint) while the pet is outside. The bag should be removed as soon as the pet is back inside. Empty fluid bags are made of heavy plastic that holds up well to repeated use.

POSTOPERATIVE INSTRUCTIONS FOR COMMON PROCEDURES

Dental Extraction

While the mouth is healing after a tooth extraction, the pet will have a soft-food diet, such as canned, semimoist pet food or dry food soaked in water until mushy. The socket will heal in 1 to 2 weeks. During the healing phase the pet may be gradually returned to its usual dry-food diet.

The client should watch for a number of specific signs. For the first day the owner may see the water in the bowl tinged red after the pet drinks. If this does not subside, the veterinarian should be notified. Long-term bleeding from the mouth indicates delayed healing, infection, or a coagulation problem. The pet rubbing or pawing at its face is an indication of pain, and the veterinarian should be notified. Crying out while eating, or refusing to eat any hard food after several days to

weeks have passed, indicates an ongoing problem. The patient that refuses to eat will not heal promptly or properly.

Feeding Tube Placement

An enteral feeding tube may be placed for many reasons to aid in the patient's nutritional support. This tube may stay in place for many weeks. Because of the critical support the feeding tube provides and the possible long-term need for the tube, the client caring for the patient at home requires detailed instructions on the tube's use and care, including the following:

1. When cleaning the area where the tube exits the skin, warm water soaks may be needed to soften any dried discharge. The discharge may be clear or slightly red tinged. Thick, cloudy, or foul-smelling discharge may indicate an infection at the site. Adding an antiseptic cleanser, such as chlorhexidine at a 1:40 dilution, helps kill microbial invaders. An antiseptic ointment can be applied, and the site is covered with a light bandage or stockinette. The end of the feeding tube should be incorporated in the bandage. The skin site should be inspected and cleaned one or two times daily.

2. During inspection of the tube, a measurement should be taken to ensure that the tube is the same length. If the tube length has changed, the tube has migrated. The tube is at continuous risk of being pulled out either by the pet chewing and tugging at it or, more gradually, by the bandage shifting and becoming tangled with the tube. An Elizabethan collar helps prevent the patient from pulling out the tube with its teeth.

3. Before and after each feeding, the tube is flushed with warm water. The end of the tube is securely plugged between feedings.

4. If the tube becomes clogged, instilling carbonated water (soft drinks, soda) repeatedly into the tube will eventually dislodge most obstructions. If the owner is unable to open the tube in this way, the veterinarian must be notified.

5. In regard to feeding, the veterinarian will have calculated the exact dietary amount that will be administered at each feeding. Commercially prepared liquid diets (e.g., CliniCare, Jevity) are mandated when the tube has a very small diameter. Gastric and esophageal tubes are often large enough in diameter that pureed canned pet foods can be used in larger patients. It is important that large chunks of food be eliminated during preparation and not be forced down the tube.
6. Liquid medications may be administered through the feeding tube. Flushing with warm water is necessary before and after medication administration as well as feeding.
7. The patient should also have food available to eat during the day. As soon as the patient is eating on its own and able to maintain its caloric needs, the feeding tube can be pulled.

Gastrointestinal Enterotomy or Anastomosis

Surgery of the gastrointestinal (GI) tract is indicated to remove foreign body obstructions, collect tissue biopsy samples, remove growths, and resect diseased areas of intestine (e.g., cancer, necrosis, intussusception). Fluid therapy is continued until the animal is drinking and not vomiting. Feeding is resumed after the animal is able to consume water without vomiting. This is usually 24 hours after surgery. Prophylactic antibiotic therapy is typically discontinued within hours postoperatively.

Animals recovering from GI surgery need to be observed with great care. If the intestinal surgical site does not hold and intestinal contents leak into the abdominal cavity, a serious infection will ensue. This complication, *peritonitis,* can occur within hours or days after surgery. Peritonitis is an extremely painful condition that responds only slightly to analgesics. The patient will also have a fever, so postoperative monitoring of body temperature is important. If the patient spikes a fever, laboratory procedures (e.g., complete blood count, CBC) may be ordered. As peritonitis progresses, fluid will accumulate in the abdominal cavity, and the patient will appear bloated. An abdominocentesis procedure may be performed

to obtain a culture sample, and abdominal ultrasound may be helpful in diagnosing peritonitis.

The owner should be instructed to monitor the patient closely for the following signs:

1. Check the abdominal incision daily for redness, swelling, discharge, and tenderness.
2. Monitor the pet's temperature twice daily, if possible. If a fever is detected, the hospital should be notified.
3. Alert the hospital if vomiting, diarrhea, constipation, or inappetence occurs.
4. Alert the hospital if the patient appears unusually lethargic or in excessive pain.
5. Alert the hospital if the patient appears bloated.

Two other postoperative concerns may not appear for weeks or months. First, the intestinal lumen may narrow due to scar formation. Second, a small, slow leak from the enterotomy site can lead to an abdominal abscess. Both complications may cause clinical signs associated with an obstruction. If an abdominal abscess has formed, clinical signs include vomiting, anorexia, lack of bowel movements, and abdominal pain.

Perianal Surgery

Surgery around and involving the anus is indicated for removal of tumors, debridement and drainage of fistulas and anal sacs, and removal of anal sacs. In addition to the general postsurgical instructions, special instructions include the following:

1. A special diet high in fiber may be prescribed to keep the stools soft. The diet may or may not be a permanent change.
2. Stool softeners such as lactulose may be prescribed for short-term therapy.
3. If diarrhea occurs, the veterinary hospital should be notified. Discontinue the stool softener, and clean the surgical site by flushing thoroughly with warm tap water. Do not scrub the site.
4. Observe the pet while passing a bowel movement. If the pet is straining or crying in pain, the veterinary hospital should be

notified. Fecal incontinence also warrants hospital contact.

Cystotomy

One major concern following bladder surgery is bladder distension. To prevent the bladder from becoming overly distended, the patient needs to be able to and allowed to empty its bladder frequently. Postoperative instructions for the owner of a pet with a procedure involving surgical incision of the bladder (cystotomy) include the following:

1. Expect bloody urine (hematuria) for 12 to 36 hours. The amount of blood in the urine should diminish as time passes. The owner can monitor the color of the urine by lining the litter box with a white paper towel or placing a white paper towel under the pet when it urinates. Blood in the urine is more easily observed when soaked into a white paper towel.
2. A special diet may be prescribed. Instructions may recommend a gradual change to the new diet by mixing the previous and new diets together for several days.
3. Antibiotic therapy may be prescribed. The choice of antibiotic may change on receiving the results of the urine culture and sensitivity test.
4. The dog should be walked outside frequently, and the amount and color of the urine should be monitored. Having the dog urinate on a white paper towel is helpful.
5. If the pet is straining to urinate or exhibiting pain when urinating, the hospital should be notified.
6. If the pet is not passing urine, it should be immediately examined. This is an emergency. Stones remaining in the bladder or blood clots in the bladder can cause obstructions.

Feline Declaw (Onychectomy)

Client instructions after an onychectomy, or declaw procedure, include the following for the feline patient:

1. Shredded paper, dried beans, or a pelleted paper product replaces clay or clumping litter.

The paper litter is less likely to leave foreign material in the surgical sites. If the paper sticks to the surgical wounds, it is easily seen and removed.
2. The cat should be restricted from jumping and running. This may mean "crating" the cat during the recuperative period.
3. If swelling of a toe is noted or the cat is non–weight bearing on one paw, the hospital should be notified.
4. Bleeding from the toes is not expected postoperatively. The hospital should be notified if bleeding from the toes occurs.
5. The cat should be kept inside for the remainder of its life.

Orthopedic Procedures

The client with a pet that underwent orthopedic surgery should receive postoperative instructions that include the following:

1. The pet will need to be confined. Dogs are walked only by leash. Cats must stay indoors during the recuperative period. Excessive activity and exercise can slow the healing process by allowing weight bearing too early or causing excessive movement of the affected joint or fracture site.
2. Dogs especially may need help standing and walking. A bath towel can be placed under the abdomen or chest to act as a sling (Figure 11-3).
3. If a bandage or cast has been applied, the owner receives specific instructions regarding its care (see earlier discussion).
4. If the patient has an external fixation device, the stainless steel pins and connecting pieces need particular attention, as follows:
   • The site where the pin exits the skin will not heal while the pin is in place. Dried discharge is cleaned from the area once or twice daily as needed. An antimicrobial ointment can be applied to the skin around the exit site.
   • The connecting pieces are covered with tape to prevent sharp edges from catching on furniture or the opposite limb.

Aural Hematoma

The major postoperative instructions for the client caring for a pet after surgery for aural hematoma are as follows:

1. The area where the drain exits the pinna needs to be cleaned of discharge. Warm water and a clean face towel or gauze work well. The drains usually stay in for 2 to 3 weeks (Figure 11-4).
2. Some animals may also need to have an infected ear canal treated with topical drops and ear cleansers. The pinna may be sore to the touch, so take extra care when instilling medication into the ear canal.
3. Some patients may have their head wrapped in a bandage. The same observations outlined earlier for extremity bandages apply to head bandages. Watch for soiling, slipping, moisture, foul odor, and skin irritation along the edges of the bandage.

Lateral Ear Canal Resection or Ablation

The ear canal is ablated, or surgically removed, when it is so chronically diseased that medical treatment is unable to establish a healthy canal.

This surgery is a last resort. The theory is that if the diseased part is removed, the pain and discomfort will disappear. Part or all of the ear canal can be removed. If the entire ear canal is removed, the pet may be rendered deaf in that ear.

The pet is usually not released to the owner's care until the need for daily bandage changes has passed and all drains have been removed. Postoperative infection may be caused by preexisting disease or contamination during surgery. Facial nerve paralysis is a well-recognized complication that usually resolves within 2 weeks. In some patients the vestibular system can be adversely affected when the entire ear canal is ablated. In these cases the pet exhibits a head tilt, nystagmus, and difficulty walking. Overall, many complications may occur, and intensive nursing care in the hospital setting is needed for a variable time after ear canal resection or ablation surgery.

The patient typically will try to scratch at the surgical site. An Elizabethan collar is an important piece of equipment used to help protect the integrity of the surgical site. Postoperative pain often drives the pet to self-trauma. Lateral ear canal resection or ear canal ablation tends to be very painful. Administration of analgesic medication and close observation of the surgical site are the owner's primary directives.

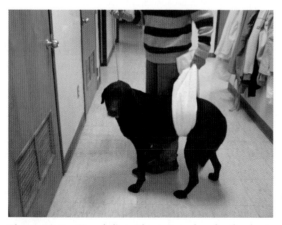

Figure 11-3   Towel sling. Place a towel under the dog's abdomen. Pull up with one or both arms. The towel sling takes some of the weight off the dog's hind end, allowing the dog to walk more easily.

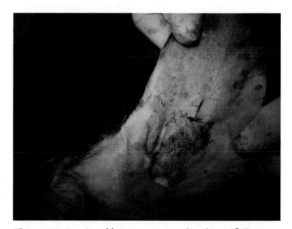

Figure 11-4   Aural hematoma repair using soft Penrose drain.

Cesarean Section

The mother and newborns are kept apart until all have completely recovered from anesthesia. The neonates are at risk of being crushed if introduced to a mother that is still heavily sedated or ataxic. Even when fully recovered, the mother may reject the newborns. The staff must watch the mother carefully for any sign of aggression toward the neonates.

The newborns should be weighed at least once daily. Each one should be steadily gaining weight every day. If any newborn is not gaining weight, it should have extra time by itself on the mammary glands. If the newborn is not nursing, the owner should be shown how to supplement the neonate's feeding with milk replacer (e.g., KMR, Esbilac).

The mother's surgical incision is at risk of irritation and injury from the mother licking or the newborns suckling. The owner should inspect the incision daily. A bloody, mucous discharge is expected from the vulva for several days post-surgically. The color of the discharge may change from red to brown as the days pass. A foul odor to the discharge is not normal, and the hospital should be notified.

It is common for the new mother to have loose stools after giving birth. The mother's appetite should be good. It is important that the new mother have plenty of high-calorie food because she must eat enough for herself and all her offspring. The new mother that is not eating will not heal promptly and cannot produce enough milk to feed the newborns.

The owner should be shown how to express milk from each mammary gland to check it for milk production and color and consistency. *Colostrum* (the first milk, generally rich in antibodies) is usually slightly yellow and sticky. After the newborns have nursed for approximately 24 hours, the milk becomes thinner and whiter. If the mammary glands stop releasing milk or become painful or red, or if the milk is thick or discolored (any color other than white), the owner must contact the veterinarian. The mother will need to be treated, and the newborns will need to be fed milk replacer. The veterinary technician often must instruct clients on how to bottle-feed or tube-feed the newborns.

Pet supply stores carry milk replacers for puppies and kittens. Bottles with nipples of appropriate size for the newborn should be purchased at the same time. Milk replacers come in canned as well as powdered forms. In *Veterinary Pediatrics: Dogs and Cats from Birth to Six Months,* Hoskins discusses the many options for supplementing the feeding of newborns. The reader is referred to this excellent reference and to Chapter 7 in this text for more details.

KEY POINTS

1. As the primary caregiver in the hospital setting, the veterinary technician is the best team member to discharge the patient to the owner's care.
2. Instructions for all postanesthesia patients address confinement, feeding, medication, possible adverse reactions, and hospital contact information.
3. The client should receive written instructions as well as a demonstration of cleaning steps for passive drains.
4. Patients with a bandage, cast, or splint need to be strictly confined. The owner needs to understand the importance of this measure.
5. The owner needs to report any change in the appearance or position of the bandage, splint, or cast to the veterinary hospital.
6. Within a week the patient that has undergone one to several tooth extractions should be pain free, and the tooth sockets should be almost healed.
7. Feeding tubes may be needed for several weeks, so the owner must care for the tube properly.
8. To assess the necessity of maintaining the feeding tube, the patient must have food available when it is ready to eat.
9. The patient exhibiting unrelenting pain hours to days after gastrointestinal surgery most likely has peritonitis.
10. The heavier and older the cat, the longer it will take for the cat to recover from declaw surgery. Confining the cat to an indoor lifestyle is imperative after onychectomy.

11. Insufficient confinement of the patient after an orthopedic procedure is the most common reason for delayed healing.
12. The bladder of the patient recovering from a cystotomy should be kept small by allowing the patient to void every few hours.
13. After aural hematoma surgery, passive drains usually remain in place for several weeks. The pinna may heal with scar tissue and significant wrinkling.
14. The patient recovering from a cesarean section must heal and also raise a litter. The newborns' feeding may need to be supplemented with milk replacer.

REVIEW QUESTIONS

1. Which of the following statements is *true* regarding postoperative, at-home nursing care?
   a. The general principles are the same regardless of what specific surgery was performed, such that every patient can be treated exactly the same when it leaves the hospital.
   b. Only the veterinarian who performed the surgery should explain postoperative nursing care to the owners at discharge.
   c. The veterinary technician knows the patient, can advocate for the patient, and can educate the owner regarding what postoperative techniques work the best for that specific animal.
   d. Well-written instructions make verbal discharge instructions unnecessary.
   e. It is best to have the patient in the examination room when discharge instructions are given to the owner.
2. Which of the following may be clinical signs of prolonged recovery from anesthesia?
   a. Lethargy.
   b. Ataxia.
   c. Depression.
   d. Both a and b.
   e. All of the above.
3. How often should the surgical site be observed once the patient is discharged to the owners?
   a. Once daily.
   b. Twice daily, as a minimum.
   c. Twice daily, as a maximum.
   d. Continuously.
   e. The surgical site does not need to be observed after the patient leaves the hospital, because the patient would not be released if this were necessary.
4. When checking the surgical site, which of the following should be noted?
   a. The number of sutures.
   b. Any swelling.
   c. Any redness or discharge from the incision.
   d. All of the above.
   e. None of the above.
5. Serous discharge tends to accumulate where a surgical drain exits the skin. What can be done to prevent this accumulation from occluding the drainage site and thereby preserve the intended function of the drain?
   a. Application of warm soaks around the exit site.
   b. Application of a thin film of petroleum jelly.
   c. Suturing the drain exit site closed.
   d. Both a and b.
   e. All of the above.
6. *True* or *False:* When a dog has a bandage, splint, or cast on a limb, it should be walked only by leash.
7. If a feeding tube becomes clogged, which of the following techniques usually resolves most occlusions?
   a. Instilling carbonated water into the tube.
   b. Instilling cold water.
   c. Instilling distilled water.
   d. Instilling coffee.
   e. Instilling IV fluids through the tube.
8. Which of the following may occur after an intestinal resection and anastomosis?
   a. Peritonitis.
   b. Narrowing of the intestinal lumen at the anastomosis site.
   c. Slow leak from the anastomosis site leading to an abdominal abscess.
   d. All of the above.
   e. Both b and c.
9. How long should hematuria be expected following a cystotomy?
   a. No longer than 12 hours.
   b. No longer than 24 hours.
   c. Up to 36 hours.
   d. Weeks after surgery.

e. Any hematuria following a cystotomy is abnormal, and the veterinarian should be alerted immediately.

10. Why should the typical clay, clumping cat litter be avoided for the first few weeks after a declaw procedure?

    a. Most cats refuse to use clumping litter after a declaw.

    b. Most cats are so clean that they refuse to use clay litter after a declaw.

    c. The clay granules tend to stick to the surgical site and can become embedded in the healing wound, leading to pain and infection.

    d. This litter is too expensive.

    e. None of the above.

11. What is another name for a declaw procedure?

    a. Orchidectomy.

    b. Onychectomy.

    c. Osteotomy.

    d. Oclawotomy.

    e. None of the above.

12. Which of the following statements regarding ear canal ablations is *true*?

    a. Postoperative infection may occur.

    b. Facial nerve paralysis is a common complication that usually resolves within 2 weeks.

    c. Head tilt, nystagmus, and difficulty walking are signs of a compromised vestibular system.

    d. All of the above.

    e. None of the above.

13. Which of the following statements regarding postoperative care of cesarean section patients is *true*?

    a. The veterinary technician should show the owner how to express milk from each mammary gland.

b. It is important that the mother eat a high-calorie diet while nursing the newborns.

c. A bloody, mucous vaginal discharge is to be expected for several days.

d. All of the above.

e. Both a and b.

ANSWERS

1. c
2. e
3. b
4. d
5. d
6. True
7. a
8. d
9. c
10. c
11. b
12. d
13. d

BIBLIOGRAPHY

Hoskins JD: *Veterinary pediatrics: dogs and cats from birth to six months,* ed 3, Philadelphia, 2001, Saunders.

McCurnin DM, Bassert JM: *Clinical textbook for veterinary technicians,* ed 5, Philadelphia, 2002, Saunders.

Praft PW: *Principles and practice of veterinary technology,* St Louis, 1998, Mosby.

PART IV

High-Volume Spay/Neuter Clinics

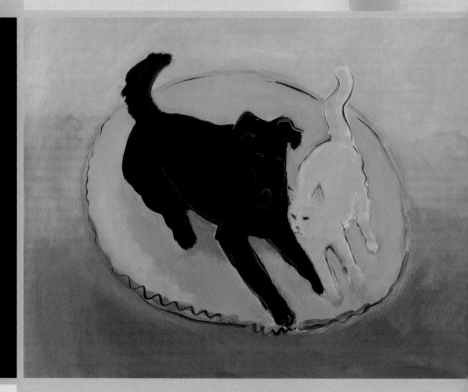

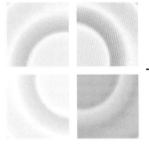

CHAPTER 12

Spay/Neuter Clinics: The Patients, Facilities, Need, and Process

James Q. Knight, Nancy Shaffran

LEARNING OBJECTIVES

After studying this chapter, the reader should be able to do the following:

- Recognize and identify the types of patients serviced by high-volume spay/neuter facilities: (1) feral cats, (2) shelter animals, (3) animals of financially fragile people, (4) animals belonging to collectors and hoarders, and (5) juvenile patients.
- Better understand the types of facilities that perform high-volume sterilization surgery, including stationary facilities, mobile surgical vans, and multi-site clinics.
- Articulate the similarities and differences between sterilization surgeries done in general practice and in high-volume settings.

- Identify the need for a high-volume sterilization service.
- Describe the special anesthesia, surgical, and postoperative considerations for the various types of patients usually seen in high-volume facilities.
- Identify the disease concerns in sterilized patients.
- Address special concerns regarding high-volume facilities and their patients, animal caretakers, staff, and the community.
- Identify and promote volunteer opportunities involving high-volume spay/neuter facilities and programs.

DEFINING THE PATIENT

Feral Cats

Although the exact numbers are unknown, many experts believe that the population of feral cats is beginning to approach that of pet cats in the United States. Because the compliance rate for spaying and neutering is much higher with pet cats, feral cats are the greatest contributor to the overpopulation of cats.

Cats can be categorized by the following descriptions:

- *Free roaming* refers to a cat that is not confined to a house or other enclosure.
- *Feral* refers to a cat that is too poorly socialized to be handled and that cannot be placed into a typical pet home; a subpopulation of free-roaming cats.
- *Abandoned* refers to a free-roaming cat that may be tame but that does not currently have an owner.

- *Stray* refers to a currently or recently owned cat that may be lost; it is usually well socialized but may become wary over time. A stray cat's kittens may be feral.

As can be seen by these definitions, a cat can be born feral or become feral because of circumstances beyond its control. These creatures, in any setting, are easily stressed by outside factors. In a veterinary medical care setting, handling, medical procedures, and inadvertent pain are additional factors that greatly increase the stress level of feral cats. To reduce this psychological stress when feral cats are in a high-volume surgical facility, veterinary technicians must take extra measures, such as covering the carriers, cages, and traps with towels or blankets to reduce visual stimuli; limiting handling and eye contact; and maintaining a quiet, peaceful environment. Physiologically, beyond the basic medical needs of cats in general, minimizing stress in feral cats also supports immune system function and helps promote healing through increased appetite and food intake, lower caloric requirements, and reduced obsession with the incision.

Shelter Animals

Generally, high-volume spay/neuter facilities treat only dogs and cats. Shelters are usually on a low, fixed budget dependent on adoption fees and donations and thus are frequent users of this surgical service. Because cost is an issue, the typical dog or cat presented from a shelter to a high-volume spay/neuter facility is already adopted or preselected as an adoptable animal. The typical adopting agency may range from a small, private rescue group (purebred rescue group or private individuals who do charitable adoptions of strays), to municipal animal control officers, to large shelters who do not have on-site surgical facilities. Occasionally, because of overloads, even large shelters with on-site veterinary services will need the additional help of a high-volume surgical facility.

Normally the needs of the shelter patient have been identified by the admitting shelter through medical examinations, behavioral and temperament testing, and evaluation, as well as the patient's history obtained from the surrendering party of a previously owned animal. Stress can play an important role for these patients as well.

Animals of Financially Fragile People

Some people are unable to pay for full-service veterinary care. Others decide, for whatever reason, that the cost of surgical sterilization is beyond their budget. Often the financial hardship is real (e.g., elderly retired person on fixed income, single parent who has lost job), or the person has too many animals to care for properly. Regardless of the societal issues involved, many animals are not sterilized because of the owner's real or perceived financial hardship. Many charitable organizations have special funds to disperse to financially needy people for spaying and neutering, but it is often necessary to put the needs of the patient and the community before the typical remuneration of the veterinary surgeon.

Animals Belonging to Collectors and Hoarders

Perhaps no situation in veterinary medicine, public health, and society in general is more shocking, disgusting, confusing, and frustrating than that of animal collectors and hoarders. News footage and newspaper headlines often describe these situations as animal "abuse" or "neglect," but it is not that simple. Often the collectors believe they are performing a great service for the animals or birds, saving them and providing a home and care.

Planned, sustained, and compassionate intervention is key to providing these animals with the help they need. Surgical sterilization can play a vital role in the intervention plan. The animal's needs become obvious once the situation is evaluated. Mobilizing available resources is extremely important because it often becomes a multidisciplinary issue. The veterinary professional fills only one of the roles in solving the problem.

Many websites and printed resources are available on animal hoarding and collecting, and the reader is encouraged to learn more about this situation.

Juvenile Patients

For more than 30 years the veterinary profession has been doing early-age surgical sterilization to help combat pet overpopulation. This trend is on the rise. Generally defined as a puppy or kitten 8 weeks or older and 2 pounds or more, the *juvenile patient* is usually presented to high-volume spay/neuter clinics by shelters, feral cat caretakers, or dealers involved with hoarders or collectors. Historically, the rate of adopted animals being surgically altered after adoption and before they reproduced was not high enough, which merely added to the pet overpopulation. Early-age sterilization, before the puppy or kitten goes to its adoptive home, helps avoid an accidental litter.

Although still somewhat controversial in the veterinary profession, juvenile surgical sterilization has gained wide acceptance, especially in the shelter industry, and has proved to be a good control measure for the prevention of pet overpopulation. The particular needs of the juvenile patient are discussed later.

Types of facilities

Stationary Facilities

Stationary high-volume sterilization facilities can range from two- or three-room buildings with a combined surgical and preparation area to modern surgical suites that incorporate state-of-the-art equipment and supplies. These facilities are usually run by not-for-profit organizations that depend on grants and donations for funding and on volunteers for the labor force. A smaller percentage of high-volume facilities are for profit, but still low cost.

One example of a stationary facility is the Luke and Lily Lerner Spay and Neuter Clinic at Tufts University School of Veterinary Medicine. In 2002, Tufts and the Massachusetts Animal Coalition (MAC) collaborated to establish and develop a modern surgical facility that would serve as a surgical training laboratory for veterinary students and help ensure that shelter animals are sterilized before adoption. During part of the school year, students receive surgical training by using shelter animals selected for adoption. On days not scheduled for student use, including the balance of the year, MAC uses the facility in its program to spay and neuter adoptable animals from their shelter partners. The benefits from this collaborative effort include (1) offering surgical training in which veterinary students can determine their patient's preoperative and postoperative health status, (2) ensuring that more animals leave the shelter for adoption already altered, (3) providing the shelter with a low-cost spay/neuter service, and (4) helping reduce pet overpopulation.

Operation Catnip, at the University of Florida Veterinary School, also utilizes the student surgery facilities once a month to sterilize an average of 150 feral cats. Using all volunteer personnel, including many students and faculty, precise protocols have been developed, and Operation Catnip has been used as a model for other programs.

A more common example of a stationary facility is the Alliance for Animals in South Boston. Founded in the mid-1980s by a neighborhood animal advocate, Alliance has served the community by providing low-cost spay and neuter services to financially fragile citizens. The facility also serves stray and feral cats throughout the Boston area, often placing them for adoption at Alliance for Animals' Cat Shelter, in another location. Although initially controversial, Alliance now offers routine veterinary services as well, making it more than a low-cost spay/neuter facility. The facility is located in a converted housing unit on two floors and consists of a reception area, preparation and cage area, small surgery room, pack preparation room, and basement with additional cages, bathroom, washer, and dryer. Alliance is a good example of making the best use of limited space and resources.

Mobile Surgical Vans

Mobile surgical facilities can range from converted recreational vehicles (RVs) to specially designed 18-wheel trucks with living quarters for four people.

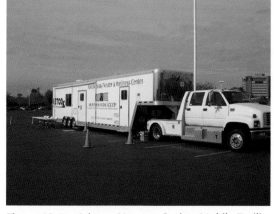

Figure 12-1   Arizona Humane Society Mobile Facility parked at a site and ready to receive clients. (Courtesy Arizona Humane Society.)

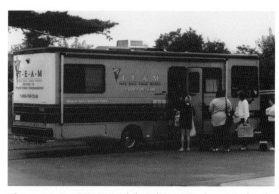

Figure 12-3   TEAM Mobile Feline Unit, an example of a converted RV, showing clients during check-in. (Courtesy Tait's Every Animal Matters, Westbrook, Conn.)

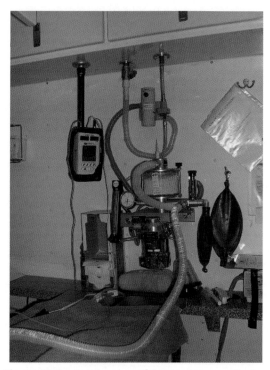

Figure 12-2   Interior view of Arizona Humane Society Mobile Facility showing the surgery room. (Courtesy Arizona Humane Society.)

In addition to two stationary high-volume spay/neuter facilities in Maricopa County, the Arizona Humane Society put its first mobile unit on the road in 1999 and began to service outlying communities, providing low-cost surgical sterilization and routine medical care for pets of financially fragile people (Figure 12-1). A second unit was added in 2002. These self-contained units have supplies and equipment of the highest quality and even sleeping quarters in the first unit. The surgery and prep areas are of adequate size, and a refrigerator, autoclave, shelving and storage, and a large bank of cages create a professional working environment (Figure 12-2). More than 8000 dogs and cats have been surgically altered in these two units.

Another example of a mobile facility is the TEAM Mobile Feline Unit, established by Tait's Every Animal Matters (TEAM) of Westbrook, Connecticut. Using a converted RV, TEAM has served the state of Connecticut since 1997, performing more than 70,000 spays and neuters for shelter, stray, feral, and owned cats (Figure 12-3). TEAM has perfected the use of limited space to provide a cage area (a rack with cat carriers instead of standard animal cages), storage and refrigeration, prep area, and surgical suite (Figure 12-4). All counter and floor space is used to create the most efficient and workable environment possible. Cats arrive at the site in the morning, are transferred to cages on the van, receive a physical examination and surgery (if healthy and stable), and are returned to the client or owner the same day. Although primarily a surgical facility, TEAM does

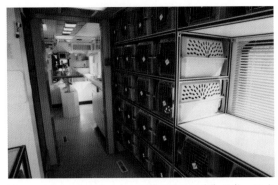

Figure 12-4   Interior view of TEAM Mobile Feline Unit showing the holding, preparation, and surgery areas. Special shelving holds standard cat carriers for the patients. (Courtesy Tait's Every Animal Matters, Westbrook, Conn.)

offer additional services as needed (e.g., rabies prophylaxis is mandatory), but clients are strongly encouraged to establish relationships with private practice veterinarians.

Multi-Site "Clinics"

The term multi-site "clinic" as used here refers to what is usually called a "feral cat clinic." Generally organized by feral cat rescue groups, the "clinic" is actually an ongoing program in which trappers are mobilized from various rescue groups and colony caretakers to bring cats to a specific facility, usually a local veterinary clinic, on a specific day. The facility often donates its time, staff, facility, and supplies for little or no compensation. The numbers of cats sterilized per "clinic" can range from 15 to 20 in a local veterinary practice to as many as 50 to 60 in programs that utilize a stationary facility and staff, especially for a feral cat clinic. Many feral cat rescue groups throughout the United States have established a regular clinic day, usually once a month, which is rotated among veterinary practices.

A variation of the clinic theme is seen with national groups such as Doris Day Animal League's Spay Day USA, in which a day per year is set aside to promote spaying and neutering, with the local practices participating. The patient pool usually consists of animals of needy clients,

although shelter animals and feral cats are also included, and often the surgery is performed for free that particular day. The number of surgeries performed depends on the particular practice.

GENERAL PRACTICE VERSUS HIGH-VOLUME STERILIZATION SURGERY

Stationary High-Volume Facilities

The main difference between sterilization surgeries in a stationary facility and those done in a traditional practice setting may be the client/patient/veterinarian relationship. The client may simply be a caretaker, a rescue group, or a shelter, and the patient is usually presented for only one reason, surgical sterilization. Client education on other issues is often provided, but definitive medical care for most conditions usually is not given. Some routine laboratory testing is required by certain facilities, but most diagnostic, preventive, and routine care is often beyond the mission and function of most stationary high-volume spay/neuter facilities.

Mobile Sterilization Facilities

The client/patient/veterinarian relationship and routine care issues are factors for the mobile surgical facility as well. A major difference between traditional facilities and mobile surgical vans, however, involves consideration of the size, age, and handling difficulty of patients and the difficulty of the procedures. Therefore, patient selection can be a challenge. Aggressive and dangerous dogs are not easily handled in a confined space and are often canceled or not even booked. In many mobile surgical facilities, cage size and space do not allow for dogs over a certain size. In some mobile facilities, only cats are seen because of the space limitations. Surgical and anesthetic risks and complications cannot be easily addressed, even with state-of-the-art protocols and equipment, because of limitations associated with space, time, personnel for postprocedural monitoring, and the added cost of overnight monitoring and care if needed. Challenging cases are usually referred to a general practitioner or stationary facility, not because of a lack of skill or expertise, but because of risks to patient and staff risk and potential complications.

Multi-Site "Clinic" Facilities

With both types of multi-site "clinics" described earlier (i.e., "feral cat clinic" and Doris Day Animal League's Spay Day USA), standards of routine care are generally determined by the hosting facilities. Depending on the patient and caretaker, more challenging cases may be handled in these traditional facilities and monitored by staff until the patient can be safely discharged. The major difference between regular client surgeries and those done for a "clinic" is the price, which is often free or drastically reduced at the clinic as a community service.

THE NEED FOR HIGH-VOLUME SPAY/NEUTER FACILITIES

The Humane Society of the United States (HSUS) estimates that in the more than 4000 animal shelters in the United States, 3 to 4 million dogs and cats are euthanized each year. This startling statistic does not even take into account the animals euthanized by municipalities and animal control officers and by private practitioners. It also does not consider stray dogs and cats that die of injury and disease with no accounting of their numbers. Further estimates indicate that a female dog and her offspring can produce 67,000 puppies in 6 years and that a female cat and her offspring can produce 420,000 kittens in 7 years. This chain can be broken by surgical sterilization. Indeed, an estimated 30% to 40% reduction in the pet animal overpopulation has already occurred because of surgical intervention.

With more responsible stewardship of dogs and cats, there would be no pet overpopulation. Just enough litters would be born to allow replacement of those animals that die, and the pet population would remain stable. There would be no need for shelters, no need for feral cat caretakers,

and no abandoned animals to reproduce themselves. Most veterinary professionals strive to achieve this goal, but until it is reached, mainly through public education and the diligent efforts of all those who care for animals, high-volume spay/neuter facilities will continue to play a major role in overpopulation reduction.

Sterilization benefits not only the patients described but also the public and the individual community, both monetarily and ethically. The veterinary profession, although sometimes at odds with high-volume (and especially low-cost) facilities, benefits as well because it is extremely difficult to make a major impact on pet overpopulation without these facilities' help. The feral cat caretaker, animal control officer, and shelter worker also benefit, with their missions fulfilled and their jobs made easier.

ANESTHESIA CONCERNS

Neutering clinics for feral cats pose two major obstacles to optimum pain management. First, feral cats can be challenging to handle preoperatively and postoperatively, making administration of analgesics difficult. Second, most programs require immediate or rapid release to the outdoors, where assessment and continued treatment is impossible.

Given these restrictions, an anesthesia protocol that minimizes contact while maximizing sedation and long-term analgesia is the best approach. One such protocol combines an alpha$_2$-adrenergic agonist (α_2-agonist), an opioid, and a dissociative anesthetic. The α_2-agonist medetomidine (Domitor) is used mainly for sedation but also has analgesic properties. Used alone, the α_2-agonist class of drug causes cardiovascular changes such as high blood pressure and low heart rate (see Chapter 1). However, if the α_2-agonist is used in a low-dose combination with other agents, these side effects are rarely seen. Likewise, a dissociative anesthetic such as ketamine (Ketaset) used alone can cause rapid heart rate and low blood pressure, but again, when used at a low dosage and combined with medetomidine and an opioid, the effects are minimized. An opioid is added to the preoperative injection to provide analgesia. Using a long-acting opioid such as buprenorphine (Buprenex) provides preemptive analgesia as well as 6 to 12 hours of postoperative pain relief.

These three classes of drugs can be combined into a single, low-volume intramuscular (IM) injection that usually provides adequate anesthesia and analgesia to perform neuter or spay. The preferred site for IM injection is the cranial thigh muscle (quadriceps), which can be easily isolated during restraint. After injection, sedation is quite rapid; most cats are ready to be neutered 5 to 8 minutes later. The cat's mucous membranes should be checked to ensure an appropriate pink color, although mild pallor is acceptable. Femoral pulses are palpated for both rate and strength. Femoral pulses should be strong and regular, and the heart rate should be greater than 100 beats/min. Typically, patients are extremely flaccid and malleable at this point and do not respond to noxious stimuli. However, some patients will display reflexive motion or an increase in heart rate or respiration on surgical manipulation of tissue. In this case a small amount of inhaled gaseous anesthesia (e.g., isoflurane) is required and can be delivered by mask or endotracheal intubation.

Occasionally, this protocol will induce one episode of vomiting almost immediately after injection. This reaction is generally limited to cats that have not been fasted appropriately.

The length of anesthesia provided by this protocol is about 45 to 90 minutes. Cats will be groggy but responsive after that point. Under ideal circumstances, patients should be allowed to recover slowly in a quiet area until they are fully awake. If adequate recovery time cannot be permitted, medetomidine can be reversed with an α_2-antagonist such as atipamezole (Antesedan) given IM at the same volume as the initial medetomidine injection. This results in more rapid anesthesia recovery but also reverses the analgesia provided by medetomidine.

The addition of a *single* preemptive dose of a nonsteroidal anti-inflammatory drug (NSAID) to the previous protocol will provide at least 24 hours of analgesia and as much as 3 days in some cats. This variation is caused by the unpredictable metabolic rate of this drug class in feline patients.

Injectable NSAIDs are most effectively used in feral cats, because they generally present close to the time of surgery. Giving an oral medication just before surgery results in unpredictable analgesia because the gastrointestinal tract is otherwise empty, and gastric motility may be altered for several hours after surgery. Injectable carprofen (Rimadyl) or meloxicam (Metacam) can be administered subcutaneously (SC), although neither is labeled for feline use. Currently, no NSAIDs are labeled for use in cats in the United States. However, NSAIDs have been labeled for use in the cat in Europe, Canada, and Australia and used routinely for many years. Based on foreign dosages and current research, pain management experts recommend the following dosages:

> Rimadyl, 2 mg/kg SC once
> or
> Metacam, 0.2 mg/kg IM on day 1, followed by
>   0.1 mg/kg IM once daily for 2 to 4 days

An example of a drug protocol when neutering feral cats is as follows:

> Medetomidine, 0.02 mg/kg IM
> Buprenorphine, 0.02 mg/kg IM
> Ketamine, 2 mg/kg IM
>   *with or without*
> Carprofen, 2 mg/kg SC

The canine patients in high-volume spay/neuter clinics are generally easier to handle than feral cats because of appropriate patient selection (see later discussion). In addition, more anesthetics and analgesics are available for dogs. For these reasons, the previous discussion on anesthesia and analgesia is limited to feral cats.

DISEASE CONCERNS

Feline Diseases

Feline panleukopenia, feline leukemia virus (FeLV), and feline immunodeficiency virus (FIV) are three diseases of major importance. However, feline respiratory diseases (e.g., rhinotracheitis, calicivirus) are probably more common and problematic in a high-volume setting. Although not usually fatal, these diseases can cause great distress in animals, can make them a surgical risk, and may spread to other cats in the facility that day.

Wounds of unknown origin can be a major problem as well, especially when dealing with feral cats. Each shelter or feral cat entity should have its own policy that effectively complies with state regulations regarding rabies exposure.

External and internal parasites are always a concern in cats, especially kittens, and most high-volume spay/neuter facilities address these concerns. With spot-on products for fleas and ticks and with injectable and liquid anthelmintics (worm-killing agents), even feral cats can be medicated for parasitic problems to facilitate their postsurgical recovery and recuperation.

Canine Diseases

Canine tracheobronchitis, or "kennel cough," can be as devastating to a shelter as the feline respiratory diseases. Although most dogs recover well from this disease, the stress of surgery and exposure of other dogs in the facility make this a major problem in a high-volume setting. Parvovirus and canine distemper virus cause other diseases of importance in shelters and high-volume settings, especially in young puppies. Laboratory testing is done to screen for (and sometimes definitively determine) the presence of endemic diseases such as heartworm, Lyme disease, and canine ehrlichiosis (*Ehrlichia* infection). As with cats, internal and external parasites can be destroyed with simple measures in dogs returning to a shelter or private owner.

Vaccinations

Currently, vaccination protocols for both dogs and cats are undergoing changes and a profession-wide review. Rather than listing particular protocols used in a high-volume spay/neuter facility, this section discusses only vaccinations in general.

For some patients and in certain facilities, no vaccinations should be given in a high-volume setting. Reasons include the stress on the immune system, the belief that traditional veterinary practices should vaccinate, and the likelihood that some patients will not receive a proper initial series. Others believe that the animal should receive at least the initial vaccinations when the opportunity presents, as with feral cats, and that some protection is better than no protection.

Almost all facilities agree in one area: *rabies prophylaxis*. As a public health concern, rabies is a disease that can easily be prevented by proper vaccination. Unless the animal is extremely debilitated, every patient whose rabies protection status is unknown or deficient typically receives a rabies vaccine, preferably before but certainly the day of surgery. Some feral cat colonies have long-standing caretakers who retrap their cats annually for physical examination and preventive medicine and who can keep their cats on a proper schedule.

Diagnostic Blood Tests

For reasons that include cost and opportunity, it is often not possible to do more than a heartworm-*Ehrlichia*-Lyme test for dogs or a FeLV-FIV test for cats, perhaps with a minimum database (MDB) of packed cell volume (PCV), total solids (TS), blood glucose (BG), and blood urea nitrogen (BUN) (see Chapter 1). Some mobile facilities, however, are not equipped for even this testing. Sending samples to an outside laboratory is not a consideration unless the facility also sees patients for routine services. This does not diminish the desirability of presurgical testing, only the opportunity.

SURGICAL CONCERNS

Patient Selection

Most patients that are poor surgical or anesthetic risks are eliminated by (1) physical findings (e.g., poor body condition, illness), (2) state of pregnancy or estrus, (3) age, (4) size, or (5) laboratory results. A veterinarian may be capable of spaying a 6-year-old dog in heat that weighs 120 pounds in a traditional practice setting, but this would not be an ideal patient for a small surgical van.

The surgical risks, time required, and recovery and follow-up problems make this dog a poor choice for most high-volume facilities.

Strict criteria should be predetermined so that patients at higher risk are not even scheduled, avoiding the stress placed on the animal, caretaker, and staff. In a high-paced environment where numbers matter, the time needed to admit, examine, and then cancel could be better spent. When making the appointment, personnel must ask the client about the patient's age, weight, temperament, and body condition, as well as any medical conditions that would affect the surgical decision. Although collecting accurate information may not be possible with feral cats, some guidelines can be established.

Surgeon Prerogatives

Basic choices such as surgical approach and suture pattern should be left to the veterinarian, within certain limits. Rigid flexibility is the key. For example, the established protocol for a feral cat clinic might call for a flank incision, but the veterinary surgeon may be uncomfortable with this approach. The type of suture material and the suture pattern used to close the incision should take into account the availability of follow-up visits (e.g., feral cats, already-adopted animals traveling long distances to new homes).

Juvenile Patients

Many veterinarians have never done early-age spays or neuters and believe that an 8- to 10-week-old patient is a poor surgical risk. Within the veterinary community there is also controversy about the long-term effects of early-age spaying and neutering on urinary incontinence and behavior. Studies need to continue on this issue, but users of high-volume facilities want early-age sterilization for their animals.

Conserving body warmth and keeping BG levels normal should always be concerns in the juvenile patient. Beyond the usual techniques for maintaining body temperature, the puppies and kittens can be kept in the same cage to allow snuggling, which helps to prevent heat loss as well as separation anxiety. Allowing a puppy or kitten to eat up to a few hours before surgery and providing food as soon as awake after surgery help to keep BG levels normal.

The surgical technique of early-age spay/neuters is simple and yields good results with few complications. Some general concerns are (1) the relatively small size of the organs, which occasionally makes them difficult to find; (2) the relatively large volume of fluid in the abdomen at this age, which may be disconcerting at first but is normal; and (3) the recovery concerns already mentioned.

Despite these concerns, early-age spaying and neutering is an acceptable method to help control the pet overpopulation, and it is being done with increasing frequency.

POSTOPERATIVE CONCERNS

Constant vigilance during the recovery period is essential, primarily because the animal is often at greatest risk during this time. In a high-volume spay/neuter clinic, the recovery team or individual needs to be especially vigilant. Patient warmth, pain and stress management, and physiologic stability require constant monitoring until the animal is fully recovered.

Often, several animals are in various states of recovery. All may not be touchable or able to be monitored with hands-on methods, especially as they return to normal consciousness. Being prepared for each patient as it comes off the table is extremely important. Every step of the recovery process, such as using and removing external heat sources, wrapping the patient in clean linens, administering fluids and timing the removal of intravenous (IV) catheters, and performing ancillary procedures, needs to be done in a precise and concise manner so that nothing is left to chance or is forgotten. A strict routine of events needs to be instituted and followed. The animal must be monitored from the moment it leaves the surgery table to the moment it is discharged to the caretaker.

Because many high-volume sterilization facilities depend on inexperienced volunteers, the protocols for all aspects of the process must be easily understood and followed. An experienced technician should be an integral part of the development of all protocols and a part of the surgery and recovery team. Each team member should be able to perform other duties, such as doing laundry and cleaning, completing medical records, and answering phones.

SPECIAL CONCERNS

Management and Planning

Planning and training for a high-volume sterilization facility will depend on the type of facility and the target patient population. Multi-site clinics may depend heavily on volunteers for much of the work needed in obtaining sites, patients, and surgical personnel. In any veterinary practice, protocols need to be established and reviewed regularly, and a high-volume facility dependent on volunteers needs thorough protocols in place. Each step of the process needs to run smoothly for the safety and well-being of the patient, caretaker, and staff and for the success of the mission. Comprehensive protocols for all aspects of the process, from the script for the initial phone call, criteria for site selection, supply lists, to the actual medical and surgical procedures, are vital to the success of the facility.

With any high-volume sterilization facility, all hands-on employees must be thoroughly trained in anesthesia and surgical procedures. The role of the veterinary technician in this regard cannot be overemphasized. The facility relies on the technician to train volunteers and inexperienced technicians, create protocols for each part of the process, and perform the direct hands-on measures with patients. The veterinarian is often focused on the surgical aspects and is relying on trained staff to ensure that other aspects of the patient's welfare are addressed properly.

Patient scheduling can be a challenge in many high-volume facilities. Initially, much time can be spent on the phone with owners, shelters, and caretakers. Mobile facilities may not have a stay-behind person and may depend heavily on an answering machine for bookings and callbacks. Often a cell phone is used on board the van to ease this burden, as well as being an emergency communication tool. Scheduling locations for the van can be challenging as well. Clinics are often held at large malls or businesses with a large parking area, and obtaining permission from the right person can be time-consuming. Safety and security, bathroom facilities, weather concerns, and other logistical problems also may need to be addressed.

Return or Release of Feral Cats

A major problem with any large collection of feral cats is identification of the individual. Many caretakers have photographs of their cats, which is helpful as long as the colony and the caretakers and feeders remain the same; however, this is seldom the case. Ways to identify animals include tattooing, microchip implanting, and ear tipping. A feral cat will likely not allow anyone close enough to scan for a microchip or look for a tattoo, so the common method of identification of a sterilized feral is tipping the left ear. *Ear tipping* involves surgically removing the tip of a cat's pinna. This can be seen easily from some distance, and if an altered animal is trapped inadvertently for sterilization, it can be released immediately.

Overnight postoperative monitoring is extremely important and certainly possible. The cat can be left in the trap or in a transfer cage, kept in a temperature-regulated building, and checked throughout the night to ensure full recovery. Every high-volume facility should have prearranged emergency veterinary coverage for cats, especially feral cats.

Proper management of a feral colony benefits the cats as well as the community. Postsurgical monitoring can be enhanced if the feeders and caretakers know their cats. Once returned to the colony, the cat usually returns to its normal routine, and any break in this routine can alert the caretaker to problems that can be addressed quickly. For more information on feral cat colonies, the reader is encouraged to search the Internet.

Fees and Services Provided

Fees in most high-volume facilities are less than the normal charges at veterinary practices in the area, and services may even be free at times. As mentioned, most high-volume spay/neuter facilities depend on grants and donations to subsidize their work. Local practitioners may resent the presence of a subsidized sterilization facility, so it is important that the facility establish a good relationship with local veterinarians to avoid problems. When possible, owners and caretakers should be screened for need, and a high-volume facility should avoid those who can afford a local practitioner.

General Impact on the Involved Parties

No one benefits more from the high-volume facility than the patient. Besides the health and behavioral benefits usually associated with spaying or neutering, health issues may be detected in animals that might not otherwise be seen by a veterinarian. These patients should always be referred to a local practitioner for definitive care, although the owner may not follow the recommendation for various reasons.

The community as a whole benefits from the reduction of unwanted births and the elimination of stray and feral cats and dogs. Complex community issues arise with animals of collectors and hoarders and involve many agencies. Many want to help in some way, and this situation provides the opportunity to volunteer or donate money. Public health concerns such as rabies are addressed as well by reducing the free-roaming animal population and vaccinating surgical cases.

The veterinary community benefits because many individuals want to do more to help solve the pet overpopulation problem, and volunteering to assist at a multi-site facility serves this purpose. The caretaker or financially fragile owner also benefits from the reduced cost and the availability of more "surgery slots."

Volunteerism

As stated, many high-volume sterilization facilities depend on volunteers for their success. Many technicians already assist at a multi-site clinic or a "feral cat day." It can be very satisfying to look back at the end of a long day at a high volume facility and realize that one has prevented thousands of unwanted births and the associated suffering.

Other ways are available to help besides the hands-on work. Truly needy clients can be referred to a high-volume facility, donations of money and supplies can be collected, and assisting in organizing and planning is helpful as well. There is also the opportunity to volunteer for work in other parts of the United States and throughout the world. Many veterinary schools are affiliated with projects in less affluent areas where students and technicians make regular visits. Many state veterinary medical associations also have national and international projects that provide routine care as well as spaying and neutering for third-world countries.

The Massachusetts Veterinary Medical Association's International Committee sponsors trips to two countries (Project Samana and Project Mazunte) and not only provides veterinary care and surgical sterilization to dogs and cats, but also works with large animals. Both projects depend heavily on veterinary technicians as part of the team and will work with the local veterinarians as well.

KEY POINTS

1. The number of feral cats in the United States is almost equal to the number of pet cats and is the major source of unwanted cats.
2. Shelter animals that are not surgically altered also contribute to pet overpopulation.
3. Collectors and hoarders of animals also contribute to pet overpopulation, although they often believe they are "saviors" and doing nothing wrong.
4. Reducing stress to the patient is important and necessary in a high-volume spay/neuter facility.
5. The veterinary community, the public, the patient, and the animal caretaker all benefit by the existence of high-volume sterilization facilities.
6. Traditional and high-volume sterilization surgeries may differ in the client/patient/veterinarian relationship, but not in the standard and quality of care.

7. High-volume spay/neuter facilities are having a major impact on the reduction of pet overpopulation.
8. With feral cats it is best to use injectable agents for all phases of anesthesia and pain medications to avoid the stress of handling.
9. A medical contraindication is the only reason for not administering pain medications in a high-volume facility.
10. High-volume spay/neuter facilities are usually limited to in-house prescreening laboratory tests.
11. Patient selection for high-volume facilities is based on many criteria, but specifically, no animal should receive surgery if there are strong medical reasons against it.
12. The increase in early-age spaying and neutering has helped to reduce dog and cat overpopulation.
13. The postoperative period is the most important part of the high-volume process, and the team should be well trained in what to expect, what to do, and how to handle postoperative monitoring and concerns.
14. Any disease that can affect a shelter or group-housing of large numbers of animals can impact a high-volume sterilization facility.
15. It is imperative from a public health standpoint to follow state guidelines regarding rabies prevention and wounds of unknown origin.
16. Concise and easily understood protocols should always be in place and should be regularly reviewed in a high-volume facility.
17. The veterinary technician plays a vital role in the planning and operations of a high-volume spay/neuter facility.

REVIEW QUESTIONS

1. Which of the following types of cat is the greatest contributor to the overpopulation of cats?
   a. Pet cats.
   b. Indoor/outdoor cats.
   c. Feral cats.
   d. Cats in catteries, such as cat breeders.
2. Animals spayed and neutered in high-volume clinics are generally from which animal population?
   a. Pets that live in house with one other pet.
   b. Feral cats.

   c. Shelter animals.
   d. All of the above.
   e. Both b and c.
3. What are the generally accepted age and weight limits for the increasing number of juvenile patients being sterilized in high-volume sterilization clinics?
   a. 12 weeks and 12 pounds.
   b. 10 weeks and 10 pounds.
   c. 2 weeks and 2 pounds.
   d. 8 weeks and 2 pounds or more.
   e. Any age and any weight.
4. *True* or *False:* Early-age (juvenile) surgical sterilization has proved to be an effective means for preventing pet overpopulation.
5. *True* or *False:* One of the major goals of high-volume spay/neuter clinics is to reduce the number of dogs and cats that cannot be placed in homes and are euthanized each year.
6. *True* or *False:* The veterinary profession has historically been at odds with high-volume spay/neuter facilities.
7. *True* or *False:* Postoperative pain management of feral cats is easy and consists of once-daily injections of anti-inflammatory drugs for 3 days after surgery.
8. *True* or *False:* It is common practice in high-volume sterilization facilities to vaccinate every animal against rabies (when the rabies protection status is unknown) on the day of surgery.
9. *True* or *False:* High-risk patients (e.g., debilitated, pregnant) are routinely selected as ideal patients to be sterilized in high-volume clinics.
10. Which of the following is the preferred method of identifying cats sterilized in high-volume spay/neuter facilities?
    a. Tattooing.
    b. Microchip implanting.
    c. Ear tipping.
    d. Neck ribbons.
    e. Reflective name tags.
11. Who benefits from the services provided by high-volume sterilization facilities?
    a. The patients.
    b. The local community.
    c. The veterinary community.
    d. All of the above.
    e. None of the above.

ANSWERS

1. c
2. e
3. d
4. True
5. True
6. True
7. False
8. True
9. False
10. c
11. d

BIBLIOGRAPHY

Cummings Karen: *ASPCA Animal Watch,* Fall 2003, p 24.
Slater Margaret R: *Community approaches to feral cats: problems, alternatives and recommendations,* Washington, DC, 2002, Humane Society Press.

Quick Reference for Common Perioperative Intravenous Infusions

INTRAVENOUS FLUID FLOW RATE

Occasionally, it is necessary to administer intravenous (IV) fluids without an infusion pump. The table below is a quick reference that allows the veterinary technician to count the number of seconds between drops of fluid (*not* the number of drops per second) into the drip chamber of the administration set to estimate the hourly infusion rate, as long as the type of fluid administration set is known.

MAINTENANCE FLUID FLOW RATE

Determining a patient's fluid flow rate is based on the following formula:

Total fluids = Maintenance fluids + Replacement fluids + Ongoing losses

Many formulas are available for calculating a patient's maintenance fluid requirements. However, a simple, easy-to-remember formula for *estimating* an animal's hourly maintenance fluid requirements

10 DROPS/ml	15 DROPS/ml	60 DROPS/ml
1 drop/sec = 360 ml/hr	1 drop/sec = 240 ml/hr	1 drop/sec = 60 ml/hr
1 drop/2 sec = 180 ml/hr	1 drop/2 sec = 120 ml/hr	1 drop/2 sec = 30 ml/hr
1 drop/3 sec = 120 ml/hr	1 drop/3 sec = 80 ml/hr	1 drop/3 sec = 20 ml/hr
1 drop/4 sec = 90 ml/hr	1 drop/4 sec = 60 ml/hr	1 drop/4 sec = 15 ml/hr
1 drop/5 sec = 72 ml/hr	1 drop/5 sec = 48 ml/hr	1 drop/5 sec = 12 ml/hr
1 drop/6 sec = 60 ml/hr	1 drop/6 sec = 40 ml/hr	1 drop/6 sec = 10 ml/hr
1 drop/7 sec = 51 ml/hr	1 drop/7 sec = 35 ml/hr	1 drop/7 sec = 8.8 ml/hr
1 drop/8 sec = 45 ml/hr	1 drop/8 sec = 30 ml/hr	1 drop/8 sec = 7.5 ml/hr
1 drop/9 sec = 40 ml/hr	1 drop/9 sec = 27 ml/hr	1 drop/9 sec = 6.7 ml/hr
1 drop/10 sec = 36 ml/hr	1 drop/10 sec = 24 ml/hr	1 drop/10 sec = 6 ml/hr

sec, Second(s); *ml/hr*, milliliters per hour.

is 1 ml/# BW, and two times (or twice) the maintenance requirement is 2 ml/# BW, where # is the abbreviation for pounds and BW is body weight.

BODY WEIGHT (POUNDS)	MAINTENANCE FLUIDS	TWICE MAINTENANCE FLUIDS
1	1 ml/hr	2 ml/hr
10	10 ml/hr	20 ml/hr
20	20 ml/hr	40 ml/hr
40	40 ml/hr	80 ml/hr
80	80 ml/hr	160 ml/hr

"SPIKING THE BAG" WITH POTASSIUM CHLORIDE

- Patients on fluid diuresis are prone to hypokalemia.
- To prevent hypokalemia, the IV fluids can be "spiked," or supplemented, with potassium chloride (KCl).
- To know how much KCl supplementation is needed, it is necessary to know the patient's serum potassium level.
- Normal serum potassium level = 3.5 to 5.5 mEq/L.
- Failure to correct hypokalemia can result in muscle weakness, lethargy, and vomiting.
- KCl *must* be given in a slow drip, diluted in another fluid.

SERUM POTASSIUM (mEq/L)	SUPPLEMENTAL POTASSIUM CHLORIDE (PER 250 ml Fluid)*
3.5-5.5 (normal)	5 mEq (20 mEq/L)
3.0-3.4	7 mEq (28 mEq/L)
2.5-2.9	10 mEq (40 mEq/L)
2.0-2.4	15 mEq (60 mEq/L)
<2.0	20 mEq (80 mEq/L)

*Never administer fluids supplemented with potassium chloride faster than twice the maintenance rate; with more potassium, adjust the rate even slower.

mEq/L, Milliequivalents per liter.

"SPIKING THE BAG" WITH DEXTROSE

- If a patient is prone to hypoglycemia, debilitated, septic, or anorectic, a dextrose supplement may be required.
- If blood glucose (BG) is less than 40 mg/dl, dextrose should be added to fluids to make a 2.5% dextrose solution.
- If BG continues to remain at or below 40 mg/dl, the solution should be increased to a 5% dextrose solution.

SIZE OF FLUID BAG*	TO MAKE 2.5% DEXTROSE SOLUTION	TO MAKE 5% DEXTROSE SOLUTION
250 ml	Add 12.5 ml of 50% dextrose.	Add 25 ml of 50% dextrose.
500 ml	Add 25 ml of 50% dextrose.	Add 50 ml of 50% dextrose.
1000 ml	Add 50 ml of 50% dextrose.	Add 100 ml of 50% dextrose.

*Before adding dextrose to fluid bag, withdraw an amount of fluid from bag equal to the amount of dextrose to be added.

HEPARINIZED SALINE ("HEP-SALINE," "FLUSH")

SIZE OF FLUID BAG OF 0.9% SODIUM CHLORIDE (NaCl)	AMOUNT OF HEPARIN [1000 UNITS/ml] TO ADD
250 ml	1.25 ml (1250 units)
500 ml	2.5 ml (2500 units)
1 liter	5 ml (5000 units)

DRUG DOSES USED TO TREAT SURGICAL PAIN IN ANIMALS

All dosages listed in the following table are referenced in the veterinary literature. However, unless otherwise stated, not all the drugs or dosages are approved by the Food and Drug Administration (FDA) for use in dogs and cats.

Nonsteroidal Anti-Inflammatory Drugs (NSAIDs)

DRUG NAME	INDICATION	DOSE	ONSET OF ACTION	DURATION OF ACTION	PRECAUTIONS
Carprofen (oral: 25-, 75-, and 100-mg tablets or chewables)	Pain and inflammation associated with arthritis and soft tissue and orthopedic surgery in dogs **FDA approved for use in dogs**	Dog: 2.2 mg/kg PO bid *or* 4.4 mg/kg PO sid	1 hr 1 hr	12 hr 24 hr	Do not use in patients with gastrointestinal (GI) or renal disease. Discontinue use if patient develops vomiting or diarrhea. NSAIDs are not recommended in hypovolemic or dehydrated patients or patients with bleeding disorders.
Carprofen (injectable: 50 mg/ml)	Postoperative pain **FDA approved for use in dogs**	Dog: 4.4 mg/kg SC, IM, or IV Cat: 1-2 mg/kg SC	1 hr	18-24 hr 48-72 hr	As above.
Deracoxib (oral: 25- and 100-mg tablets)	Control of pain and inflammation associated with orthopedic surgery and chronic pain (osteoarthritis) **FDA approved for use in dogs**	Postoperatively: 3-4 mg/kg PO sid for 7 days Chronic pain: 1-2 mg/kg PO sid	1 hr	24 hr	As for carprofen. Do not use in patients less than 4 pounds or 16 weeks of age (see listing on label).
Etodolac (oral: 150- and 300-mg tablets)	Control of pain and inflammation associated with osteoarthritis **FDA approved for use in dogs**	Dog: 10-15 mg/kg PO sid	1 hr	24 hr	As for carprofen. Not recommended for dogs weighing less than 5 kg.
Ketoprofen (oral: 25-, 50-, and 75-mg capsules; 5-, 10-, and 20-mg tablets)	Postoperative pain	Dog: 1 mg/kg PO sid Cat: 1 mg/kg PO sid	1 hr	18-24 hr	As for carprofen. Do not use before surgery. Do not use parenterally for more than 3 days or orally more than 5 days.
Ketoprofen (injectable: 100 mg/ml)	Postoperative pain **FDA approved for use in horses for inflammation and pain associated with**	Dog:1-2 mg/kg SC sid Cat: 1-2 mg/kg SC sid	1 hr	18-24 hr	As for carprofen. Do not use before surgery. Do not use parenterally for more than 3 days or orally more than 5 days.

musculoskeletal disorders

Drug	Indication	Dose	Onset	Duration	Comments
Meloxicam (oral solution: 1.5 mg/ml)	Postoperative and chronic pain (not labeled for postoperative use, only for osteoarthritis) **FDA approved for use in dogs**	Dog: 0.2-0.3 mg/kg PO sid for 1 day, then 0.1 mg/kg PO sid Cat: 0.2 mg/kg PO on day 1, followed by 0.1 mg/kg PO sid for 2-4 days, then 0.1 mg/cat PO sid	1 hr	18-24 hr	As for carprofen. Loading dose can be by injection or oral administration.
Meloxicam (injectable: 5 mg/ml)	Postoperative and chronic pain in dogs	Dog: 0.2 mg/kg IM sid	1 hr	18-24 hr	As for carprofen. Loading dose can be by injection or oral administration.
Tepoxalin (oral: 30-, 50-, 100-, and 200-mg disintegrating tablets)	Control of pain associated with osteoarthritis in dogs over 3 kg **FDA approved for use in dogs**	Dog: 10 mg/kg PO sid; 20 mg/kg once on initial dose	1 hr	18-24 hr	Tablets in foil blister packs. Administer with food or water; place in mouth for a minimum of 4 seconds to allow tablet to dissolve.

Alpha$_2$-Adrenergic Agonists

Drug	Indication	Dose	Onset	Duration	Comments
Medetomidine*† (injectable: 1 mg/ml)	Sedative, analgesic **FDA approved for use in dogs**	Dog: 10-60 µg/kg IM	20 min	1.0-3.0 hr	Do not use in patients with underlying cardiopulmonary or renal disease.
		5.0-10 µg/kg IV	3 min	0.5-1.5 hr	The lower IV dose is to be used as adjunct to opioid analgesia or as premedication before anesthesia.
		Cat: 20-80 µg/kg IM	20 min	1.0-3.0 hr	Even lower doses may be used for anxiety and dysphoria (see Sedatives below).
		5.0-10 µg/kg IV	3 min	0.5-1.5 hr	
Xylazine*† (injectable: 20 and 100 mg/ml)	Sedative, analgesic **FDA approved for use in dogs and cats**	Dog: 0.1-0.5 mg/kg IM, SC	20 min	0.5 hr	Do not use in patients with underlying cardiopulmonary or renal disease.
		0.05-0.1 mg/kg IV	1 min	20 min	The low IV dose is to be used as an adjunct to opioid analgesia, not by itself.
		Cat: 0.1-0.5 mg/kg IM, SC	20 min	0.5 hr	
		0.05-0.1 mg/kg IV	1 min	20 min	

Continued

Opioids

DRUG NAME	INDICATION	DOSE	ONSET OF ACTION	DURATION OF ACTION	PRECAUTIONS
Morphine (oral: 10-, 15-, and 30-mg tablets)	Acute and cancer-related pain	Dog: 0.5-4 mg/kg PO tid or qid Cat: 0.25-1.0 mg/kg PO tid or qid	1 hr	3-4 hr	Higher doses may induce sedation or dysphoria.
Morphine (oral sustained-release: 15-, 30-, 60-, 100-, and 200-mg tablets)	Acute and cancer-related pain	Dog: 0.5-4.0 mg/kg PO bid or qid Cat: not recommended because of size of tablets that should not be scored	1 hr	8-12 hr	Higher doses may induce sedation or dysphoria. Increase frequency of administration before increasing dose if duration is insufficient.
Morphine (injectable: preservative free: 1 mg/ml)	Perioperative and acute pain	Dog: 0.5-2.2 mg/kg SC, IM 0.1-0.5 mg/kg IV (slowly) Cat: 0.1-0.5 mg/kg SC, IM 0.05-0.1 mg/kg IV (slowly)	15 min 1 min 15 min 1 min	3-6 hr 1 hr 3-6 hr 1 hr	IV administration should be avoided in dogs that are not normovolemic and normotensive because morphine may induce histamine release and vasodilation.
Hydromorphone (injectable: 2 mg/ml)	Perioperative and acute pain	Dog: 0.1-0.2 mg/kg SC, IM 0.03-0.1 mg/kg IV Cat: 0.05-0.1 mg/kg SC, IM 0.01-0.025 mg/kg IV	20 min 1 min 20 min 1 min	3-4 hr 30-45 min 3-4 hr 30-45 min	Hydromorphone is less likely to induce vomiting or hypotension than morphine.
Fentanyl (injectable: 50 µg/ml)	Perioperative and acute pain	Dog: 10 µg/kg SC 2-5 µg/kg IV loading dose, followed by 5-20 µg/kg/hr CRI intraoperatively;	20 min 1 min Continuous	40-60 min 15-30 min Continuous	Duration may be variable from individual to individual because of variations in liver metabolism.

			Onset	Duration	
Fentanyl (transdermal: 25-, 50-, 75-, and 100-µg/hr patches)	Acute and chronic pain	2-5 µg/kg/hr perioperatively Cat: usually no SC or IM administration 1-2 µg/kg IV loading dose followed by 5-20 µg/kg/hr CRI Dog and cat: 3-5 µg/kg/hr	1 min Continuous 12-24 hr	15-30 min Continuous 72 hr	Most cats can tolerate a 25-µg/hr patch. Fentanyl patches alone should not be relied on for relief of acute postoperative pain.
Butorphanol (oral: 1-, 5-, and 10-mg tablets)	Pain associated with surgical procedures **FDA approved for use in dogs as antitussive**	Dog: 1.0-4.0 mg/kg PO Cat: 0.5-2.0 mg/kg PO	0.5 hr	1-4 hr	Oral butorphanol usually will not achieve the same degree of analgesia as morphine, hydromorphone, or fentanyl.
Butorphanol (injectable: 2 and 10 mg/ml)	Pain associated with trauma and surgical procedures **FDA approved for use in cats**	Dog: 0.2-0.8 mg/kg SC, IM; 0.1-0.4 mg/kg IV Cat: 0.1-0.4 mg/kg SC, IM; 0.05-0.2 mg/kg IV	20 min 1 min 20 min 1 min	1-2 hr 45 min 4 hr 45-60 min	Injectable butorphanol usually will not achieve the same degree of analgesia as morphine, hydromorphone, or fentanyl.
Buprenorphine (injectable: 0.3 mg/ml)	Acute and perioperative pain	Dog: 0.01-0.03 mg/kg SC, IM, IV Cat: 0.005-0.01 mg/kg SC, IM, IV or 0.01-0.02 mg/kg buccal/sublingual	45-60 min	6-12 hr 6-12 hr 6-8 hr	Cats tolerate buccal administration well. Due to its high affinity for the mu receptor, buprenorphine is virtually impossible to reverse. Injectable buprenorphine usually will not achieve the same degree of analgesia as morphine, hydromorphone, or fentanyl.

Continued

DRUG NAME	INDICATION	DOSE	ONSET OF ACTION	DURATION OF ACTION	PRECAUTIONS
Local Anesthetics					
Lidocaine (injectable: 20 mg/ml)	Acute pain	Dog: 1-2 mg/kg infiltration or epidurally;	2 min	60 min	Epidural administration will result in hindlimb motor paralysis.
		2 mg/kg IV, followed by 20-50 µg/kg/min for continuous systemic analgesia	2 min	Continuous	
Bupivacaine (injectable: 5 and 7.5 mg/ml) (Marcaine)	Acute pain	Dog and cat: 1-2 mg/kg infiltration;	10-20 min	6-8 hr	Inadvertent IV injection can result in cardiac arrest.
		0.1-0.75 mg/kg epidurally	10-20 min	6-8 hr	Low concentrations or doses administered epidurally can potentially block sensory nerves without resulting in hindlimb motor paralysis.
Other Drugs					
Tramadol (oral: 50-mg tablets)	Acute and cancer-related pain	Dog: 8-10 mg/kg PO sid;	1 hr	24 hr	Tramadol has opioid-like effects without being a controlled substance.
		2-5 mg/kg PO bid or tid;	1hr	8-12 hr	
		0.2-0.4 mg/kg IV	1 min	4-6 hr	
		Cat: 0.1-0.2 mg/kg IV; oral dose unknown	1 min	4-6 hr	
Ketamine (microdose: 100 mg/ml)	Prevention and treatment of "wind-up" (central hyper-sensitization)	Dog and cat: 0.5 mg/kg IV, followed by 10 µg/kg/min during surgery and 2 µg/kg/min for 24 hr after surgery	1 min	Continuous	Does not provide analgesia directly but helps prevent and treat wind-up caused by NMDA receptor antagonist activity. Potential for CNS excitation when ketamine given alone.
Amantidine (oral: 100-mg capsule; 10-mg/ml liquid)	Prevention and treatment of "wind-up"	Dog and cat: 3 mg/kg PO sid	1 hr	24 hr	Does not provide analgesia directly but helps prevent and treat wind-up caused by NMDA receptor antagonist activity.
Gabapentin (oral: 100-, 300-, and	Neuropathic pain	Dog and cat: 1.25-10 mg/kg PO sid	1 hr	24 hr	Does not provide analgesia directly but may help control abnormal neural processing in patients with

400-mg tablets)

peripheral and central neuropathic pain and chronic pain.

Sedatives and Anxiety-Dysphoria–Relieving Drugs

Drug		Dose	Onset	Duration	Comments
Acepromazine (injectable: 10 mg/ml)	Provides sedation **FDA approved for use in dogs**	Dog and cat: 0.01-0.2 mg/kg SC, IM, IV	10-20 min	4-6 hr	May last considerably longer in geriatric patients and those with liver disease. Should be avoided in patients with a history of seizures or who are currently hypotensive or dehydrated.
Acepromazine (oral:10- and 25-mg tablets)	Provides sedation **FDA approved for use in dogs**	Dog and cat: 0.5 mg/kg PO	30-60 min	As above. 6-12 hr	
Diazepam or midazolam (injectable: 5 mg/ml)	Relieves anxiety	Dog and cat: 0.1-0.2 mg/kg IV; 0.1-0.2 mg/kg/hr CRI	1 min Continuous	20-60 min Continuous	May cause excitement instead of sedation in younger animals.
Medetomidine (injectable: 1 mg/ml)	Provides sedation **FDA approved for use in dogs**	Dog and cat: 0.5-3.0 μg/kg IV	3 min	20-60 min	To be avoided in patients with cardiopulmonary or renal disease. Low IV dose is to be used as an adjunct to opioid analgesia and to help relieve anxiety; not intended for use alone.
Xylazine (injectable: 20 and 100 mg/ml)	Provides sedation **FDA approved for use in dogs and cats**	Dog and cat: 0.05-0.1 mg/kg IV	1 min	20 min	As for medetomidine.

Data from Dr. Jamie Gaynor and other members of the Companion Animal Pain Management Consortium.

NOTE: Some of the dosages in this table are based on the authors' personal experiences and observations. These doses may differ from those approved by the FDA. Veterinarians should ensure that their actions in administering drugs are in accordance with the latest legislation and standards of good practice.

*Alpha$_2$-agonists have significant sedative effects. Sedation lasts longer than analgesia and frequently may be two to five times longer. The combination of alpha$_2$-agonists with opioids or anesthetics *greatly* enhances the levels of central nervous system depression and level of analgesia unless dosages are adjusted. There is an effective ceiling effect of alpha$_2$-agonists. Dosages above the effective level result in increased duration of effect.

†Duration of analgesic varies with dosage and route of administration. Intravenous (IV) administration generally results in a more rapid onset and shorter duration, whereas subcutaneous (SC) administration usually results in a slower onset and longer duration than listed above for intramuscular (IM) administration. The CVM-approved dosage of medetomidine in dogs as a sole agent is 750 μg/body surface area (m^2) IV or 1000 μg/m^2 IM. For convenience, this relates to a dosage range of 30 to 80 μg/kg for most dogs, with smaller dogs requiring the higher dosage. Medetomidine at 5 and 10 μg/kg IM has been evaluated as a preanesthetic to propofol anesthesia. Alpha$_2$-agonists may be reversed with atipamezole, 25 to 300 μg/kg IM.

PO, Orally; *IV*, intravenously; *IM*, intramuscularly; *SC*, subcutaneously; *sid*, once daily; *bid*, twice daily; *tid*, three times daily; μg, micrograms; *CRI*, constant-rate infusion; *CNS*, central nervous system.

SAMPLE SURGICAL ANALGESIA PROTOCOLS

The following protocols are taken from the Pfizer Animal Health Pain Management Toolkit. These protocols were created by the Companion Animal Pain Management Consortium (CAPMC) and include drugs and dosages that may or may not be approved by the FDA for use in animals. However, all drugs and dosages are referenced in the veterinary literature and have been used by one or more members of the CAPMC for treatment of acute or chronic pain in animals. Two protocols are offered for each procedure, without preference for protocol A or B. These protocols are meant to serve as examples of good surgical analgesia practice.

SURGICAL PROCEDURE	ANTICIPATED DEGREE OF PAIN	PROTOCOL A	PROTOCOL B
Canine ovario-hysterectomy (OHE)	Moderate	*Premedication* Acepromazine, 0.02 mg/kg SC Buprenorphine, 0.01 mg/kg SC ± Atropine, 0.01-0.04 mg/kg SC Carprofen, 4 mg/kg SC *Postoperative analgesia* Incisional block: bupivacaine, 1.5 mg/kg (with 1:200,000 epinephrine) Carprofen, 4 mg/kg PO sid for 3 or 4 days, starting day after surgery	*Premedication* Medetomidine, 0.005-0.010 mg/kg IM Morphine, 0.5-1.0 mg/kg IM *or* Hydromorphone, 0.2 mg/kg IM ± Atropine 0.01-0.04 mg/kg IM Carprofen, 4 mg/kg SC *Postoperative analgesia* Repeat dose of opioid 4-6 hours after initial dose, or sooner if needed. Carprofen, 4 mg/kg PO sid for 3-4 days, starting 24 hours after initial dose
Canine castration	Mild to moderate	As for OHE.	As for OHE.
Feline OHE	Moderate	*Premedication* Medetomidine, 0.02 mg/kg IM Hydromorphone, 0.05 mg/kg IM ± Atropine 0.01-0.04 mg/kg IM *Postoperative analgesia* Incisional block: bupivacaine, 1.5 mg/kg (with 1:200,000 epinephrine) NSAID (see previous table on drug doses for recommendations)	*Premedication* Medetomidine, 0.02 mg/kg IM Buprenorphine, 0.02 mg/kg IM Ketamine, 2 mg/kg IM ± Carprofen, 1-2 mg/kg SC *Postoperative Analgesia* Repeat buprenorphine 6-8 hours (IM or buccal) after initial dose. On discharge (postop day 1): buprenorphine, 0.02 mg/kg (buccal) q8-12h for 1 day, followed by 0.01 mg/kg q8-12h for 2-3 days

SURGICAL PROCEDURE	ANTICIPATED DEGREE OF PAIN	PROTOCOL A	PROTOCOL B
Feline castration	Mild to moderate	*Premedication* Medetomidine, 0.02 mg/kg IM Buprenorphine, 0.02 mg/kg IM Ketamine, 2 mg/kg IM ± Carprofen, 1-2 mg/kg SC	As for OHE, but may omit the postoperative opioid.
Feline onychectomy	Moderate to severe	*Premedication* Medetomidine, 0.02 mg/kg IM Hydromorphone, 0.05 mg/kg IM ± Atropine 0.01-0.04 mg/kg IM *Additional intraoperative analgesia* Declaw block: lidocaine (1.5 mg/kg) + bupivacaine (1.5 mg/kg) *Postoperative analgesia* Hydromorphone, 0.05 mg/kg SC q3h for duration of supervised hospitalization Carprofen, 1-2 mg/kg SC (once) Buprenorphine, 0.02 mg/kg (buccal) q8-12h starting 3 hours after last dose of hydromorphone	*Premedication* Apply fentanyl patch, 25 µg/hr (may cover half the absorptive surface of patch in cats <10 kg). Medetomidine, 0.02 mg/kg IM Morphine, 0.2-0.5 mg/kg IM ± Atropine 0.01-0.04 mg/kg IM *Additional intraoperative analgesia* Declaw block: bupivacaine, 1-2 mg/kg *Postoperative analgesia* Morphine, 0.2-0.5 mg/kg IM q4h for up to two doses Remove fentanyl patch within 3-5 days.
Canine abdominal exploratory (e.g., GDV repair, splenectomy)	Moderate to severe	*Premedication* Morphine, 0.5-1.0 mg/kg or Hydromorphone, 0.2 mg/kg IM ± Atropine, 0.01-0.04 mg/kg IM *Postoperative analgesia* Incisional block: bupivacaine, 1.5 mg/kg (with 1:200,000 epinephrine) Morphine, 0.05-0.2 mg/kg/*hr* (CRI) Oral morphine, 0.5-1.0 mg/kg after discontinuation of CRI (see drug chart for dosing interval)	*Premedication* Morphine, 0.5-1.0 mg/kg IM or Hydromorphone, 0.2 mg/kg IM Fentanyl patch (refer to drug dose table for dosing) ± Atropine 0.01-0.04 mg/kg IM *Additional intraoperative analgesia* Repeat preoperative opioid at half-dose to full dose as needed (IV or IM). *Postoperative analgesia* Repeat morphine or hydromorphone q4h for 12-24 hours. NSAID therapy for 7-10 days after discharge (if not a gastrointestinal procedure).

Continued

SURGICAL PROCEDURE	ANTICIPATED DEGREE OF PAIN	PROTOCOL A	PROTOCOL B
Feline abdominal exploratory (e.g., cystotomy, linear foreign body removal)	Moderate to severe	*Premedication* Hydromorphone, 0.05 mg/kg IM ± Medetomidine, 0.02 mg/kg IM ± Atropine 0.01-0.04 mg/kg IM *Postoperative analgesia* Incisional block: bupivacaine, 1.5 mg/kg (with 1:200,000 epinephrine) Hydromorphone, 0.03-0.05 mg/kg/*hr* (CRI) Buprenorphine, 0.02 mg/kg (buccal) q8-12h starting immediately after discontinuation of hydromorphone CRI	*Premedication* Morphine epidural (0.1 mg/kg) Morphine, 0.25 mg/kg IM ± Medetomidine, 0.02 mg/kg IM ± Atropine 0.01-0.04 mg/kg IM Apply fentanyl patch, 25 µg/hr *Postoperative analgesia* May need to repeat morphine IM once or twice until fentanyl patch becomes effective.
Canine repair of ruptured cranial cruciate ligament or other hindlimb orthopedic procedure (e.g., repair of femoral fracture)	Moderate to severe; can be severe to excruciating	*Premedication* Acepromazine, 0.01-0.04 mg/kg SC Morphine, 1.0 mg/kg SC ± Atropine 0.01-0.04 mg/kg SC Carprofen, 4 mg/kg SC *Additional intraoperative analgesia* Epidural: morphine (0.1 mg/kg) + bupivacaine (1.0 mg/kg) Bupivacaine, 1.0-2.0 mg/kg intra-articularly *Postoperative analgesia* Morphine, 1.0 mg/kg SC, 4 hours after initial dose Carprofen, 4 mg/kg PO sid starting day after surgery for 7-10 days	*Premedication* Medetomidine, 0.005-0.010 mg/kg IM Hydromorphone, 0.2 mg/kg IM ± Atropine 0.01-0.04 mg/kg IM Carprofen, 4 mg/kg SC Appropriate-size fentanyl patch applied 12 hours preoperatively. *Additional intraoperative analgesia* Bupivacaine, 1.0-2.0 mg/kg intra-articularly *Postoperative analgesia* Hydromorphone, 0.2 mg/kg IM 4 hours after initial dose Carprofen, 4 mg/kg PO sid starting day after surgery for 7-10 days
Canine radius/ulna fracture repair or other forelimb orthopedic procedure	Moderate to severe; can be severe to excruciating	Same as hindlimb orthopedic procedure, but omit epidural and intra-articular block. *Additional intraoperative analgesia* Brachial plexus block: bupivicaine, 1.0-2.0 mg/kg (for procedures distal to elbow)	Same as hindlimb orthopedic procedure, but omit epidural. *Additional intraoperative analgesia* Lidocaine, 0.025-0.050 mg/kg/*min* (CRI) Repeat preoperative opioid at half-dose to full dose as needed (IV or IM).

SURGICAL PROCEDURE	ANTICIPATED DEGREE OF PAIN	PROTOCOL A	PROTOCOL B
Feline radius/ulna fracture repair or other forelimb orthopedic procedure	Moderate to severe; can be severe to excruciating	*Premedication* Medetomidine, 0.02 mg/kg SC Hydromorphone, 0.05 mg/kg SC ± Atropine 0.01-0.04 mg/kg IM *Additional intraoperative analgesia* Brachial plexus block: bupivicaine, 1.0-2.0 mg/kg (for procedures distal to elbow) *Postoperative analgesia* Carprofen, 1-2 mg/kg SC (once) Buprenorphine, 0.02 mg/kg (buccal) q8-12h starting 4-6 hours after initial dose of hydromorphone	*Premedication* Acepromazine, 0.05-0.1 mg/kg IM Morphine, 0.25 mg/kg IM ± Atropine, 0.01-0.04 mg/kg IM ± Carprofen, 1-2 mg/kg SC (once) Fentanyl patch, 25 µg/hr *Additional intraoperative analgesia* Consider ketamine CRI (0.002 mg/kg/min). *Postoperative analgesia* May need to repeat morphine IM once or twice until fentanyl patch becomes effective.

Data from Dr. James S. Gaynor, DVM, MS, DACVA.

See previous table on drug doses for abbreviations; *q8-12,* every 8 to 12 hours; *GDV,* gastric dilatation and volvulus; *NSAID,* non-steroidal anti-inflammatory drug.

Sample Calculations for Constant-Rate Infusion of Analgesics

Constant pain requires constant-rate infusion (CRI) of analgesics. The following sample calculations offer examples of how to determine the number of milliliters (ml) of the different analgesics to add to different sizes of fluid bags in delivering a CRI of analgesics through an IV drip.

Overview

1. Give an initial loading dose as a bolus to the desired effect.
2. Begin a CRI of one of the analgesics discussed below either in a syringe pump or as an IV drip.
3. Monitor for signs of inadequate pain control.
   a. Evaluate the following *behavioral categories* hourly while the patient is receiving CRI.

Posture
- Painful signs: hunched back, tense muscles, anxious facial expression, withdrawn, cowering.
- Managed pain: grooming, sleeping in normal posture.

Vocalization
- Painful signs: whining, whimpering, growling, distressful yowling.
- Managed pain: quiet, purring.

Mobility
- Painful signs: unable to lie quietly (restless) *or* unwilling/reluctant to get up or move.
- Managed pain: gets up, sits, lies down, walks willingly.

Response to touch (specifically, palpation of wound if present)

- Painful signs: trembling, guarding wound, baring teeth.

- Managed pain: affectionate, relaxed.
  b. Evaluate the following *physiologic parameters* hourly while the patient is receiving CRI.
- Temperature, pulse, respiration.
- Mucous membrane color and capillary refill time.
- Blood pressure.
  c. Titrate delivery rate accordingly (increase if painful).
  or
  d. Unrelenting pain may need to be treated with a combination CRI of morphine, lidocaine, and ketamine.

4. Monitor for signs of excessive dosing.
   - Dysphoria.
   - Central nervous system (CNS) depression.
     a. Titrate delivery rate accordingly (decrease or discontinue).
     or
     b. Consider an opioid antagonist if an opioid was administered.

Fentanyl

Loading dose
- Canine: 2 to 5 micrograms per kilogram body weight (µg/kg) intravenously (IV)
- Feline: 1 to 2 µg/kg IV
- Give to effect.

Constant-rate infusion (using 10-pound [10#] cat as example)

1. Determine the hourly flow rate of IV fluids for the patient.
   - For the following example, maintenance fluid flow rate will be used as the hourly rate, as calculated by the following formula: 1 ml/pound (#)/hour (hr).
   - In this example the patient is a 10# domestic short-hair cat.
   - $10\# \times (1 \text{ ml}/\#/\text{hr}) = 10 \text{ ml/hr}$
   - Hourly IV fluid flow rate = **10 ml/hr**

2. Determine the hourly analgesic dose rate.
   - Fentanyl CRI dose range for cats: **5 to 20 µg/kg/hr.** NOTE: The low end of the given

dose range is appropriate for postoperative, awake analgesia. The high end of the given dose range is more appropriate for intraoperative analgesia when very little inhaled anesthesia is desired.
- Convert # to kg: $10\# \times (1 \text{ kg}/2.2\#) = 4.5 \text{ kg}$.
- Calculate the lower and upper limits of the dose range:
  —$4.5 \text{ kg} \times (5 \text{ µg/kg}) = 23 \text{ µg}$
  —$4.5 \text{ kg} \times (20 \text{ µg/kg}) = 90 \text{ µg}$
- Range = 23 to 90 µg/hr
- Select a dose in the calculated range based on the patient's level of pain and purpose of analgesia (awake vs. intraoperative).
  —For this example, select **23 µg/hr.**

3. Determine how many units of analgesic per ml of IV fluids.
   - In this case, using fentanyl, the units are micrograms (µg).
   - Use hourly IV fluid flow rate determined in step 1 in the formula below.
   - $(23 \text{ µg/hr}) \times (1 \text{ hr}/10 \text{ ml}) = \textbf{2.3 µg/ml of IV fluids}$

4. Determine how many units of analgesic to add to a liter (L) bag of fluids.
   - In this case, using fentanyl, the units are µg.
   - $(2.3 \text{ µg/ml}) \times (1000 \text{ ml/L}) = \textbf{2300 µg/L}$
     —If using 500-ml bag of fluids, add 1150 µg of fentanyl to half-liter ($\frac{1}{2}$-L) bag of fluids.
     —If using 250-ml bag of fluids, add 575 µg of fentanyl to this fluid bag.

5. Determine how many ml of analgesic to add to bag of fluids. NOTE: Before adding analgesia to fluid bag, remove equal volume of fluid from bag of diluent.

   - Need to obtain concentration of analgesic off vial; in this case, fentanyl = [50 µg/ml].
   - $(2300 \text{ µg}) \times ([ml/50 \text{ µg}]) = \textbf{46 ml}$ of fentanyl, which should be added to a liter bag.
     —Or add 23 ml of fentanyl to a half-liter bag (500 ml) of fluids.
     —Or add 11.5 ml of fentanyl to a 250-ml bag of fluids.
     —Or connect patient to a syringe pump of fentanyl and deliver IV fluids separately.

Morphine

- Monitor for signs of histamine release (pruritus, hypotension) whenever administering morphine IV.
- Morphine analgesia continues for approximately 30 minutes after CRI has been discontinued.
- Dysphoria associated with morphine may be alleviated with a low dose of a sedative.

Loading dose
- Canine: 0.2 to 0.5 mg/kg IV
- Feline: 0.05 to 0.1 mg/kg IV
- Give to effect.

Constant-rate infusion (using 50# dog as example)

1. Determine the hourly fluid flow rate of IV fluids for the patient.
   - For the following example, maintenance fluid flow rate will be used as the hourly rate, as calculated by the following formula: 1 ml/#/hr.
   - In this example the patient is a 50# dog.
   - $50\# \times (1 \text{ ml}/\#/\text{hr}) = 50 \text{ ml/hr}$
   - Hourly IV fluid flow rate = **50 ml/hr**

2. Determine the hourly analgesic dose rate.
   - Morphine CRI dose range for canines: **0.1 to 0.3 mg/kg/hr**
   - Convert # to kg: $50\# \times (1 \text{ kg}/2.2\#) = 23 \text{ kg}$.
   - Calculate the lower and upper limits of the dose range:
     —$23 \text{ kg} \times (0.1 \text{ mg/kg}) = 2.3 \text{ mg}$
     —$23 \text{ kg} \times (0.3 \text{ mg/kg}) = 6.9 \text{ mg}$
   - Range = 2.3 to 6.9 mg/hr
   - Select a dose in the calculated range based on patient's level of pain.
     —For this example, select **5 mg/hr.**

3. Determine how many units of analgesic per ml of IV fluids.
   - In this case, using morphine, the units are milligrams (mg).
   - Use hourly IV fluid flow rate determined in step 1 in the formula below.
   - $(5 \text{ mg/hr}) \times (1 \text{ hr}/50 \text{ ml}) = $ **0.1 mg/ml of IV fluids**

4. Determine how many units of analgesic to add to liter (L) bag of fluids.
   - In this case, using morphine, the units are mg.
   - $(0.1 \text{ mg/ml}) \times (1000 \text{ ml/L}) = $ **100 mg/L**
     —If using a 500-ml bag of fluids, add 50 mg of morphine to half-liter bag of fluids.
     —If using 250-ml bag of fluids, add 25 mg of morphine to this fluid bag.

5. Determine how many ml of analgesic to add to bag of fluids. NOTE: Before adding analgesia to fluid bag, remove an equal volume of fluid from bag of diluent.
   - Need to obtain concentration of analgesic off vial; in this case, morphine = [15 mg/ml].
   - $(100 \text{ mg}) \times ([\text{ml}/15 \text{ mg}]) = $ **6.7 ml** of morphine, which should be added to a liter bag.
     —Or add 3.4 ml of morphine to a half-liter bag (500 ml) of fluids.
     —Or add 1.7 ml of morphine to a 250-ml bag of fluids.
     —Or connect patient to a syringe pump of morphine and deliver IV fluids separately.

Lidocaine

Loading dose
- Canine: 2 mg/kg IV
- Give to desired effect.
- Feline: not recommended for use in cats.

Constant-rate infusion (using 50# dog as example)
1. Determine the hourly fluid flow rate.
   - For the following example, maintenance fluid flow rate will be based on the formula 1 ml/#/hr.
   - In this example the patient is a 50# dog.
   - $50\# \times (1 \text{ ml}/\#/\text{hr}) = 50 \text{ ml/hr}$
   - Hourly IV fluid flow rate = **50 ml/hr**

2. Determine the hourly analgesic dose rate.
   - Lidocaine CRI dose range for canines: **20-50 µg/kg/*min***
   - Convert # to kg: $50\# \times (1 \text{ kg}/2.2\#) = 23 \text{ kg}$.
   - Calculate the lower and upper limits of the dose range:
     —$23 \text{ kg} \times (20 \text{ µg/kg}) = 460 \text{ µg}$
     —$23 \text{ kg} \times (50 \text{ µg/kg}) = 1150 \text{ µg}$
   - Range = 460 to 1150 µg/min

- Select a dose in the calculated range based on patient's level of pain.
  - —For this example, select 600 μg/min.
- Convert the minute rate to an hourly rate
  - —(600 μg/min) × (60 min/hr) = 36,000 μg/hr
  - —Note: 36, 000 μg = 36 mg.
  - —Hourly rate = **36 mg/hr**

3. Determine how many units of analgesic per ml of IV fluids.
   - In this example, using lidocaine, the units are now in milligrams (mg).
   - Use hourly IV fluid flow rate determined in step 1.
   - (36 mg/hr) × (1 hr/50 ml) = **0.72 mg/ml**

4. Determine how many units to add to a liter (L) bag of fluids.
   - In this example, using lidocaine, the units are now in mg.
   - (0.72 mg/ml) × (1000 ml/L) = **720 mg/L**
     - —If using a 500-ml bag of fluids, add 360 mg of 2% lidocaine to this half-liter bag of fluids.
     - —If using a 250-ml bag of fluids, add 180 mg of 2% lidocaine to that bag of fluids.

5. Determine how many ml of analgesic to add to a bag of fluids. NOTE: Before adding analgesia to fluid bag, remove an equal volume of fluid from bag of diluent.
   - Need to obtain concentration of analgesic off vial; in this case, 2% lidocaine = [20 mg/ml].
   - (720 mg) × ([ml/20 mg]) = **36 ml** of lidocaine to a liter bag
     - —Or add 18 ml to a half-liter bag of fluids.
     - —Or add 9 ml to a 250-ml bag of fluids.
     - —Or connect patient to a syringe pump of lidocaine and deliver IV fluids separately.

Ketamine

Loading dose
Canine and feline: 0.5 mg/kg IV
Give to desired effect.
Intraoperative dose
- Canine and feline: 10 μg/kg/*min*
Constant-rate infusion (up to 24 hours postoperatively) (using 10# cat as example)

1. Determine hourly fluid flow rate.
   - For the following example, maintenance fluid flow rate will be based on the formula 1 ml/#/hr.
   - In this example the patient is a 10# cat.
   - 10# × (1 ml/#/hr) = 10 ml/hr
   - Hourly IV fluid flow rate = **10 ml/hr**

2. Determine hourly analgesic dose rate.
   - Postoperative ketamine CRI dose for felines: **2 μg/kg/*min***
   - Convert # to kg: 10# × (1 kg/2.2#) = 4.5 kg
   - Calculate the minute rate of ketamine:
     - —(4.5 kg) × (2 μg/kg) = 9 μg/min
   - Convert the minute rate to an hourly rate:
     - —(9 μg/min) × (60 min/hr) = 540 μg/hr
   - Hourly dose = **540 μg/hr**

3. Determine how many units of analgesic per ml of IV fluids.
   - In this example, using ketamine, the units are in micrograms (μg).
   - Use hourly IV fluid flow rate determined in step 1 in the formula below.
   - (540 μg/hr) × (1 hr/10 ml) = **54 μg/ml**

4. Determine how many units to add to a liter (L) bag of IV fluids.
   - Note shift from *μg* to *mg* in this example.
   - (54 μg/ml) × (1000 ml/L) = 54,000 μg/L
     - —Note: 54,000 μg = 54 mg.
   - Add **54 mg** of ketamine to a liter bag of fluids.
     - —Or add 27 mg to a half-liter bag of fluids.
     - —Or add 13.5 mg to a 250-ml bag of fluids.

5. Determine how many ml of ketamine to add to bag of fluids.
   - Need to know concentration of ketamine, in this case [100 mg/ml].
   - (54 mg) × ([ml/100mg]) = 0.54 ml
   - Add **0.54 ml** of ketamine to a liter bag of fluids.
     - —Or add 0.27 ml of ketamine to a half-liter bag of fluids.
     - —Or add 0.14 ml of ketamine to a 250-ml bag of fluids.
     - —Or connect patient to a syringe pump of ketamine and deliver IV fluids separately.

Selected Product and Manufacturer Contact Information

ANESTHESIA MACHINES AND SUPPLIES

North American Drager anesthesia machine, North American Drager, Telford, Pa.

Matrix anesthesia machine, MDS Matrix, Orchard Park, N.Y.

Ohmeda anesthesia machine, Datex Ohmeda, Madison, Wis.

Moduflex, Dispomed, Joliette (Quebec), Canada; 450-759-9395

ANESTHESIA MONITORING DEVICES

Cardell BP Monitor, Minrad, Inc, Buffalo, N.Y.

Anesthesia monitoring devices, SurgiVet, Waukesha, Wis.

Doppler monitor, Parks Medical Electronics, 19460 SW Shaw, Aloha, OR 97007; 800-547-6427

APM audio patient monitor, A.M. Bickford, 12318 Big Tree Rd, Wales Center, NY 14169; 800-795-3062

ECG/BP Criticare CSI 8100, Criticare Systems, Inc, Waukesha, Wis.; 800-458-4615

BODY HEAT CONSERVATION UNITS

Hard pad, Hallowell Engineering and Manufacturing Corp, Pittsfield, Mass.

Warm water blanket: T/Pump and B'Air Hugger Convection warming system, Gaymar Industries, 10 Centre Dr, Orchard Park, NY 14127; 800-828-7341, 716-662-2551

SnuggleSafe: Lenric International Ltd, Rudford Industrial Estate Ford, ARUNDEL BN18 0BD/UK, T/ + 44 (0)1903 730811, F/ + 44 (0)1903 726486; www.LenricC21.com

STERILIZATION AND DISINFECTING SUPPLIES

Hydrogen peroxide sterilizer, Sterrad 100S, Advanced Sterilization Products, Johnson & Johnson, New Brunswick, N.J.

Ethylene oxide sterilizer, Anderson Products, Haw River, N.C.

Cidex-OPA, Advanced Sterilization Products, Johnson & Johnson, Division of Ethicon, Inc, Irvine, CA 92618

Endozime, The Ruhof Corp, Bio-Med Division, Mineola, N.Y.

Chlorhexidine 2% surgical scrub and solution, Vet Solutions, PO Box 210037, Bedford, TX 76095; 817-285-8500

Roccal-D-Plus alkyl dimethylbenzyl ammonium chloride; benzalkonium chloride; quaternary ammonium chlorides, Pharmacia & Upjohn (Pfizer), Kalamazoo, Mich.; 800-253-8600

Surgical instrument soap, Haemo-Sol, Inc, 7301 York Rd, Baltimore MD 21204; 800-821-5676

Ultrasonic cleaner solution, Metrex Research Corp, 28210 Wick Rd, Romulus, MI 48174

Disinfectant foam, Precise, Caltech Industries, Inc, Midland, MI 48648; 800-234-7700

BIOPSY SUPPLIES

Bio Pince full-core biopsy instrument, Medical Device Technologies, Gainesville, Fla.

Tru-cut biopsy needle, Allegiance Healthcare Corp, McGraw Park, Ill.

Jamshidi bone marrow biopsy needle, Allegiance Healthcare Corp, McGraw Park, Ill.

SURGICAL SUPPLIES AND APPLIANCES

Clippers and accessories, Oster Co, McMinnville, Tenn.

Sabre 2400 cautery unit, ConMed Corp, Englewood, Calif.

Suction machine, Ohio Medical Products, Madison, Wis.

TA 30 internal staples, U.S. Surgical, Norwalk, Conn.

Skin stapler, Appose ULC, U.S. Surgical, Norwalk, Conn.

Monocryl suture, Ethicon, Inc, Somerville, N.J.

Nylon suture, Ethicon, Inc, Somerville, N.J.

PDS suture, Ethicon, Inc, Somerville, N.J.

Tissue adhesive, 3M Corp, 3M Center, St Paul, MN 55144

Sandbags and other positioning devices, R.P. Kincheloe Co (RPKCO.com), 4501 W. Mockingbird Lane, Dallas, TX 75209; 214-956-9729, 214-351-2338 (fax)

Weck-Cel Surgical Spears, Xomed Surgical Products, Inc, Jacksonville, Fla.

Surgery light (80Z9), ALM Getinge USA, Inc, Rochester, N.Y.; 800-475-9040

ORTHOPEDIC SURGICAL SUPPLIES AND APPLIANCES

Cruciate Repair System, Securos, Inc, Charlton, Mass.

Orthopedic power tools, 3M Co, St Paul, Minn.

Orthopedic instruments, Synthes (USA), West Chester, Pa.

External fixation (KE, SK, Ring Fixator), Imexx Veterinary, Inc, Longview, Texas

Interlocking Nail (I.N.), Innovative Animal Products, Division of Gauthier Medical, Inc, Rochester, Minn.

Internal fixation (plates and screws), Synthes Inc, (USA), West Chester, Pa.

Orthopedic power drills, 3M Mini and Max Drivers, Linvatec (subsidiary of CONMED), Largo, Fla.; 800-237-0169

LASER SURGERY SUPPLIES

Accu Vet V25 Fiber-Coupled Diode Laser System, Accu Vet (Lumenis), Bothell, Wash.

Accu Vet Novapulse LX-20SP CO_2 Laser, Accu Vet (Lumenis), Bothell, Wash.

ENDOSCOPY AND LAPARASCOPY

Endoscopy Support Services, Brewster, N.Y. 10509

Laparoscopy equipment, Carl Storz Veterinary Endoscopy, Inc, Goleta, Calif.

Olympus America, Melville, NY 11747

Pentax Precision Instrument Corp, Orangeburg, NY 10962-2699

MISCELLANEOUS SUPPLIES

Feeding tube diets, Clinicare, Abbott Labs, 100 Abbott Park Rd, Abbott Park, IL 60064; 847-937-6100

Red rubber catheters (feeding tubes and urinary catheters), Kendall Co, 15 Hampshire St, Mansfield, MA 02048; 800-962-9888

Argyle Bubble Connector, Kendall Co, Mansfield, Mass.

Elizabethan collar (E-collar): Jorgensen Laboratories, Inc, 1450 N Van Buren Ave, Loveland, CO 80538; 800-525-5614

Teat cannula, Dr Larson's, PO Box 39, Spring Valley, WI 54767

INDEX

Page numbers followed by f indicate figures; t, tables;
b, boxes.